Neonatology
at a Glance

KU-740-223

Trust Library
Central Manchester University Hospitals
Education South
Oxford Road
Manchester M13 9WL

This book is to ~ ~turr ~d ~ or bef~

WITHDRAWN

This title is also available as an e-book.
For more details, please see
www.wiley.com/buy/9781118767436
or scan this QR code:

Neonatology at a Glance

Editors

TOM LISSAUER, MB, BChir, FRCPCH
Honorary Consultant Neonatologist
Imperial College Healthcare Trust
London, UK

AVROY A. FANAROFF, MD, FRCPE, FRCPCH
Eliza Henry Barnes Professor of Neonatology
Rainbow Babies & Children's Hospital
Emeritus Professor of Pediatrics
Case Western Reserve University School of Medicine
Cleveland, Ohio, USA

LAWRENCE MIALL, MBBS, BSc, MMedSc, FRCPCH
Consultant Neonatologist
Leeds Children's Hospital
Leeds, UK
Honorary Senior Lecturer, University of Leeds
Leeds, UK

JONATHAN FANAROFF, MD, JD
Co-Medical Director, Neonatal Intensive Care Unit
Director, Rainbow Center for Pediatric Ethics
Rainbow Babies & Children's Hospital
Cleveland, Ohio, USA

Associate Editors

NICHOLAS HOQUE, MBBS, BSc, PhD, MRCPCH
Consultant Neonatologist (Locum)
Chelsea and Westminster NHS Trust
London, UK

MOIRA A. CROWLEY, MD
Co-director, Neonatal ECMO Program
Rainbow Babies & Children's Hospital
Assistant Professor of Pediatrics
Case Western Reserve University School of Medicine
Cleveland, Ohio, USA

Third Edition

WILEY Blackwell

This edition first published 2016 © John Wiley & Sons, Ltd
Second edition © 2011 by Blackwell Publishing Ltd
First edition © 2006 by Blackwell Publishing Ltd

Registered Office
John Wiley & Sons, Ltd, The Atrium, Southern Gate, Chichester, West Sussex, PO19 8SQ, UK

Editorial Offices
350 Main Street, Malden, MA 02148-5020, USA
9600 Garsington Road, Oxford, OX4 2DQ, UK
The Atrium, Southern Gate, Chichester, West Sussex, PO19 8SQ, UK

For details of our global editorial offices, for customer services, and for information about how to apply for permission to reuse the copyright material in this book please see our website at www.wiley.com/wiley-blackwell.

The right of Tom Lissauer, Avroy A. Fanaroff, Lawrence Miall and Jonathan Fanaroff to be identified as the authors of the editorial material in this work has been asserted in accordance with the UK Copyright, Designs and Patents Act 1988.

All rights reserved. No part of this publication may be reproduced, stored in a retrieval system, or transmitted, in any form or by any means, electronic, mechanical, photocopying, recording or otherwise, except as permitted by the UK Copyright, Designs and Patents Act 1988, without the prior permission of the publisher.

Wiley also publishes its books in a variety of electronic formats. Some content that appears in print may not be available in electronic books.

Designations used by companies to distinguish their products are often claimed as trademarks. All brand names and product names used in this book are trade names, service marks, trademarks or registered trademarks of their respective owners. The publisher is not associated with any product or vendor mentioned in this book.

Limit of Liability/Disclaimer of Warranty: While the publisher and author(s) have used their best efforts in preparing this book, they make no representations or warranties with respect to the accuracy or completeness of the contents of this book and specifically disclaim any implied warranties of merchantability or fitness for a particular purpose. It is sold on the understanding that the publisher is not engaged in rendering professional services and neither the publisher nor the author shall be liable for damages arising herefrom. If professional advice or other expert assistance is required, the services of a competent professional should be sought.

Library of Congress Cataloging-in-Publication Data

Neonatology at a glance / edited by Tom Lissauer, Avroy A. Fanaroff, Lawrence Miall, Jonathan Fanaroff ; associate editors, Nicholas Hoque, Moira A. Crowley. – Third edition.
       p. ; cm. – (At a glance series)
    Includes index.
    ISBN 978-1-118-76743-6 (pbk.)
    I. Lissauer, Tom, editor.   II. Fanaroff, Avroy A., editor.   III. Miall, Lawrence, editor.   IV. Fanaroff, Jonathan M., editor.
 V. Series: At a glance series (Oxford, England).
    [DNLM: 1. Infant, Newborn. 2. Infant Care. 3. Infant, Newborn, Diseases–therapy. 4. Neonatology–methods.
 WS 420]
    RJ251
    618.92'01–dc23
                                                                    2015008082
A catalogue record for this book is available from the British Library.

Set in 9.5/11.5pt Times by SPi Global, Pondicherry, India
Printed and bound in Singapore by Markono Print Media Pte Ltd

1   2016

Contents

Trust Library
Central Manchester University Hospitals
Education South
Oxford Road
Manchester M13 9WL

Preface

This book provides a concise, illustrated overview of neonatal medicine. We have divided all of neonatology into only 83 topics, with each covered in one or occasionally two or three double pages. This has been a challenging exercise; it would have been easier to write a longer book, but this format has forced us to identify the most important points and omit unnecessary details. The book has been designed to facilitate learning and to make it more enjoyable. Modern education emphasizes visual impact and this is reflected in this book. The layout, photographs and illustrations have been chosen to assist learning and make the book attractive, stimulating and interesting. In addition, there are specific aids to learning, with boxes to highlight key points and questions and answers.

The book covers the wide range of common or important neonatal clinical conditions and their management. It also puts neonatology into context, with sections on its history, epidemiology, perinatal medicine and a global overview, together with the care of the normal newborn and how to recognize the sick infant. The challenging topics of ethical issues, research, quality assurance, evidence-based medicine, palliative and end-of-life care, autopsy and neonatal outcome are also considered. Practical procedures are described, including neonatal resuscitation and neonatal transport; descriptions of cranial ultrasound, amplified EEG, neuroimaging and echocardiography have been included to inform the practicing clinician about them even if they do not perform these procedures themselves.

The book is written for pediatric interns and residents, medical students, neonatal nurse practitioners, neonatal nurses, therapists and midwives who care for newborn babies either on a neonatal unit or with their mothers in the normal newborn nursery (postnatal wards). For neonatologists, pediatricians and nurse tutors it will be a useful aid to teaching. Whilst the book describes the salient features of intensive care, such as stabilizing the sick infant and respiratory support, it is not a manual of neonatal intensive care, of which there are many.

The book has been a collaborative project between editors and contributors from both North America and the UK. Where practices differ between the two sides of the Atlantic this has been acknowledged and described. This collaboration has been highly educational and hugely enjoyable for the editors and contributors as well as improving the book by forcing us to concentrate on the principles of practice instead of the details.

This new edition has allowed us to update and revise the book. New topics have been added, such as amplified EEG and perinatal neuroimaging.

Another new and innovative development is video clips to enhance the teaching capacity of the book, which have been produced by Dr Lawrence Miall. To help ensure that the book has been thoroughly revised and updated, the editorial team has been enlarged and now includes Drs Lawrence Miall and Jonathan Fanaroff as Editors and Drs Nicholas Hoque and Moira Crowley as Associate Editors.

We would like to thank our many colleagues who have given their time to revise or review chapters and offer advice on improvements. Others have willingly contributed photographs and other images that enhance the book immensely. We are grateful to the many doctors, nurses and therapists whose positive comments about the book encouraged us to produce this third edition. We would also like to thank our families for allowing us to spend so much time over many years on this project.

Tom Lissauer
Avroy A. Fanaroff
Lawrence Miall
Jonathan Fanaroff

Contributors

The Editors are indebted to the following for writing or reviewing chapters for this edition, many of whom also contributed to previous editions of the book:

Mark Anderson
Consultant Paediatrician, Newcastle upon Tyne Hospitals NHS Trust, Newcastle upon Tyne, UK
Pharmacology

Tomoki Arichi
Centre for the Developing Brain, King's College London, St Thomas' Hospital, London, UK
Department of Bioengineering, Imperial College London, UK
Perinatal neuroimaging

Denis Azzopardi
Professor of Neonatal Medicine, Centre for the Developing Brain, King's College London, UK
Amplitude-integrated electroencephalography (aEEG)

Hannah Blencowe
Research Fellow, London School of Hygiene and Tropical Medicine, London, UK
Global neonatology

A David Edwards
Chair in Paediatrics and Neonatal Medicine, Centre for the Developing Brain, King's College London, UK
St Thomas' Hospital, London, UK
Department of Bioengineering, Imperial College London, UK
Perinatal neuroimaging

Afif EL-Khuffash
Consultant Neonatologist, The Rotunda Hospital, Dublin, Ireland
Children's University Hospital, Temple Street, Dublin, Ireland
Patent ductus arteriosus and Echocardiography

Sharon English
Consultant Neonatologist, Leeds Children's Hospital, Leeds, UK
Palliative and end-of-life care

Cath Harrison
Consultant Neonatologist, Embrace Paediatric and Neonatal Transport Service, Sheffield Children's Hospital and Leeds Children's Hospital, Leeds, UK
Transport of the sick newborn infant

Kathryn Johnson
Consultant Neonatologist, Leeds Children's Hospital, Leeds, UK
Maternal drugs affecting the fetus and newborn infant

Larissa Kerecuk
Consultant Paediatric Nephrologist, Birmingham Children's Hospital, Birmingham, UK
Renal and urinary tract anomalies diagnosed prenatally, Renal and urinary tract disorders, Genital disorders

Mark Kilby
Professor of Fetal Medicine, School of Clinical & Experimental Medicine, The College of Medical & Dental Sciences, University of Birmingham, Birmingham, UK
Department of Fetal Medicine, Birmingham Women's Foundation Trust, Birmingham, UK
Perinatal Medicine – Part 2

Joy Lawn
Professor and Director of MARCH Centre, London School of Hygiene and Tropical Medicine, London, UK
Global neonatology

David Lissauer
Lecturer, Department of Fetal Medicine, Birmingham Women's Foundation Trust, Birmingham, UK
Perinatal medicine – Part 2

Hermione Lyall
Consultant in Paediatric Infectious Diseases, Imperial College Healthcare Trust, London, UK
Congenital infection, Neonatal infection, Specific bacterial infections, Viral infections

Neil Marlow
Professor of Neonatal Medicine, UCL Institute for Women's Health, London, UK
Epidemiology, Outcome of preterm infants, Follow-up of high-risk infants

Richard J. Martin
Director, Division of Neonatology, Drusinsky–Fanaroff Chair in Neonatology, Rainbow Babies & Children's Hospital, Cleveland, Ohio, USA
Apnea, bradycardia and desaturations

Patrick McNamara
Associate Professor of Paediatrics and Physiology, University of Toronto, Toronto, Canada
Staff Neonatologist & Associate Scientist, Hospital for Sick Children, Toronto, Canada
Patent ductus arteriosus and Echocardiography

Liz McKechnie
Consultant Neonatologist, Leeds Children's Hospital, Leeds, UK
Pain

Naaz Merchant
Consultant Neonatologist, West Hertfordshire NHS Trust, Watford Hospital, Watford, UK
Honorary Senior Clinical Lecturer, Centre for the Developing Brain, King's College London
Amplitude-integrated electroencephalography (aEEG)

Sam Oddie
Consultant Neonatologist, Bradford Royal Infirmary, Bradford, UK
Stabilizing the sick newborn infant

Irene Roberts
Professor of Paediatric Haematology, Weatherall Institute of Molecular Medicine, University of Oxford, Oxford, UK
Anemia and polycythemia, Neutrophil and thrombotic disorders, Coagulation disorders

Robert Tulloh
Professor of Paediatric Cardiology, Bristol Congenital Heart Centre, Bristol Royal Hospital for Children, Bristol, UK
Cardiac disorders

Chakrapani Vasudevan
Consultant Neonatologist, Bradford Royal Infirmary, Bradford, UK
Seizures and stroke, Neurological examination

Inga Warren
Consultant Therapist in Neonatal Developmental Care, Imperial College Healthcare Trust, London UK
Developmental care, Admission to the neonatal unit, Pain, Discharge from hospital

We would like to thank Dr Sheila Berlin, Assistant Professor of Radiology, Rainbow Babies & Children's Hospital, Cleveland, Ohio, USA for providing a range of radiographs, Professor Brian Fleck, Consultant Paediatric Ophthalmologist, Royal Hospital for Sick Children, Edinburgh, UK for commenting on the sections on Retinopathy of prematurity and Vision and Dr Jeanette Kraft, Consultant Radiologist, Leeds Children's Hospital, Leeds, UK for commenting on the section on Cranial ultrasound, Dr David Clark, Professor and Chairman, The Children's Hospital, Albany, New York, USA, and Dr Alan Spitzer, Senior Vice President and Director, The Center for Research and Education, Pediatric Medical Group, Sunrise, Florida, USA, for contributing photographs and Dr Carlos Sivit, Professor of Radiology and Director of Pediatric Radiology, Rainbow Babies & Children's Hospital, Cleveland, Ohio, USA for providing many of the cranial ultrasound photographs.

We also would like to thank contributors or reviewers to the first two editions; we have often drawn extensively upon their contributions:

Ricardo J. Rodriguez
Associate Editor, first edition

Michael Weindling
Associate Editor, first edition

Karel Allegaert
Pharmacology

Nancy Bass
Cerebral hemorrhage and periventricular leukomalacia, Seizures and strokes, Neural tube defects and hydrocephalus, The hypotonic infant

Monica Bhola
Intubation and chest drains, Common practical procedures, Umbilical catheters and intraosseous cannulation, Central venous catheters and exchange transfusions

Paula Bolton-Maggs
Anemia and polycythemia, Coagulation disorders

Bernie Borgstein
Hearing

Subarna Chakravorty
Anemia and polycythemia, Neutrophil and thrombotic disorders, Coagulation disorders

Hugo Devlieger
Pharmacology

George Haycock
Kidney and urinary tract disorders: antenatal diagnosis, Kidney and urinary tract disorders

Susan Izatt
Neonatal resuscitation

Helen Kingston
Birth defects and genetic disorders

Carolyn Lund
Skin

Cheryl Jones
Congenital infection, Neonatal infection, Specific bacterial infections, Viral infections

Sam Lissauer
Intubation and chest drains, Common practical procedures, Umbilical catheters

Neil McIntosh
Ethics, Research and consent

Maggie Meeks
Common problems of term infants, Common practical procedures, Central venous catheters

Simon Newell
Growth and nutrition

Mary Nock
Jaundice

Michael Reed
Pain

Sam Richmond
Adaptation to extrauterine life, Neonatal resuscitation, Stabilizing the sick newborn infant

Clare Roberts
Vision

Jonathan Stevens
Transport of the sick newborn infant, Central venous catheters and exchange transfusions, Umbilical catheters and intraosseous cannulation, Chest tubes and exchange transfusions

Eileen Stork
Bone and joint disorders

Nim Subhedar
Respiratory support, Lung development and surfactant, Respiratory distress syndrome

Dharmapuri Vidyasagar
Milestones in neonatology

Deanne Wilson-Costello
Outcome of very low birthweight infants, Follow-up of high-risk infants

Qin Yao
Neonatal resuscitation

How to use this textbook

Features contained within this textbook

Each topic is presented in a double-page spread with clear, easy-to-follow diagrams supported by succinct explanatory text.

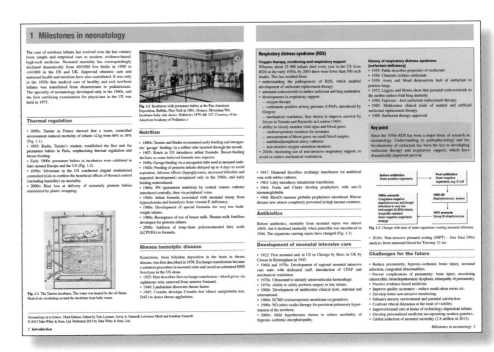

Key points

- Although clinicians sometimes refer to TORCH (toxoplasmosis, other, rubella, cytomegalovirus, herpes) screening, a range of different tests is required.
- Collect samples as soon as possible after birth to optimize chances of diagnosis.

Key point boxes highlight points to remember.

Question

What is the long-term significance of a low Apgar score (3 or less)?

An infant with a low Apgar score at 1 minute but responding rapidly to resuscitation has an excellent prognosis.

An infant with a low Apgar score beyond 10 minutes of age in spite of adequate resuscitation is at markedly increased risk of neurologic damage resulting in cerebral palsy; the longer the score remains low, the greater the risk.

Question boxes offer additional clinical insight.

Your textbook is full of **photographs, illustrations and tables.**

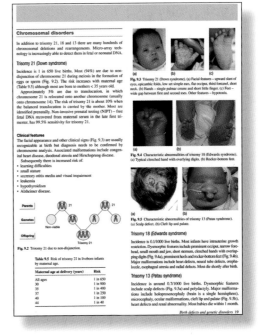

The anytime, anywhere textbook

Wiley E-Text

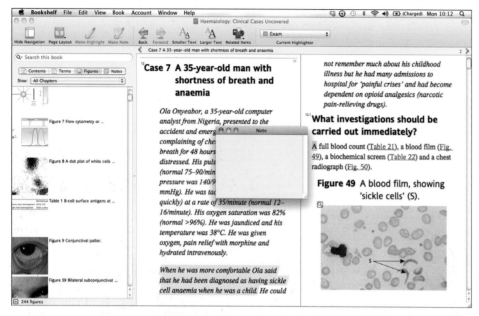

Wiley E-Text
Powered by VitalSource®

Your book is also available to purchase as a **Wiley E-Text: Powered by VitalSource** version – a digital, interactive version of this book which you own as soon as you download it.

Your **Wiley E-Text** allows you to:

Search: Save time by finding terms and topics instantly in your book, your notes, even your whole library (once you've downloaded more textbooks)

Note and Highlight: Colour code, highlight and make digital notes right in the text so you can find them quickly and easily

Organize: Keep books, notes and class materials organized in folders inside the application

Share: Exchange notes and highlights with friends, classmates and study groups

Upgrade: Your textbook can be transferred when you need to change or upgrade computers

The **Wiley E-Text** version will also allow you to copy and paste any photograph or illustration into assignments, presentations and your own notes.

To access your Wiley E-Text:

- Visit **www.vitalsource.com/software/bookshelf/downloads** to download the Bookshelf application to your computer, laptop, tablet or mobile device.

- Open the Bookshelf application on your computer and register for an account.

- Follow the registration process.

The VitalSource Bookshelf can now be used to view your Wiley E-Text on iOS, Android and Kindle Fire!

- **For iOS:** Visit the app store to download the VitalSource Bookshelf: http://bit.ly/17ib3XS

- **For Android and Kindle Fire:** Visit the Google Play Market to download the VitalSource Bookshelf: **http://bit.!y/ BSAAGP** You can now sign in with the email address and password you used when you created your VitalSource Bookshelf Account.

Full E-Text support for mobile devices is available at: **http://support.vitalsource.com**

CourseSmart

CourseSmart gives you instant access (via computer or mobile device) to this Wiley-Blackwell e-book and its extra electronic functionality, at 40% off the recommended retail print price. See all the benefits at: **www.coursesmart.com/students**

Instructors … receive your own digital desk copies!
CourseSmart also offers instructors an immediate, efficient, and environmentally friendly way to review this book for your course.

For more information visit **www.coursesmart.com/instructors**.

With CourseSmart, you can create lecture notes quickly with copy and paste, and share pages and notes with your students. Access your **CourseSmart** digital book from your computer or mobile device instantly for evaluation, class preparation, and as a teaching tool in the classroom.

Simply sign in at **http://instructors.coursesmart.com/bookshelf** to download your Bookshelf and get started. To request your desk copy, hit 'Request Online Copy' on your search results or book product page.

We hope you enjoy using your new book. Good luck with your studies!

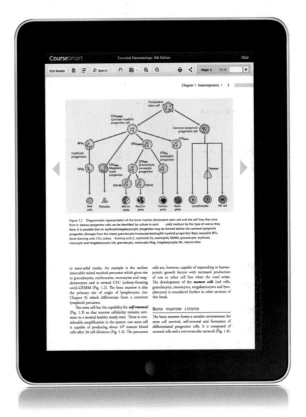

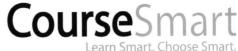

About the companion website

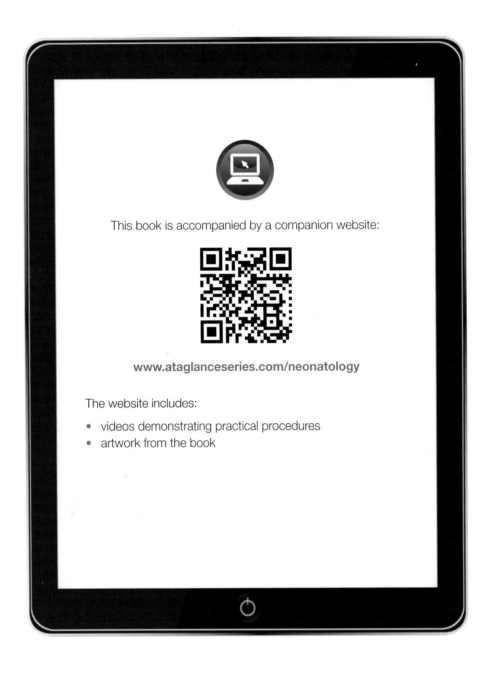

This book is accompanied by a companion website:

www.ataglanceseries.com/neonatology

The website includes:

- videos demonstrating practical procedures
- artwork from the book

1 Milestones in neonatology

The care of newborn infants has evolved over the last century from simple and empirical care to modern, evidence-based, high-tech medicine. Neonatal mortality has correspondingly declined dramatically from 40/1000 live births in 1900 to <4/1000 in the US and UK. Improved obstetric care and maternal health and nutrition have also contributed. It was only in the 1950s that medical care of healthy and sick newborn infants was transferred from obstetricians to pediatricians. The specialty of neonatology developed only in the 1960s, and the first certifying examination for physicians in the US was held in 1975.

Thermal regulation

- 1890s: Tarnier in France showed that a warm, controlled environment reduced mortality of infants <2 kg from 66% to 38% (Fig. 1.1).
- 1893: Budin, Tarnier's student, established the first unit for premature babies in Paris, emphasizing thermal regulation and breast-feeding.
- Early 1900s: premature babies in incubators were exhibited in fairs around Europe and the US (Fig. 1.2).
- 1950s: Silverman in the US conducted elegant randomized controlled trials to confirm the beneficial effects of thermal control (including humidity) on mortality.
- 2000s: Heat loss at delivery of extremely preterm babies minimized by plastic wrapping.

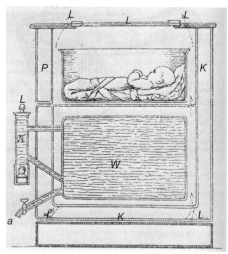

Fig. 1.1 The Tarnier incubator. The water was heated by the oil flame. Heated air circulating around the incubator kept baby warm.

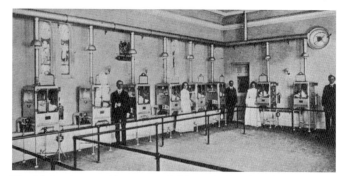

Fig. 1.2 Incubators with premature babies at the Pan-American Exposition, Buffalo, New York in 1901. (Source: Silverman WA. Incubator-baby side shows. *Pediatrics* 1979; **64**: 127. Courtesy of the American Academy of Pediatrics.)

Nutrition

- 1880s: Tarnier and Budin recommend early feeding and intragastric 'gavage' feeding via a rubber tube inserted through the mouth.
- 1907: Rotch in US introduces infant formula. Breast-feeding declines as some believed formula was superior.
- 1940s: Gavage feeding via a nasogastric tube used in neonatal units.
- 1940s: Feeding of preterm infants delayed up to 4 days to avoid aspiration. Adverse effects (hypoglycemia, increased bilirubin and impaired development) recognized only in the 1960s, and early feeding reintroduced.
- 1960s: PN (parenteral nutrition) introduced by central venous catheter, then via peripherally inserted (PICC) lines.
- 1960s: Infant formula associated with neonatal tetany from hypocalcemia and hemolysis from vitamin E deficiency.
- 1980s: Development of special formulas for very low birth-weight infants.
- 1980s: Resurgence of use of breast milk. Human milk fortifiers developed for preterm infants.
- 2000s: Addition of long-chain polyunsaturated fatty acids (LCPUFA) to formula.

Rhesus hemolytic disease

Kernicterus, from bilirubin deposition in the brain in rhesus disease, was first described in 1938. Exchange transfusions became a common procedure in neonatal units and saved an estimated 8000 lives/year in the US alone.

- 1925: Hart describes first exchange transfusion – blood given via saphenous vein, removed from anterior fontanel.
- 1940: Landsteiner discovers rhesus factor.
- 1945: Coombs develops Coombs test (direct antiglobulin test, DAT) to detect rhesus agglutinins.

Neonatology at a Glance, Third Edition. Edited by Tom Lissauer, Avroy A. Fanaroff, Lawrence Miall and Jonathan Fanaroff.
© 2016 John Wiley & Sons, Ltd. Published 2016 by John Wiley & Sons, Ltd.

- 1947: Diamond describes exchange transfusion via umbilical vein with rubber catheter.
- 1963: Liley introduces intrauterine transfusion.
- 1964: Freda and Clarke develop prophylaxis with anti-D immunoglobulin.
- 1968: Rho(D) immune globulin prophylaxis introduced. Rhesus disease now almost completely prevented in high income countries.

Antibiotics

Before antibiotics, mortality from neonatal sepsis was almost 100%, but it declined markedly when penicillin was introduced in 1944. The organisms causing sepsis have changed (Fig. 1.3).

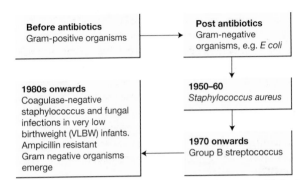

Fig. 1.3 Change with time of main organisms causing neonatal infection.

Respiratory distress syndrome (RDS)

History of respiratory distress syndrome (surfactant deficiency)

- 1955: Pattle describes properties of surfactant.
- 1956: Clements isolates surfactant.
- 1959: Avery and Mead demonstrate lack of surfactant in preterm lungs.
- 1972: Liggins and Howie show that prenatal corticosteroids to the mother induce fetal lung maturity.
- 1980: Fujiwara – first surfactant replacement therapy.
- 1985: Multicenter clinical trials of natural and artificial surfactant replacement therapy.
- 1989: Surfactant therapy approved.

Oxygen therapy, monitoring and respiratory support

Whereas about 25 000 infants died every year in the US from RDS in the early 1950s, by 2003 there were fewer than 500 such deaths. This has resulted from:
- understanding the pathogenesis of RDS, which enabled development of surfactant replacement therapy
- antenatal corticosteroids to induce surfactant and lung maturation
- developments in respiratory support:
  - oxygen therapy
  - continuous positive airway pressure (CPAP), introduced by Gregory
  - mechanical ventilators, first shown to improve survival by Swyer in Toronto and Reynolds in London (1965)
- ability to closely monitor vital signs and blood gases:
  - cardiorespiratory monitors for neonates
  - measurement of blood gases on small blood samples
  - umbilical/peripheral artery catheters
  - non-invasive oxygen saturation monitors.
- 2010s: increasing use of non-invasive respiratory support to avoid or reduce mechanical ventilation.

Key point

Since the 1950s RDS has been a major focus of research in neonatology. Understanding its pathophysiology and the biochemistry of surfactant has been the key to developing surfactant therapy and respiratory support, which have dramatically improved survival.

Development of neonatal intensive care

- 1922: First neonatal unit in US in Chicago by Hess; in UK by Crosse in Birmingham in 1945.
- 1960s and 1970s: Development of regional neonatal intensive care units with dedicated staff, introduction of CPAP and mechanical ventilation.
- 1970s: Ultrasound to identify intraventricular hemorrhage.
- 1970s: Ability to safely perform surgery in tiny infants.
- 1980s: Development of multicenter clinical trials, national and international.
- 1980s: ECMO (extracorporeal membrane oxygenation).
- 1990s: NO (nitric oxide) therapy for persistent pulmonary hypertension of the newborn.
- 2000s: Mild hypothermia shown to reduce morbidity of hypoxic–ischemic encephalopathy.
- 2010s: Non-invasive prenatal testing (NIPT) – free fetal DNA analysis from maternal blood for Trisomy 21 etc.

Challenges for the future

- Reduce prematurity, hypoxic–ischemic brain injury, neonatal infection, congenital abnormalities.
- Prevent complications of prematurity: brain injury, necrotizing enterocolitis, bronchopulmonary dysplasia, retinopathy of prematurity.
- Practice evidence-based medicine.
- Improve quality assurance – reduce medication errors etc.
- Develop better non-invasive monitoring.
- Enhance nursery environment and parental satisfaction.
- Confront ethical dilemmas at the limit of viability.
- Improve/extend care at home of technology-dependent infants.
- Develop personalized medicine incorporating modern genetics.
- Global reduction of neonatal mortality (2.8 million in 2013).

2 Epidemiology

Epidemiology is the study of the patterns, causes and effects of disease in a defined population. In perinatal medicine the focus is on the prevalence and causes of illness and death and long-term disability in mothers, the fetus and newborn infants.

These indicators are valuable as measures of the health of a region or country and allow comparisons between them and monitoring of changes over time.

Definitions

Newborn infant
- **Preterm:** <37 completed weeks of gestation.
- **Term:** 37–41 completed weeks of gestation.
- **Post-term:** ≥42 completed weeks of gestation.
- **Low birthweight (LBW):** <2500 g.
- **Very low birthweight (VLBW):** <1500 g.
- **Extremely low birthweight (ELBW):** <1000 g.

Mortality
- **Maternal mortality ratio:** the number of maternal deaths (during pregnancy and within 42 days postpartum) per 100 000 live births.
- **Stillbirth:** Variable definitions. In US, fetal death (no signs of life) ≥20 weeks' gestation. In the UK, fetus born with no signs of life after 24 weeks. For international comparison, WHO recommend defining stillbirth rate as fetal deaths >1000 g or >28 completed weeks per 1000 total births.
- **Perinatal mortality rate (PMR):** stillbirths plus early neonatal deaths (up to 6 completed days of life) per 1000 live and stillbirths (adjusted as above for international comparisons).
- **Neonatal mortality rate (NMR):** deaths in the first 4 weeks (27 completed days) of life per 1000 live births.
- **Post-neonatal mortality rate:** deaths from 28 days until 1 year per 1000 live births.
- **Infant mortality rate:** deaths in the first year of life per 1000 live births.

Stillbirths (5.2 per 1000 total births)		Early neonatal deaths (2.6 per 1000 live births)	
Unexplained antepartum fetal death	76%	Immaturity	46%
Intrapartum 'asphyxia' or 'trauma'	7%	Congenital malformation	22%
Congenital malformation	7%	Intrapartum causes	12%
Infection	3%	Infection	7%
Other	7%	Other	13%

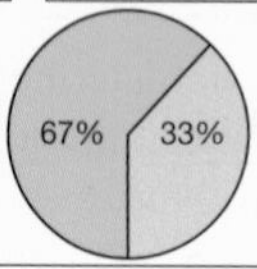

Fig. 2.1 Causes of perinatal mortality in UK (Confidential Enquiry into Maternal and Child Health, 2009).

Births

There are 4 million births per year in the US (population 315 million) and 813 000 in the UK (population 64 million). The mean age of a mother giving birth has risen to 26 years in the US and to 29 years in the UK (average age at first child 28 years). There has been a steady rise in the birth rate for women in their thirties and forties. Increased use of assisted reproduction has led to a rise in multiple birth, particularly twins, with increased risk of mortality.

Maternal mortality

The huge reduction in deaths directly and indirectly related to pregnancy is one of the most dramatic improvements in health outcomes in high income countries. In the US, maternal mortality declined from 582/100 000 live births in 1936 to a nadir of 11.5/100 000 in 1990. This is due to reduced mortality from puerperal sepsis following the development of antibiotics, improved obstetric care, availability of blood and blood products, and better maternal health, including fewer pregnancies per woman. However, maternal mortality in the US has subsequently risen to 18/100 000 in the last 5 years possibly due to an increase in chronic health conditions, including congenital heart disease. It was 12/100,000 live births in the UK in 2010.

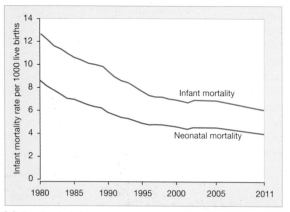

Fig. 2.2 Decline in infant and neonatal mortality in the US since 1980 (CDC 2013).

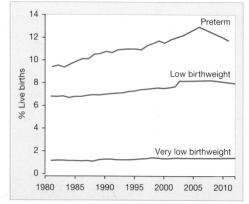

Fig. 2.3 Percentage of live births born preterm, low bithweight (<2.5 kg) and very low birthweight (<1.5 kg) since 1980 in the US (CDC 2013).

Neonatology at a Glance, Third Edition. Edited by Tom Lissauer, Avroy A. Fanaroff, Lawrence Miall and Jonathan Fanaroff.
© 2016 John Wiley & Sons, Ltd. Published 2016 by John Wiley & Sons, Ltd.

Table 2.1 Birthweight distribution and neonatal mortality.

Birthweight (g)	Births (%)	Neonatal mortality rate (per 1000 live births)
>2500	91.7	0.8
2000–2499	5.2	5.6
1500–1999	1.6	17
<1500	1.5	209

Perinatal mortality

The causes of perinatal mortality are shown in Fig. 2.1. The risk to the infant of perinatal death is about 100 times that for the mother. In the US, the perinatal mortality fell from 13/1000 live and still-births in 1980 to 6/1000 in 2011. The decline has occurred not only because of advances in neonatal care, but also from improved maternal health, nutrition and obstetric care.

Neonatal mortality

Neonatal mortality rate in the US and England and Wales have declined markedly over the last 30 years (Fig. 2.2). This has been achieved in spite of the rise in the proportion of preterm deliveries, the main determinant of neonatal mortality (Fig. 2.3 and Table 2.1).

Epidemiologic data collection

Neonatal epidemiologic data are gathered through several systems including national vital registration (birth and death certification) and rapid reporting audit systems (e.g. confidential enquiries). There are also special collaborative neonatal databases such as the Vermont–Oxford Neonatal Network, NICHD (National Institute of Child Health and Human Development) Neonatal Research Network, the Canadian Neonatal Network and the National Neonatal Audit Program in England and Wales, which are used for benchmarking across a large number of neonatal units. Particularly informative are the population-based datasets (Fig. 2.4), that combine obstetric and neonatal data with outcome information.

Infant mortality

The marked reduction in infant mortality since 1980 is shown in Fig 2.2. With the decline in deaths from infectious diseases since the 1900s and more recently from sudden infant death syndrome, over two-thirds of infant deaths are in the neonatal period, and even after the first month of life many deaths are related to neonatal problems. Sixty-six percent of all infant deaths occur in the 8.3% of infants born with low birthweight; 52% of infant deaths are among the 1.5% very low birthweight infants. Complications of preterm birth and congenital abnormalities are the largest contributors to both neonatal and infant deaths.

Both preterm birth prevalence and mortality risk in the US are influenced by ethnicity; the infant mortality rate of infants of black mothers is over twice that of infants of white or Hispanic mothers. The difference in the UK is similar.

Outcome of extremely preterm infants – the EPICure studies

Two countrywide epidemiological studies of infants at the limit of viability have been undertaken – the first in babies <26 weeks of gestation in the UK in 1995 and the second in babies born <27 weeks in England during 2006.

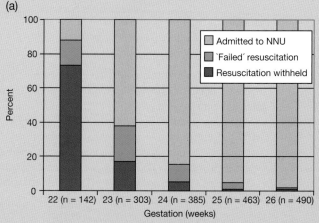

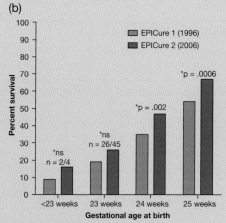

Fig. 2.4 (a) Results of labor ward management for extremely preterm births, England 2006. (Source: EPICure 2; www.epicure.ac.uk.) (b) Gestation–specific mortality rates for babies admitted for neonatal intensive care in England in 1995 and 2006. (Sources: Costeloe K. *et al. Pediatrics* 2000; **106**: 659–671; www.epicure.ac.uk.)

3 Perinatal medicine

Perinatal medicine aims to provide a 'seamless' care pathway for the fetus and infant with complex problems from before and during pregnancy, through labor and delivery into the neonatal period. This requires expertise that is highly specialized, rapidly advancing and multidisciplinary. In many countries this involves close collabora-tion between specialists in maternal–fetal medicine, high-risk obstetrics, neonatology and pediatrics. Such care is usually provided centrally as a tertiary service, although some services are available locally or as 'shared care' (Fig. 3.1).

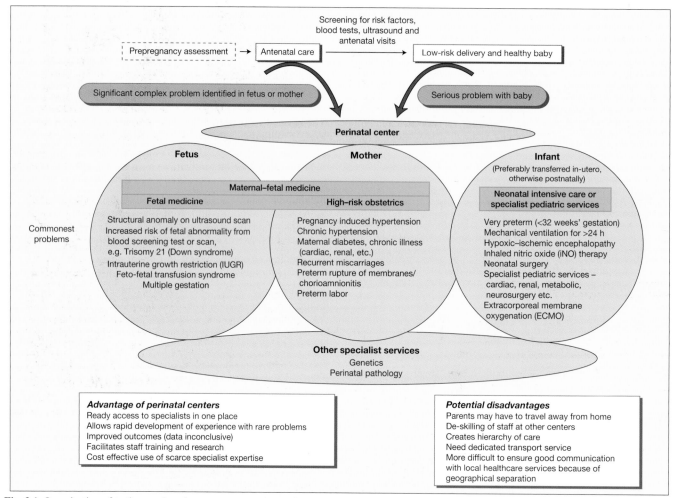

Fig. 3.1 Organization of tertiary perinatal care.

Neonatal involvement in perinatal care

An increasing number of conditions requiring specialist neonatal or pediatric care are recognized antenatally. This allows counseling (both obstetric and pediatric), multidisciplinary discussion and transfer, if necessary, to a perinatal center. Parents require discussion of complex information about their baby's condition and management options, often on multiple occasions and with several healthcare professionals; these may include neonatologists, specialist pediatricians and pediatric surgeons. Interpretation of antenatal ultrasound scans may be difficult and defining prognosis may be problematic. This is facilitated by multidisciplinary team (MDT) meetings of relevant specialists, which may include fetal medicine, obstetrics, genetics, neonatology and pediatric surgery. Other pediatric specialists such as those involved in urology, neurosurgery, otolaryngology (ENT), orthopedics and pediatric medical specialties may also be involved.

Neonatology at a Glance, Third Edition. Edited by Tom Lissauer, Avroy A. Fanaroff, Lawrence Miall and Jonathan Fanaroff.
© 2016 John Wiley & Sons, Ltd. Published 2016 by John Wiley & Sons, Ltd.

Examples of perinatal care

Significant fetal abnormality diagnosed on prenatal ultrasound.

An example is an omphalocele (Fig. 3.2). Another is a diaphragmatic hernia, requiring antenatal planning for infant to be transferred for ECMO (Fig. 3.3) and neonatal surgery.

Fetus diagnosed with supraventricular tachycardia (SVT)
The mother is treated with oral flecainide (transplacental therapy) to control the fetal heart rate and rhythm and prevent heart failure. Performed in conjunction with pediatric/perinatal cardiologists. The neonate is delivered in a cardiac center to optimize medical management and radio-ablation of an accessory conduction pathway.

However, specialist assessment and counseling need to be prompt to allow parents to make informed choices, including termination of pregnancy, in order to keep within national legal boundaries.

Information about less severe problems identified antenatally also needs to be communicated to the neonatology and specialist pediatric teams so that appropriate assessment and follow-up are arranged postnatally.

Neonatal Networks

The different levels of care required by newborn infants are shown in Fig 3.4. As it is not possible or efficient to provide all levels of care in every hospital, neonatal or perinatal (including maternity) networks working across hospital boundaries have been developed. Their aim is to improve care for mother and baby by facilitating collaborative working, unified protocols and minimizing geographic variations in care.

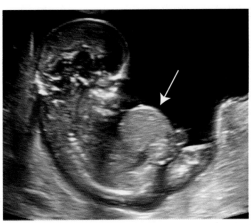

Fig. 3.2 Significant fetal abnormalities detected on prenatal ultrasound screening, such as the omphalocele (arrow) shown , will need to be assessed in a perinatal center to allow review by a fetal medicine specialist, neonatologist and pediatric surgeon, counseling with parents and planning for delivery and management.

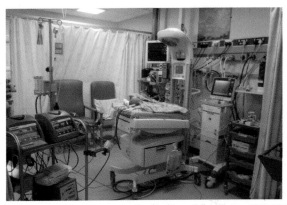

Fig. 3.3 An infant on extracorporeal membrane oxygenation (ECMO), which is provided at only a relatively small number of specialist centers.

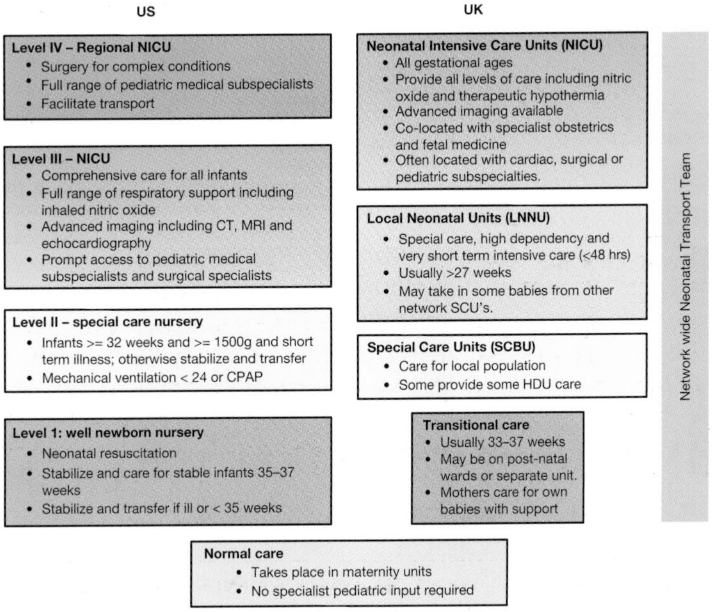

US

Level IV – Regional NICU
- Surgery for complex conditions
- Full range of pediatric medical subspecialists
- Facilitate transport

Level III – NICU
- Comprehensive care for all infants
- Full range of respiratory support including inhaled nitric oxide
- Advanced imaging including CT, MRI and echocardiography
- Prompt access to pediatric medical subspecialists and surgical specialists

Level II – special care nursery
- Infants >= 32 weeks and >= 1500g and short term illness; otherwise stabilize and transfer
- Mechanical ventilation < 24 or CPAP

Level 1: well newborn nursery
- Neonatal resuscitation
- Stabilize and care for stable infants 35–37 weeks
- Stabilize and transfer if ill or < 35 weeks

UK

Neonatal Intensive Care Units (NICU)
- All gestational ages
- Provide all levels of care including nitric oxide and therapeutic hypothermia
- Advanced imaging available
- Co-located with specialist obstetrics and fetal medicine
- Often located with cardiac, surgical or pediatric subspecialties.

Local Neonatal Units (LNNU)
- Special care, high dependency and very short term intensive care (<48 hrs)
- Usually >27 weeks
- May take in some babies from other network SCU's.

Special Care Units (SCBU)
- Care for local population
- Some provide some HDU care

Transitional care
- Usually 33–37 weeks
- May be on post-natal wards or separate unit.
- Mothers care for own babies with support

Network wide Neonatal Transport Team

Normal care
- Takes place in maternity units
- No specialist pediatric input required

Fig. 3.4 Levels of neonatal care.

4 Prepregnancy care, prenatal screening and fetal medicine

Prepregnancy care

To optimize the chances of a healthy baby, mothers are advised:
- Attend clinic for prenatal care.
- Avoid or cease maternal smoking, alcohol, drug misuse, medication (unless essential) prior to conception.
- Toxoplasmosis exposure – avoid eating undercooked meat (and wear gloves when handling cat litter).
- *Listeria* infection – avoid unpasteurized dairy products and soft ripened cheeses, e.g. brie.
- Folic acid supplements preconceptually to 12 weeks – to reduce risk of neural tube defects and cardiac malformations in countries without folic acid fortification of foods, as in the UK and Europe. Higher dose if previous baby with neural tube defect.
- Avoid eating shark, swordfish, marlin and limit tuna as high levels of mercury. Limit oily fish as contain pollutants.
- Optimize management of pre-existing maternal medical conditions such as diabetes and hypertension.

Pregnancies at increased risk of fetal abnormality need to be identified:
- previous child with congenital anomaly
- family history of an inherited disorder, consanguineous
- parents known carriers of an autosomal recessive disorder
- parents from ethnic group with specific risk, e.g. Ashkenazi Jews (Tay–Sachs disease, a neurodegenerative disorder)
- parent with known balanced chromosomal rearrangement.

Prenatal screening

Maternal blood

The routine screening tests vary geographically, but include:
- maternal blood group, antibodies against rhesus (D) and other red cell incompatibilities
- hepatitis B (surface and e-antigen status)
- syphilis serology, rubella, HIV infection
- screening for chromosomal anomalies (see below)
- hemoglobin electrophoresis.

Ultrasound

Ultrasound screening is recommended for all mothers before 20 weeks. Usually involves two ultrasound scans:
- a late first-trimester scan (11 weeks to 13 weeks 6 days)
- a mid-trimester scan (18 to 22 weeks).

Ultrasound screening allows:
- Gestational age calculation, optimal at late first trimester scan.
- Multiple pregnancy to be identified – number of fetuses and the chorionicity (number of placentae and amniotic sacs).
- Structural malformations – up to 80% of major congenital malformations can be identified.
- Screening for trisomy 21 (Down syndrome). First trimester – nuchal translucency measurement combined with serum maternal hormones. Second trimester – four fetoplacental and maternal hormones in serum, adjusted for maternal age. Confirmed on amniocentesis or chorionic villous sampling. Detects about 90% with trisomy 21, but 3–5% false positive rate and 1% risk of fetal loss.
- Non-invasive prenatal testing (NIPT) – fetal DNA from maternal blood for trisomies, Rhesus, gender.
- Fetal growth monitoring – by serial measurement of fetal head size (biparietal diameter and head circumference), abdominal circumference and femur length.
- Amniotic fluid volume assessment to identify:
  (i) oligohydramnios – may result in pulmonary hypoplasia and limb and facial deformities
  (ii) polyhydramnios – associated with maternal diabetes, fetal bowel obstruction, CNS anomalies and multiple births.
- Doppler ultrasound measurement of flow/velocity waveforms – maternal and fetal circulation (if indicated).

Screening – Group B streptococcal, chlamydia, cystic fibrosis

In US but not UK. If at high risk of cystic fibrosis, a panel of common gene mutations is used.

Examples of structural malformations identified on ultrasound (Figs 4.1–4.3) **(see videos: Fetal echocardiogram 1, Fetal echocardiogram 2, Fetal myelomeningocele)**

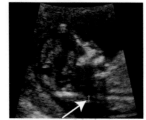

Fig. 4.1 Increased nuchal translucency associated with trisomy 21 (Down syndrome).

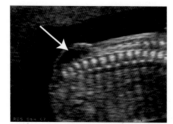

Fig. 4.2 Sacral myelocele. (Courtesy of Dr Venkhat Rahman.)

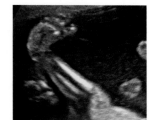

Fig. 4.3 Talipes equinovarus.

Neonatology at a Glance, Third Edition. Edited by Tom Lissauer, Avroy A. Fanaroff, Lawrence Miall and Jonathan Fanaroff.
© 2016 John Wiley & Sons, Ltd. Published 2016 by John Wiley & Sons, Ltd.

Fetal medicine

Fetal medicine (Fig. 4.4) may allow:
- identification of congenital abnormalities (structural and chromosomal) with varying specificity and sensitivity of detection.
- therapy (either indirectly or directly) to be given for a limited but increasing number of conditions, (e.g. fetal arrhythmias, intrauterine blood transfusion for severe rhesus disease)

- optimal multidisciplinary discussion to impart information on prognosis and allow parents to make informed decisions including option of termination of pregnancy for severe disorders
- optimal obstetric management of the fetus, e.g. timing of delivery
- neonatal management to be planned in advance, e.g. counseling and transfer to specialty center.

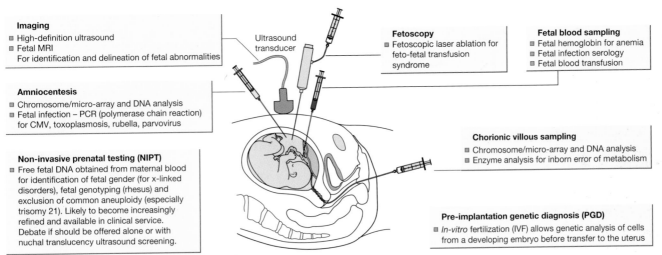

Imaging
- High-definition ultrasound
- Fetal MRI
  For identification and delineation of fetal abnormalities

Ultrasound transducer

Fetoscopy
- Fetoscopic laser ablation for feto-fetal transfusion syndrome

Fetal blood sampling
- Fetal hemoglobin for anemia
- Fetal infection serology
- Fetal blood transfusion

Amniocentesis
- Chromosome/micro-array and DNA analysis
- Fetal infection – PCR (polymerase chain reaction) for CMV, toxoplasmosis, rubella, parvovirus

Chorionic villous sampling
- Chromosome/micro-array and DNA analysis
- Enzyme analysis for inborn error of metabolism

Non-invasive prenatal testing (NIPT)
- Free fetal DNA obtained from maternal blood for identification of fetal gender (for x-linked disorders), fetal genotyping (rhesus) and exclusion of common aneuploidy (especially trisomy 21). Likely to become increasingly refined and available in clinical service. Debate if should be offered alone or with nuchal translucency ultrasound screening.

Pre-implantation genetic diagnosis (PGD)
- *In-vitro* fertilization (IVF) allows genetic analysis of cells from a developing embryo before transfer to the uterus

Fig. 4.4 Techniques in fetal medicine and their indications.

Fetal surgery

Creates media headlines as cutting-edge technology. However, the results are generally poor as the malformations justifying fetal surgery are severe, and the risk of premature labor is high. Now practiced only in a few centers and mainly restricted to randomized trials. Cases must be carefully selected.

Open fetal surgery
Randomized trial (MOMS) for myelomeningocele showed fetal surgery after hysterotomy (uterus opened at 19–25 weeks' gestation) reduced the need for shunting and improved motor outcomes at 30 months. But uterine scarring and increased risk of preterm births.

Fetoscopic/minimally invasive fetal surgery
Fetal endoscopic tracheal occlusion (FETO) for congenital diaphragmatic hernia. As fetal tracheal obstruction promotes lung growth, this is replicated by inflating a balloon in the trachea, inserted at fetoscopy. Randomized controlled trial (TOTAL) shows slightly improved lung function in infancy though increased rate of preterm delivery and survival not improved (see Chapter 38).

Catheter shunts
(i) For fetal pleural effusions, usually a chylothorax (lymphatic fluid) – inserted under ultrasound guidance (Fig. 4.5). Reduces risks of fetal death from hydrops and pulmonary hypoplasia. Neonatal course often satisfactory.

(ii) Congenital bladder neck obstruction – vesicoamniotic shunting. Controversial. A randomized controlled trial (PLUTO) showed shunt improved perinatal survival but did not reduce morbidity from renal disease or death at 2 years.

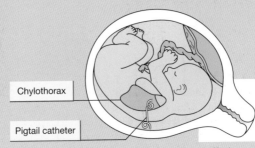

Chylothorax

Pigtail catheter

Fig. 4.5 Fetus with pigtail catheter to drain a pleural effusion.

5 Maternal medical conditions

Diabetes mellitus

Maternal insulin-dependent diabetes (type 1) is associated with increased perinatal morbidity and mortality, mainly from congenital malformations and intrauterine death. These can both be reduced by tight blood glucose control from preconception onwards. Multidisciplinary management and close prenatal surveillance are required.

Fetal problems

• Congenital malformations. The overall risk is 6% (four times normal) with particularly increased risk of cardiac malformations and caudal regression syndrome (sacral agenesis).
• Macrosomia (Fig. 5.1). Maternal hyperglycemia results in fetal hyperinsulinemia, which promotes growth. Depending upon pre-pregnancy and gestational control of blood glucose; up to 25% of infants of diabetic mothers are macrosomic, with a birthweight >4 kg, compared with 8% of infants of non-diabetic mothers.
• Macrosomia predisposes to cephalopelvic disproportion and increased risk of delivery-related complications, both to the mother (cesarean section and forceps delivery) and the fetus, including birth injuries.
• Intrauterine growth restriction (IUGR). Threefold increase, usually associated with maternal microvascular disease.
• Polyhydramnios.
• Preterm labor. Occurs in 10%, either natural or induced.
• Sudden intrauterine death in third trimester. Less common with good diabetic control and induction at about 38 weeks.

Neonatal problems

• Check for malformations and birth injuries.
• Hypoglycemia is common in first 48 h due to residual hyperinsulinism. Monitor blood glucose before feeds until >45 mg/dL

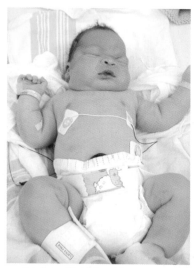

Fig. 5.1 Macrosomic infant with birthweight 4.8 kg at 38 weeks' gestation. There is excess adipose tissue and organomegaly (liver and heart).

(>2.6 mmol/L). Hypoglycemia is often prevented by early, frequent feeding, but may require gavage (nasogastric) feeds or intravenous glucose. Mothers can express breast milk before delivery in preparation. Hypocalcemia and hypomagnesemia are often present.
• Polycythemia – plethoric appearance. Occasionally requires partial exchange transfusion.
• Hyperbilirubinemia.
• Respiratory distress syndrome – increased risk from delayed maturation of surfactant.
• Hypertrophic cardiomyopathy – uncommon. Rarely causes outflow tract obstruction, treated with beta-blockers.
• Renal vein thrombosis – rare.

Type 2 and gestational diabetes

The prevalence of type 2 diabetes is increasing. May be associated with neonatal macrosomia, hypoglycemia and polycythemia. Also increases future risk of diabetes in later life.

Maternal red blood cell alloimmunization

Maternal antibody is formed to fetal red blood cell antigens, (e.g. rhesus D, anti-Kell and anti-c). Rhesus disease was a major cause of fetal and neonatal morbidity and mortality, but prophylaxis with anti-D has significantly reduced risks of alloimmunization; most are now anti Kell and anti-c.

Rhesus hemolytic disease

Etiology (Fig. 5.2)
Presentation
• Antibodies (usually anti-D, c or Kell) found on routine antenatal antibody screen at first visit and 28 and 34 weeks.
• Previous pregnancy affected with hemolytic disease, fetal hydrops or stillbirth.
• Fetal hydrops on ultrasound.
• Detection of fetal anemia by Doppler ultrasound screening (middle cerebral artery blood flow increased for gestational age).
• Maternal polyhydramnios.
• Neonatal – jaundice, anemia, hydrops, hepatosplenomegaly.

Prenatal management
• Increasing antibody levels on maternal blood screening – refer to specialist center if necessary.
• Fetal rhesus genotyping can be determined non-invasively through free fetal DNA detection in maternal plasma.
• Monitor with serial ultrasound for fetal anemia (usually by serial middle cerebral artery Doppler blood flow) and signs of hydrops.
• Measure fetal hematocrit (from cordocentesis; if fetal anemia).
• Intrauterine blood transfusion – blood injected directly into umbilical vein under ultrasound guidance.
• Elective preterm delivery if necessary.

Neonatology at a Glance, Third Edition. Edited by Tom Lissauer, Avroy A. Fanaroff, Lawrence Miall and Jonathan Fanaroff.
© 2016 John Wiley & Sons, Ltd. Published 2016 by John Wiley & Sons, Ltd.

Etiology

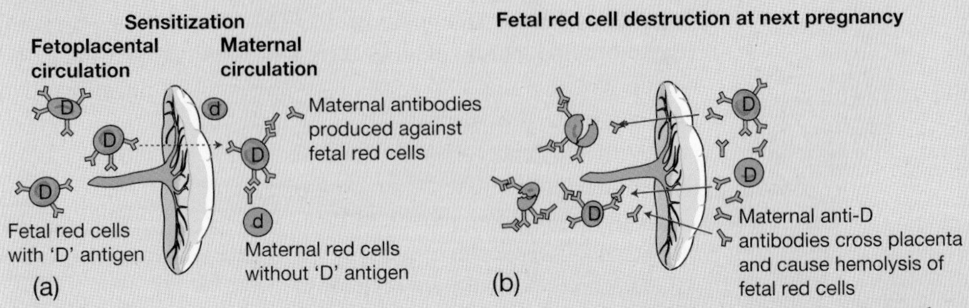

Fig. 5.2 (a) A small number of Rhesus positive fetal red cells enter the Rhesus negative maternal circulation and antibodies are formed. This usually occurs at delivery, but also at miscarriages, placental abruption, from blood transfusions and occasionally during normal pregnancies. (b) On re-exposure to fetal red cells at subsequent pregnancy, maternal antibodies cross the placenta and bind to fetal cells, causing hemolysis (see Table 5.1).

Table 5.1 Effect of hemolysis.

Fetus	Infant
Anemia	Anemia
Hepatosplenomegaly	Hyperbilirubinemia
Hydrops (edema, ascites)	Hepatosplenomegaly
Death	Kernicterus, death

Key point

Over 50% of maternal red cell alloimmunization is now due to rarer red cell antigens (Kell and c).

Postnatal management

- Check cord blood for blood type, hemoglobin, bilirubin and direct antibody test (DAT).
- Monitor bilirubin closely as level may increase rapidly and cause high-frequency deafness or kernicterus.
- Start intensive phototherapy, adequate fluid balance and give IVIG (immunoglobulin) and perform an exchange transfusion if severe anemia or rapidly rising bilirubin concentration.
- Often need 'top up' blood transfusion for anemia within first 3 months of age until antibodies are depleted.

Prevention

Anti-D gammaglobulin has almost eliminated rhesus disease. It is given to rhesus-negative mothers during pregnancy, after potentially sensitizing events and after delivery.

About 15% percent of white women are rhesus-negative (smaller percentage of black and Asian women); less than 2% of them become sensitized from inadequate or failed prophylaxis.

Perinatal alloimmune thrombocytopenia

Analogous to rhesus disease – maternal antibodies directed against paternally inherited fetal platelets (Human Platelet Antigen (HPA)-1a and 5b). It affects 1 in 5000 births. May occur in first pregnancy. Intracranial hemorrhage may occur secondary to fetal thrombocytopenia. If identified from a previously affected infant with intracranial hemorrhage, prevention options are mainly maternal infusions of intravenous immunoglobulin (IVIG) and maternal glucocorticoid therapy and delivery by cesarean section.

Severe thrombocytopenia after birth is treated with platelets that are negative for the platelet antigen. IVIG may reduce need for repeated platelet transfusions.

Other maternal medical conditions (Table 5.2)

Table 5.2 Other maternal medical conditions that may affect the infant.

Maternal condition	Significance for the infant
Maternal hyperthyroidism	If mother is controlled on treatment, fetus and infant are usually unaffected. Rarely causes: • Transient hyperthyroidism – fetal tachycardia, and neonatal hyperthyroidism (1–3%) – tachycardia, heart failure, vomiting, diarrhea and poor weight gain (despite good intake), jitteriness, goiter and exophthalmos (protuberant eyes). Treated for 2–3 months • Transient hypothyroidism – from maternal drug therapy
Maternal hypothyroidism	Mothers treated with thyroxine; neonatal problems are rare. Worldwide; commonest cause is iodine deficiency. Important cause of congenital hypothyroidism, leading to short stature and severe learning difficulties. Rarely seen in North America or Western Europe as iodine deficiency rare and identified on newborn biochemical screening
Autoimmune thrombocytopenic purpura (AITP)	Maternal autoantibodies against platelet surface antigens cross the placenta and cause fetal thrombocytopenia. Most fetuses unaffected. Main risk is maternal or fetal bleeding at delivery. Infants with severe thrombocytopenia or petechiae at birth should be given intravenous immunoglobulin. Platelet transfusions are reserved for severe thrombocytopenia or active bleeding because of the anti-platelet antibodies. The platelet count declines over the first few days before increasing

6 Intrauterine growth restriction

Importance

The prenatal identification of intrauterine growth restriction (IUGR) is important because it allows:
• timely delivery of the fetus with chronic hypoxia, who is at risk of intrauterine death
• early identification of serious fetal abnormalities and fetal infection.

The neonate is at risk of:
• preterm delivery
• birth asphyxia
• hypoglycemia because of poor reserves of glycogen and other energy sources, e.g. fat
• polycythemia from intrauterine hypoxia
• hypothermia
• increased mortality, especially if also preterm.

During childhood most show catch-up growth, but some remain short and thin. There is a slight increase in risk of learning difficulties with IUGR, depending upon underlying etiology and gestation at birth.

Definition

IUGR is the failure of a fetus to achieve his or her genetic growth potential. Most will also be small for gestational age (SGA), although the two terms are not synonymous.

SGA means that the infant is below a particular weight centile for gestation; the 10th centile is most often chosen, but the 3rd or other centiles are also used (Fig. 6.1). The higher the centile chosen, the higher the proportion of infants included who are normal but small; the lower the centile used the higher the proportion with a pathologic cause. The fetus may have growth failure but may not be SGA as their weight is still above the 10th centile. For this reason a prenatal combination of ultrasound features are utilized to identify IUGR in the fetus:
(a) estimated fetal weight or fetal abdominal circumference less than 10th centile for gestation, i.e. SGA
(b) a 'reduced' fetal growth velocity (change in abdominal circumference <1 standard deviation over 14 days)
(c) the presence of oligohydramnios
(d) abnormal cerebroplacental ratio (of middle cerebral artery to umbilical artery pulsitility index) or absent or reversed end diastolic velocity on Doppler insonation. The presence of two or more of these conditions places the fetus at 'high risk' from IUGR.

Etiology

Maternal

• Undernutrition, e.g. famine in developing countries, eating disorders.
• Maternal hypoxia, e.g. cyanotic heart disease, chronic respiratory disease, high altitude.
• Drugs, e.g. cigarettes (Fig. 6.2), alcohol, illicit drug use.

Placental

• Reduced maternal uterine vascular supply – pre-eclampsia, chronic maternal disease, e.g. hypertension, diabetes mellitus, renal disease.
• Placental vascular thrombosis and/or infarction, e.g. maternal lupus anticoagulant, antiphospholipid syndrome, sickle cell disease.
• Unequal sharing of uteroplacental vascularity – multiple gestation.

Fetal

• Chromosomal disorders, e.g. trisomy 18 and other syndromes.

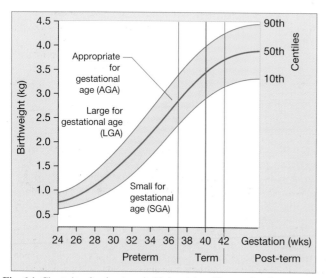

Fig. 6.1 Chart showing increase in birthweight with gestational age. Most small for gestational age fetuses or infants are constitutionally small.

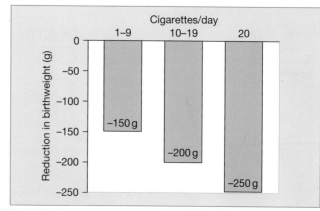

Fig. 6.2 Reduction of birthweight with maternal smoking.

Neonatology at a Glance, Third Edition. Edited by Tom Lissauer, Avroy A. Fanaroff, Lawrence Miall and Jonathan Fanaroff.
© 2016 John Wiley & Sons, Ltd. Published 2016 by John Wiley & Sons, Ltd.

- Structural malformations.
- Congenital infection – CMV, toxoplasmosis, rubella.

Pathophysiology

Traditionally, IUGR has been classified as symmetric or asymmetric, though in clinical practice there is considerable overlap and this distinction is no longer important prenatally.

- **Symmetric** – growth failure affecting weight, head and length. Caused by fetal factors, e.g. chromosomal disorders, syndromes or congenital infection. May be accompanied by polyhydramnios if there is reduced fetal swallowing of amniotic fluid, e.g. trisomy 21 (Down syndrome) or gastrointestinal obstruction. The infant is likely to continue to be small throughout childhood.
- **Asymmetric** – growth failure with head (reflecting brain) growth relatively preserved. Classically caused by uteroplacental insufficiency with reduced oxygen transfer to the fetus. Fetal adaptation to hypoxia is to preserve blood supply to the vital organs, i.e. the brain, myocardium and adrenal glands, at the expense of the kidney, gastrointestinal tract and liver, limbs and subcutaneous tissues. This is reflected in maintained head growth but reduced abdominal circumference from reduced glycogen stores in the liver and oligohydramnios from reduced urine production. If it progresses, it results in fetal acidemia and fetal death.

Management

Management is intensive fetal surveillance to maximize gestation without compromising the fetus (Fig. 6.3).

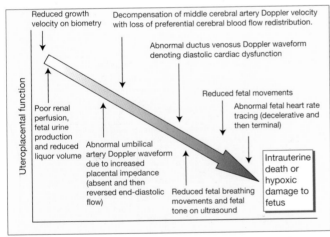

Fig. 6.3 Consequences of progressive uteroplacental failure with increasing base excess and worsening fetal blood pH (acidemia) which may result in intrauterine death. Progression may not follow sequentially.

- Establish if there is a fetal cause by detailed ultrasound scanning for fetal anomalies and karyotype if indicated.
- Monitor fetal growth and well-being from measurements of growth parameters, biophysical profile (amniotic fluid volume, fetal movement, fetal tone, fetal breathing movements, fetal heart activity) and Doppler blood flow velocity (umbilical, ductus venosus and middle cerebral artery). Timing of delivery will depend on gestational age, if growth ceases or there is an abnormal biophysical profile or significant abnormality of the Doppler flow velocity waveform (Figs 6.4 and 6.5).

Postnatal

- After birth, monitor for hypoglycemia and polycythemia and examine for dysmorphic features or congenital infection.

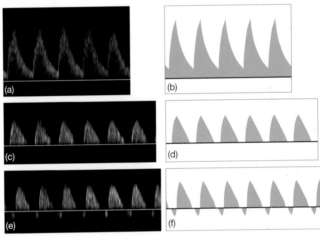

Fig. 6.4 Umbilical artery Doppler waveforms and diagrammatic representation. Normal (a and b), absent end-diastolic velocity (c and d), reversed end diastolic velocity (e and f). Doppler signals from the umbilical artery give information about fetoplacental blood velocities. Increased blood flow velocities in the fetal middle cerebral artery and absent or reversed flow in diastole in the fetal aorta indicate fetal hypoxia.

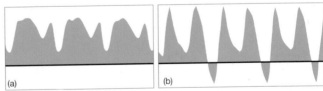

Fig. 6.5 Doppler flow velocity waveform of the ductus venosus showing (a) normal and (b) reversed flow during atrial contraction. In the second-trimester growth-restricted fetus, this represents cardiac decompensation. It is a better predictor of stillbirth than umbilical artery Doppler alone.

7 Multiple births

The incidence of spontaneous multiple gestation is:
- 1 in 89 for twins
- 1 in 89^2 (1 in 8000) for triplets
- 1 in 89^3 (1 in 700 000) for quadruplets.

However, the number of multiple gestations has increased because of fertility enhancing therapies and the older age of childbearing. As a result, 1 in 64 births in the UK is a multiple birth; in the US it is 1 in 58 births. The rate of twin pregnancies has increased markedly since 1980, and was 15.3 per 1000 live births in the UK in 2012 (Fig. 7.1) and 16.8 per 1000 live births in the US in 2013. The number of triplets and higher order births rose markedly in the 1990s but has declined since then, following changes in assisted reproductive therapy practices.

Twins may:
- have their own chorionic sac and placenta (dichorionic, 67%)
- share a chorionic sac and placenta (monochorionic, 33%).

Ultrasound can show whether twins share a placenta (chorionicity) but not if they are identical (zygosity), which can often only be determined through DNA testing (Fig. 7.2).

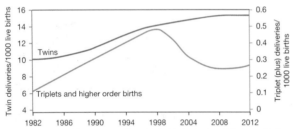

Fig. 7.1 Change in the number of multiple births in the UK since 1980. There has been a marked increase in number of twin deliveries. The number of triplets and higher order deliveries increased markedly during the 1990s but have subsequently decreased. Changes in the US have followed a similar pattern, but at a higher rate for triplet and higher order births.

Pregnancy complications

The main pregnancy complications of twins are:
- **Preterm delivery.** The increased prematurity rate (Table 7.1) is responsible for the increase in perinatal mortality, which for twins is six times that of singletons. Monochorionic twins are at particularly increased risk of iatrogenic preterm delivery. In very high order pregnancies, selective fetal reduction reduces the rate of preterm delivery and perinatal mortality.
- **Intrauterine growth restriction (IUGR).** Severe IUGR, with inter-twin estimated fetal weight difference of >20%, affects 20% of dichorionic twins and 40% of monochorionic twins. If one twin has IUGR, the potential benefits of early delivery for that twin has to be weighed against the prematurity-related complications of the normally grown twin.
- **Congenital abnormalities.** In dichorionic twins the risk is twice normal, as there are two infants. However, in monochorionic twins the risk is four times normal. Anomalies may be discordant or concordant. There is a particularly increased risk of congenital heart disease.
- **Twin–twin transfusion syndrome (TTTS).** This occurs in approximately 10% of monochorionic twin pregnancies due to placental arteriovenous anastomoses. The 'donor' has low perfusion pressures, growth restriction, oliguria and oligohydramnios. The recipient twin experiences hypervolemia, which may result in high-output cardiac failure, polyuria and polyhydramnios. Before 26 weeks' gestation, this may result in preterm labor or intrauterine death in up to 90% if untreated. Potential *in utero* treatment includes fetoscopic laser therapy to divide the placental blood vessels or periodic drainage of the amniotic fluid (amniodrainage). The latter is utilized in relatively mild disease presenting after 26 weeks' gestation. Such cases require prenatal evaluation in a perinatal center by a fetal medicine subspecialist. Even when successfully treated, the infants may have anemia–polycythemia sequence (TAPS), where the hemoglobin difference at birth is >5 g/dL, and 5–10% of survivors have neurologic morbidity.

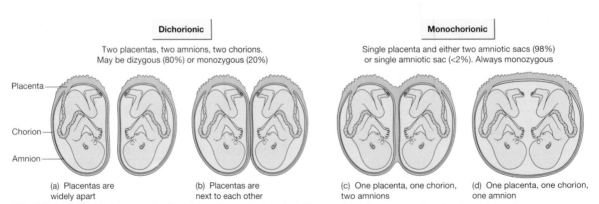

Fig. 7.2 Relationship between chorionicity and zygosity in twins. Placentation of monozygotic twins depends on the stage at which the split occurs. Early splits are dichorionic, later splits are monochorionic.

Neonatology at a Glance, Third Edition. Edited by Tom Lissauer, Avroy A. Fanaroff, Lawrence Miall and Jonathan Fanaroff.
© 2016 John Wiley & Sons, Ltd. Published 2016 by John Wiley & Sons, Ltd.

Table 7.1 Peak gestation and mean birthweight for singleton and multiple births.

	Peak gestation (weeks)	Birthweight (mean, kg)
Singleton	40	3.5
Twins	37	2.5
Triplets	34	1.8
Quadruplets	32	1.4

• **Death of a fetus.** Intrauterine death of one twin may result in preterm labor. In monochorionic twins (with associated placental anastomoses) there may be blood loss from the live to the dead twin, leading to hypovolemia, severe anemia, neurologic impairment (15–20%) or death of the surviving twin (20%). Mono-amniotic twins (Fig 7.2d) risk cord entanglement leading to hypoxia of one or both twins.

• **Conjoined twins.** If twinning of monozygotic twins occurs very late (>14th day) they may be conjoined, with fused skin or organs. Monozygotic twins may also demonstrate "mirroring" where they have opposite asymmetry of certain features.

Neonatal complications

For multiple preterm births, the immediate problem may be to identify sufficient intensive care capacity.

Apart from prematurity, other immediate medical problems may be twin–twin transfusion syndrome (anemia may require blood or exchange transfusion); polycythemia (may require exchange transfusion), IUGR and congenital malformations. Mortality of twins is over five times greater than for single births, for triplets it is increased 10-fold and for quadruplets more than 20-fold.

Families of multiple births may need additional assistance and support:

• Feeding – it is more difficult, but often possible, to breast-feed twins fully, but is usually not possible for higher order births.

• Practical – with their care and housework (requires about 200 h/week for triplets in infancy!); may require help to be able to leave the house (Fig. 7.3).

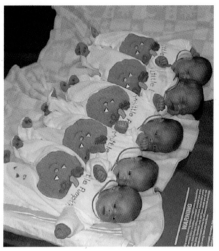

Fig. 7.3 Quintuplets. Multiple births look endearing but families may need assistance with their care.

• Emotional – can be exhausting to provide care.

• Privacy – loss of privacy as a couple, and increased rate of separation and divorce.

• Financial – considerable additional costs (cannot hand down clothes or equipment), may need to move to larger living space.

• Increased incidence of parental depression, especially if there was fetal or neonatal loss (when every birthday or other achievement of the survivor is a reminder that the co-twin died).

• Behavioral – problems in other siblings are increased threefold.

• Development – reduced opportunities for mother–infant interaction, as mothers are busy and often tired. Increased risk of delayed language development and poor attention span. Although multiple births may provide companionship, affection and stimulation between each other, they may also engender domination, dependency and jealousy. The rate of disability is increased, e.g. the cerebral palsy rate for twins is 7 per 1000 live births and for triplets 27 per 1000 live births, compared to 1.6 per 1000 live births in singletons. This is mainly related to prematurity.

There are local and national support groups for parents of multiple births.

8 Preterm delivery

Up to 12% of deliveries in developed countries are preterm. In the US, 11.5% of births were preterm in 2012. In the UK, 7.2% of births were preterm, but only 5.9% in Sweden and Japan (Fig. 8.1). The increase in the proportion of infants born preterm in the US since 1980 is shown in Fig 2.3.

Causes

Neonates may be born preterm following:
• spontaneous labor with intact membranes – 40 to 45%
• preterm premature rupture of the membranes (PPROM) – 25 to 30%
• labor induction or cesarean delivery for maternal or fetal indications – 30 to 35%.
   The main causes are shown Fig. 8.2.

Epidemiological risk factors

There are many risk factors which are poorly understood but generally predispose the mother to infection or inflammation.
   These include:
• Previous preterm delivery – twofold increased risk, increasing for each additional preterm delivery.
• Short inter-pregnancy interval of <6 months – more than doubles the risk.
• Maternal age – increased risk if <20 or >35 years old.
• Maternal nutrition – low BMI (body mass index) increases risk of spontaneous preterm birth. Obese mothers are more likely to have preterm births for medical indications, particularly pre-eclampsia and diabetes mellitus.
• Ethnicity – whereas the preterm rate in the US is 10–11% in White or non-Hispanic mothers, it is 16–18% in Black mothers.

Women from south Asia have high rates of low-birthweight infants rather than preterm delivery.
• Multiple births – result in 15–20% of preterm births. Early delivery is recommended for monochorionic twins by 36 weeks in the UK, 37 weeks in US.
• High levels of maternal psychological or social stress – increased risk – generally less than twofold.
• Smoking – increased risk – less than twofold.
• Substance misuse.
• Socio-economic deprivation – inter-relationship poorly defined.
• Maternal health – infections, either localized, i.e. ascending infection, or generalized, e.g. malaria.

Prevention

Strategies to prevent preterm labor include:
• Progesterone – given prophylactically from 24 weeks, reduces preterm birth and perinatal mortality in those at high risk of preterm labor, e.g. previous preterm birth or short cervix identified on ultrasound, but not multiple births.
• Cervical 'cerclage' – purse-string suture to maintain closure of the maternal cervix. Benefit uncertain, but often offered if multiple preterm births, mid-trimester fetal losses or cervix is shortening. Non-surgical 'cervical pessary' is being investigated.
• Genital infections, e.g. bacterial vaginosis, where overgrowth of anaerobic vaginal organisms displaces normal lactobacillus species. Remains controversial, may be treated.
• Cessation of maternal smoking.
• Reduction in multiple births by limiting embryo transfer in IVF treatment.
• Reduction in elective preterm deliveries – (see below).
   However, the potential impact of these interventions to reduce the proportion of infants born preterm is relatively small.

Management

Antenatal corticosteroids

Maternal corticosteroids administered before preterm birth reduce rates of respiratory distress syndrome by 44%, intraventricular hemorrhage by 46% and neonatal death by 31%. Also associated with a reduction in necrotizing enterocolitis, respiratory support, intensive care admissions and systemic infections in the first 48 hours of life (see Fig. 67.2).
   A single course is administered to mothers at risk of preterm birth up to 35 weeks of gestation. In the UK it is also offered to women having an elective cesarean section prior to 39 weeks' gestation to reduce the risk of respiratory morbidity.

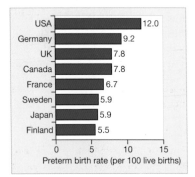

Fig. 8.1 Preterm birth rate in different countries in 2010, showing the high rate in the US and moderately high rate in the UK. (Adapted from Chang HH *et al.* Preventing preterm births: analysis of trends and potential reductions with interventions in 39 countries with very high human development index. Lancet 2013;381:223–34.)

Neonatology at a Glance, Third Edition. Edited by Tom Lissauer, Avroy A. Fanaroff, Lawrence Miall and Jonathan Fanaroff.
© 2016 John Wiley & Sons, Ltd. Published 2016 by John Wiley & Sons, Ltd.

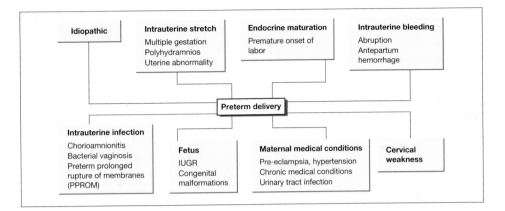

Fig. 8.2 Causes of prematurity. (IUGR, intrauterine growth restriction; PPROM, preterm prolonged rupture of the membranes.)

Preterm premature rupture of the membranes (PPROM)

Affects 2–3% of pregnancies, but is associated with 25–30% of preterm deliveries. Increases neonatal morbidity and mortality due to prematurity, infection and pulmonary hypoplasia. Associated with ascending maternal infection from the lower genital tract; about one-third have positive amniotic fluid cultures. Antibiotics reduce chorioamnionitis and neonatal infection. The decision to deliver or manage expectantly requires balancing of risk of intrauterine infection compared with neonatal risks from prematurity. If <=34 weeks, corticosteroids are usually given. Beyond 34 weeks' delivery is usually indicated.

Tocolysis

Used to suppress uterine contractions. No clear evidence that any improve outcomes, but widely used to try to suppress contractions to enable completion of course of antenatal corticosteroids or allow maternal transfer to a perinatal center.

Magnesium sulfate

Offered to mothers shortly before preterm delivery at 24–32 weeks' gestation to reduce the risk of cerebral palsy. Several trials have shown a 30–40% reduction in cerebral palsy rates, (number needed to treat 63 to prevent one case of cerebral palsy).

Delivery

The aim is to prolong pregnancy for as long as possible while ensuring the safety of the mother and fetus.

1. Extreme preterm delivery (<28 weeks)

   Deciding about the timing of a preterm delivery is most difficult at the limit of viability (22–26 weeks) and should involve the obstetrician, neonatologist and parents. Decision-making is helped by a detailed assessment of fetal well-being including assessment of amniotic fluid volume, fetal heart rate monitoring, Doppler studies, fetal growth, gestation and predicted birthweight (with estimates of their accuracy). This should also be informed by knowledge of outcomes at these early

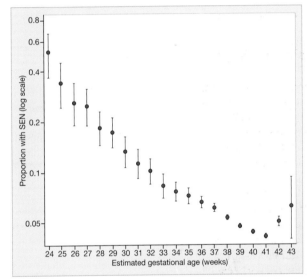

Fig. 8.3 Prevalence of special educational needs (SEN) by gestational age at birth, showing increased proportion even at 34–39 weeks compared with full-term births. Data based on 407 503 school-aged children in Scotland in 2005. (Source: MacKay D.F. *et al. PLoS Medicine* 2010; **7**(6): e1000289.)

gestational ages. National and international data are available, but will need to be modified according to the circumstances. Delivery of high-risk infants should occur at a perinatal center to avoid subsequent transfer and separation of the infant and mother.

2. Delivery at 34–38 weeks

   Although much of the attention of neonatologists (and a significant proportion of this book) is focused on the extremely preterm infant, attention has recently turned to outcomes of infants delivered at 34–38 weeks. These infants have an increase in respiratory morbidity and increased length of stay in hospital compared with full term infants born at 39–<41 weeks. Although the neurodisability rate is highest in extremely preterm infants, rates are higher in these infants than those born at full term (Figs 8.3 and 38.2). There has been a marked reduction in the number of infants delivered before 39 weeks' gestation in the US following new guidelines.

9 Birth defects and genetic disorders

The underlying etiologies of congenital anomalies and mechanisms by which they arise are shown in Table 9.1 and Figure 9.1. When confronted with a neonate with a congenital anomaly, there are a number of questions to ask (Table 9.2), features to look for (Table 9.3) and investigations to consider (Table 9.4). This evaluation process to establish a diagnosis is also appropriate when congenital anomalies are identified prenatally on antenatal ultrasound.

Table 9.1 Causes of congenital anomalies.

Teratogenic	Environmental agents during pregnancy – infections, drugs (particularly anticonvulsants), alcohol and radiation
Sporadic or multifactorial	Many single birth defects occur as isolated cases with low recurrence risk. These may be polygenic or due to faults in developmental pathways
Single-gene disorders	May be family history or previous pregnancy losses. Many multiple malformation syndromes follow autosomal recessive inheritance, but consider X-linked recessive disorders in males and new dominant mutations in isolated cases
Chromosomal	Usually cause multiple congenital malformations and learning difficulties

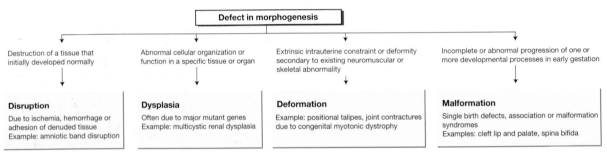

Fig. 9.1 Mechanisms of birth defects.

Question. What history is needed?

Table 9.2 What to ask about in history.

Parental age and health
Previous reproductive history
Family history of congenital anomalies
Consanguinity
Maternal medications, drugs, alcohol, and other potential teratogens
Complications during pregnancy
Ultrasound screening and further investigations

Question. What to look for on clinical exam?

Table 9.3 What to look for.

Growth parameters	Intrauterine growth restriction, overgrowth, microcephaly
Movement and posture	Hypotonia, contractures, seizures
Minor anomalies	Features with little cosmetic or functional significance. The presence of 2 or more should prompt a search for major anomalies
Major birth defects	May represent an association (defects occurring together more often than by chance alone), e.g. VACTERL (vertebral, anal atresia, cardiac, tracheo-esophageal fistula, renal and limb)
	May represent a sequence (one initial malformation resulting in the development of others, e.g. renal agenesis resulting in Potter sequence)
	May represent a syndrome (defects occurring together which have a common, specific etiology)
Dysmorphic features	Unusual or distinctive external appearance of the face, hands, feet, etc.

Question. Which investigations to consider?

Table 9.4 Investigations to consider.

Clinical photographs	Provide a valuable record, especially if the phenotype changes with time
Chromosome analysis	Order chromosome analysis (karyotype) in all babies with multiple malformations or dysmorphic features. Consider requesting comparative micro-array test to analyze chromosomes in more detail.
Biochemical analysis	Examples are calcium (for suspected Williams syndrome or DiGeorge syndrome) and creatine kinase (for suspected congenital muscular dystrophy)
Skeletal survey	Suspected skeletal dysplasia, such as achondroplasia
Echocardiography	Suspected congenital heart disease
Renal ultrasound	If renal anomalies suspected, e.g. in some chromosomal disorders
Brain CT/MRI/ultrasound scan	Suspected CNS malformation
Specific gene tests	Specific disorders, e.g. cystic fibrosis, spinal muscular atrophy type 1

Neonatology at a Glance, Third Edition. Edited by Tom Lissauer, Avroy A. Fanaroff, Lawrence Miall and Jonathan Fanaroff.
© 2016 John Wiley & Sons, Ltd. Published 2016 by John Wiley & Sons, Ltd.

Chromosomal disorders

In addition to trisomy 21, 18 and 13 there are many hundreds of chromosomal deletions and rearrangements. Micro-array technology is increasingly able to detect them in fetal or neonatal DNA.

Trisomy 21 (Down syndrome)

Incidence is 1 in 650 live births. Most (94%) are due to non-disjunction of chromosome 21 during meiosis in the formation of eggs or sperm (Fig. 9.2). The risk increases with maternal age (Table 9.5) although most are born to mothers < 35 years old.

Approximately 5% are due to translocation, in which chromosome 21 is relocated onto another chromosome (usually onto chromosome 14). The risk of trisomy 21 is about 10% when the balanced translocation is carried by the mother. Most are identified prenatally. Non-invasive prenatal testing (NIPT) – free fetal DNA recovered from maternal serum in the late first trimester has 99.5% sensitivity for trisomy 21.

Clinical features

The facial appearance and other clinical signs (Fig. 9.3) are usually recognizable at birth but diagnosis needs to be confirmed by chromosome analysis. Associated malformations include congenital heart disease, duodenal atresia and Hirschsprung disease.

Subsequently there is increased risk of:
- learning difficulties
- small stature
- secretory otitis media and visual impairment
- leukemia
- hypothyroidism
- Alzheimer disease.

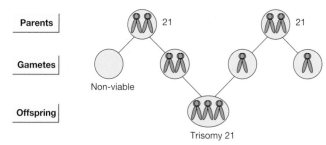

Fig. 9.2 Trisomy 21 due to non-disjunction.

Table 9.5 Risk of trisomy 21 in liveborn infants by maternal age.

Maternal age at delivery (years)	Risk
All ages	1 in 650
30	1 in 900
35	1 in 400
37	1 in 250
40	1 in 100
44	1 in 40

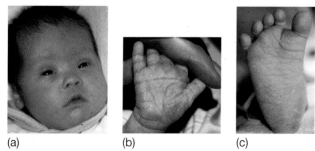

Fig. 9.3 Trisomy 21 (Down syndrome). (a) Facial features – upward slant of eyes, epicanthic folds, low set simple ears, flat occiput, third fontanel, short neck. (b) Hands – single palmar crease and short little finger. (c) Feet – wide gap between first and second toes. Other features – hypotonia.

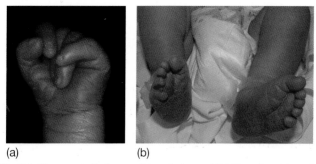

Fig. 9.4 Characteristic abnormalities of trisomy 18 (Edwards syndrome). (a) Typical clenched hand with overlying digits. (b) Rocker-bottom feet.

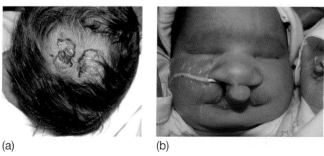

Fig. 9.5 Characteristic abnormalities of trisomy 13 (Patau syndrome). (a) Scalp defect. (b) Cleft lip and palate.

Trisomy 18 (Edwards syndrome)

Incidence is 0.1/1000 live births. Most infants have intrauterine growth restriction. Dysmorphic features include prominent occiput, narrow forehead, small mouth and jaw, short sternum, clenched hands with overlapping digits (Fig. 9.4a), prominent heels and rocker-bottom feet (Fig. 9.4b). Major malformations include heart defects, neural tube defects, omphalocele, esophageal atresia and radial defects. Most die shortly after birth.

Trisomy 13 (Patau syndrome)

Incidence is around 0.7/1000 live births. Dysmorphic features include scalp defects (Fig. 9.5a) and polydactyly. Major malformations include holoprosencephaly (brain is a single hemisphere), microcephaly, ocular malformations, cleft lip and palate (Fig. 9.5b), heart defects and renal abnormality. Most babies die within 1 month.

10 Maternal drugs affecting the fetus and newborn infant

Fetuses are often exposed to one or more of the following potential toxins:
- over-the-counter medications
- prescription drugs
- diagnostic agents (e.g. X-rays)
- recreational drugs, e.g. cigarettes, alcohol or illicit drugs
- herbal and vitamin supplements
- environmental exposure (e.g. pollutants).

The potential consequences for the fetus are listed in Table 10.1.

Table 10.1 Potential consequences for the fetus or infant of perinatal drug exposure.

Intrauterine growth restriction
Intrauterine death or miscarriage
Recognizable patterns of congenital anomalies
Maladaptation to extrauterine life
Neonatal withdrawal syndrome
Toxic effects from drugs excreted into breast milk
Delayed effects on neurodevelopment and behavior

Maternal smoking

In the fetus, maternal cigarette smoking is associated with:
- increased risk of miscarriage, abruption and stillbirth
- reduction in birthweight, by an average of 170 g at term with severity of intrauterine growth restriction (IUGR) related to number cigarettes smoked per day.

In the infant it is associated with:
- increased risk of sudden infant death syndrome (SIDS)
- increased wheezing in childhood.

Alcohol

Encompasses a spectrum of effects (fetal alcohol spectrum disorder, FASD) from mild growth deficiency and neurodevelopmental problems to the classical appearance of fetal alcohol syndrome (Fig. 10.1). Advice to pregnant women from the American Academy of Pediatrics and the Department of Health in the UK is to avoid alcohol completely. Although the effect of occasional, mild alcohol ingestion or occasional binge drinking is not known, there is no safe lower limit for exposure.

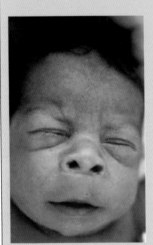

Features of fetal alcohol syndrome:
- Characteristic facies
  - saddle-shaped nose
  - maxillary hypoplasia
  - absent philtrum (ridges between the nose and upper lip)
  - thin upper lip
- Symmetric growth failure – severe, persistent
- Cardiac defects (40–50%)
- Behavior problems – irritable in infancy, hyperactive in childhood
- Developmental delay – average I.Q. 63

Fig. 10.1 Features of fetal alcohol syndrome. (Photograph courtesy of Dr David Clark.)

Neonatal withdrawal (abstinence) syndrome

- Serious problem because of widespread use of narcotics and other drugs of dependency during childbearing years.
- Situation often complicated by multiple drug use.
- Mothers on heroin are often encouraged to embark upon opiate replacement therapy (ORT) such as methadone or buprenorphine.
- Increased risk of blood-borne viruses (hepatitis B and C and HIV) if intravenous drug user.
- Onset of clinical features in infant:
  - heroin <2 days old but can be delayed past one week
  - methadone 1–3 days but can be delayed up to 2 weeks.

Clinical assessment

This must be done systematically and repeatedly (6-hourly) (Table 10.2). It is facilitated by using a scoring system (e.g. Finnegan's score) to determine whether therapy is required. Meconium or infant hair can be analyzed to determine drug exposure during pregnancy but has clinical limitations.

Treatment

Infants who persistently demonstrate features of withdrawal are treated with an oral opiate, usually morphine sulfate, with gradual dose reduction titrated against clinical signs and symptoms. Breast feeding should usually be encouraged for mothers on a stable methadone regimen, as concentration in breast milk is low.

Table 10.2 Clinical features of opiate withdrawal.

Irritability	Vomiting
Scratching	Diarrhea
Wakefulness	Yawning
Shrill cry	Hiccoughs
Tremors	Salivation
Hypertonicity	Stuffy nose
Seizures	Sneezing
Unexplained pyrexia >38 °C	Sweating
Tachypnea (rate >60/min)	Dehydration

Neonatology at a Glance, Third Edition. Edited by Tom Lissauer, Avroy A. Fanaroff, Lawrence Miall and Jonathan Fanaroff.
© 2016 John Wiley & Sons, Ltd. Published 2016 by John Wiley & Sons, Ltd.

Multidisciplinary monitoring of the health and social situation of the mother and infant is required before and after delivery.

Cocaine

Cocaine causes problems from direct transfer of the drug rather than withdrawal:
• placental infarction which may lead to IUGR or placental abruption and antepartum hemorrhage leading to fetal death
• neurobehavioral features - irritability, tremor, high pitched cry on day 1–3 of life.

Medicines

Relatively few medicines produce recognizable patterns of malformation in the fetus (Table 10.3). Adverse effects may not be recognized if they are subtle or have delayed presentation, e.g. diethylstilbestrol (DES) was given for threatened miscarriage in mothers for 30 years before an association with clear-cell adenocarcinoma of the vagina and cervix in female adolescent or adult offspring was identified.

Pregnant women should avoid taking prescribed and over-the-counter medications whenever possible. For prescribed drugs, the benefits must outweigh the risks and appropriate maternal and fetal surveillance should be undertaken.

Key point

Consider drug withdrawal (abstinence) if an infant has suggestive clinical features and no cause has been identified.

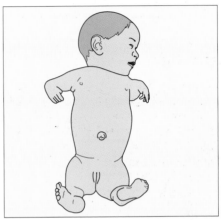

Fig. 10.2 Severe limb shortening (phocomelia, 'like a seal') from maternal thalidomide therapy, which was widely marketed (except in US) for morning sickness from 1957. Teratogenic effects only recognized several years later.

Table 10.3 Some recognizable patterns of malformation or neonatal problems following maternal drug ingestion.

Time in pregnancy	Drug	Malformations/problems	Drug	Malformations/problems
Organogenesis (<8 weeks' gestation)	**Thalidomide**	Short limbs (Fig. 10.2) Absent auricles, deafness	**Folic acid inhibitors** (methotrexate) as cytotoxic therapy	Fetal syndrome – microcephaly, neural tube defects, short limbs
	Anticonvulsants: • carbamazepine • valproic acid (sodium valproate) • hydantoins (phenytoin)	Fetal carbamazepine/valproate/ hydantoin syndrome – midfacial hypoplasia, CNS, limb and cardiac malformations Developmental delay Autistic spectrum disorder with valproic acid	**Coumarin** (warfarin)	Fetal coumarin (warfarin) syndrome – nasal hypoplasia, microcephaly, hydrocephalus, optic atrophy, congenital heart defects, stippled epiphyses, purpuric rash
Pregnancy (>8 weeks' gestation)	**Antithyroid drugs** (iodides, propylthiouracil)	Goiter Congenital hypothyroidism	**Tetracyclines**	Hypoplasia of tooth enamel, yellow–brown staining of teeth
	Androgens	Masculinization of female	**β-Blockers and hypoglycemic agents**	Neonatal hypoglycemia Poor fetal growth
	Aspirin/non-steroidal anti-inflammatory drugs	Closure of ductus arteriosus in fetus		
Labor and delivery	**Opiate analgesia**	Respiratory depression at birth		

11 Congenital infection

The term 'congenital infection' applies to infections acquired *in utero* (Fig. 11.1) whereas 'neonatal infection' is acquired shortly before or at delivery or postnatally (see Chapter 40).

Most congenital infections are viral, but other significant causes include toxoplasmosis and (in terms of world-wide prevalence) syphilis.

Maternal infection is usually primary, i.e. it is a first infection, when there is lack of maternal immunity. Risk of infection from recurrent maternal infection (e.g. with CMV or HSV) is usually markedly lower than from a primary infection. Maternal infection may be asymptomatic or associated with mild symptoms. Diagnoses may be made antenatally or postnatally (Table 11.1). The placenta may play an important role in diagnosing congenital infection.

Key points

- Although clinicians sometimes refer to TORCH (toxoplasmosis, other, rubella, cytomegalovirus, herpes) screening, a range of different tests is required.
- Collect samples as soon as possible after birth to optimize chances of diagnosis.

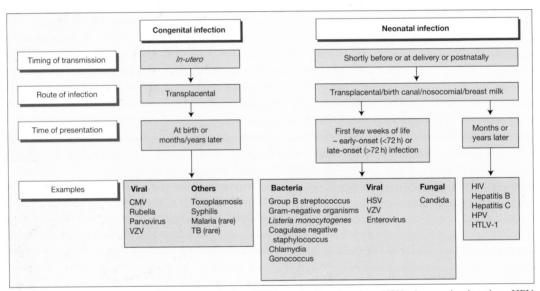

Fig. 11.1 Congenital and neonatal infections. (CMV – cytomegalovirus; VZV – varicellazoster virus; HSV – herpes simplex virus; HPV – human papilloma virus; HTLV-1 – human T-cell leukemia virus 1.)

Diagnosis (Table 11.1)

Table 11.1 Diagnosis of congenital infection.

Antenatal	Postnatal
Maternal	**Infant**
History (e.g. rash, 'flu-like' illness, contact)	Culture/PCR – blood, urine, CSF, stool, nasopharyngeal aspirate, saliva, skin lesions
Screening serology – seroconversion (IgG, IgM, IgA), or low avidity IgG to identify if infection was recent	CT or MRI head – for calcification, microcephaly
	Ophthalmologic assessment – for retinitis
Culture/PCR of lesion, e.g. cervical herpes, blood, urine	Paired serology – for comparison with maternal titers (IgG, IgM, etc.), but production of IgM may be delayed in the neonate
Fetal	**Placenta**
Ultrasound or fetal MRI scanning for anomalies	Histology/microscopic dark-field examination for spirochetes in syphilis, culture/PCR
Amniocentesis for fluid or fetal blood sample for serology/platelet count/PCR	

PCR, polymerase chain reaction.

Neonatology at a Glance, Third Edition. Edited by Tom Lissauer, Avroy A. Fanaroff, Lawrence Miall and Jonathan Fanaroff.
© 2016 John Wiley & Sons, Ltd. Published 2016 by John Wiley & Sons, Ltd.

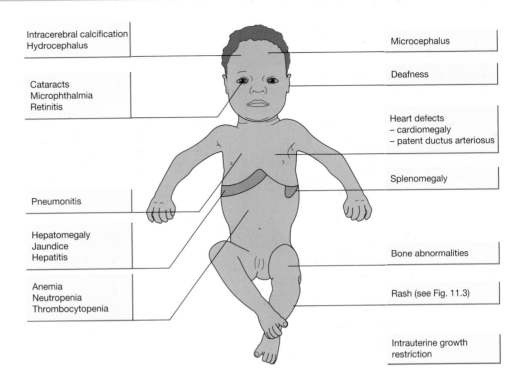

Fig. 11.2 The symptomatic infant.

Clinical features

Congenital infections may precipitate pregnancy loss or preterm delivery. The clinical features of the symptomatic infant are shown in Fig. 11.2.

Key point

It is not possible to reliably differentiate between CMV, toxoplasmosis, rubella or syphilis either by prenatal ultrasound or physical examination of the neonate.

Congenital cytomegalovirus (CMV) infection

- Commonest congenital infection in the US and UK (0.5–1/1000 live births).
- 1–2% of mothers seroconvert during pregnancy.
- Overall mother-to-infant transmission rate is 40%.
- May be reactivated during pregnancy
- May be transmitted postnatally in breast milk or blood transfusions.

Infected infants

- 5–10% severely affected (Fig. 11.2). Poor prognosis for abnormalities detectable on prenatal ultrasound/*in utero* MRI. These include significant intrauterine growth restriction (IUGR), central

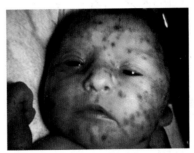

Fig. 11.3 Blueberry muffin rash in rubella and sometimes CMV.

nervous system abnormalities (including ventriculomegaly), renal abnormality and oligohydramnios. In infants, on postnatal CT or MRI scan, they include microcephaly and periventricular calcification (Fig. 11.4),
- 80–90% asymptomatic at birth, but 10–15% of them are at risk of sensorineural hearing loss.
- Most common infectious cause of sensorineural hearing loss.

Diagnosis

- Viral DNA (by PCR amplification) from amniotic fluid, fetal blood, or infant's blood, urine, CSF or saliva collected at less than 3 weeks of age.

Treatment

For infants with CNS involvement, antiviral therapy with oral valganciclovir for 6 months has been shown to improve hearing and neuroevelopmental outcome in a randomized controlled trial.

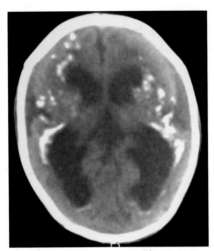

Fig. 11.4 Postnatal CT scan of the brain showing intracranial calcification from congenital CMV infection. The calcification may be identified on antenatal ultrasound.

Other points

- No vaccine yet for seronegative mothers.
- Infected infants may excrete CMV in urine for many months.
- All infected infants should be followed regularly for late-onset sensorineural hearing loss until school age.

Question

Should babies with congenital CMV infection be isolated when on the neonatal unit?

No. About 1% of infants in newborn nurseries excrete CMV, but most are asymptomatic. Pregnant staff are potentially at risk, though most are immune. Attention to hand-washing is the key to preventing infection of caregivers, and should be strictly adhered to when touching any baby.

Congenital toxoplasmosis

- Usually after primary maternal infection in pregnancy.
- Seronegative mothers are most at risk from poorly cooked meat. Small risk from handling feces of recently infected cats or ingesting contaminated soil from unwashed vegetables.
- The transmission rate and treatment are shown in Table 11.2 though this is controversial. The earlier in pregnancy the mother is infected the more severely the fetus is affected.
- The clinical features of the symptomatic infant are shown in Fig. 11.2. Subclinical disease includes retinitis (Fig. 11.5), epilepsy and learning difficulties.
- Treatment of infants with congenital infection – pyrimethamine and sulfadiazine plus folinic acid for prolonged duration.

Table 11.2 Transmission rate and treatment of toxoplasmosis.

Trimester	Transmission rate (%)	Clinical features	Treatment
First	15	35% die before birth, 40% severely affected	Preventative – maternal spiramycin if <18 weeks
Second	40	90% subclinical disease at birth; clinical manifestations may present years later	If severely affected – with antibiotics (pyrimethamine and sulfadiazine) and folinic acid

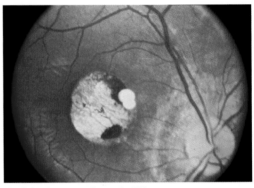

Fig. 11.5 Retinitis from toxoplasmosis. This may present many years later.

Rubella

- Prevented by maternal vaccination. Now very rare in immunized populations.
- The earlier in pregnancy the mother is infected the more severely the fetus is affected.
- Clinical features are shown in Fig. 11.2.
- There is no effective treatment.

Congenital syphilis

In the US, a marked increase in incidence occurred in the 1980s, especially among drug users, but it has since declined. In the UK it is extremely rare. Antenatal screening on maternal blood is performed routinely. If active infection is diagnosed or suspected, the mother should be treated. Treatment more than 4 weeks before delivery prevents congenital infection.

- Transmission rate during primary infection in pregnancy is 100%.
- Without treatment there is 40% abortion/stillbirth/perinatal death.
- Prenatally, is associated with severe IUGR in developing countries.
- Clinical features are shown in Fig. 11.2. Those specific to congenital syphilis include a characteristic rash and desquamation on the soles of the feet (Fig. 11.6) and hands (Fig. 11.7) and bone lesions (Fig. 11.8).

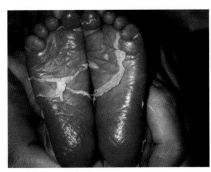

Fig. 11.6 Characteristic rash and desquamation on the feet in congenital syphilis. (Courtesy of Dr Hermione Lyall.)

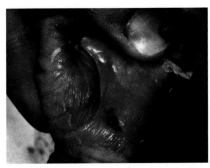

Fig. 11.7 Characteristic rash and desquamation on hands in congenital syphilis. (Courtesy of Dr Hermione Lyall.)

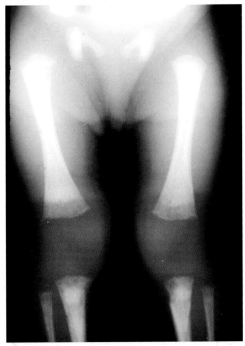

Fig. 11.8 X-rays in congenital syphilis showing bilateral metaphyseal lucency of the long bones and destruction of the medial proximal metaphysis of the left tibia.

• Treatment antenatally and/or postnatally is with penicillin. Effectiveness of treatment is monitored serologically.

• If the mother has not received adequate treatment or if there is physical, laboratory or radiographic evidence of disease, treat. If there is any doubt, treat directly.

Varicella: chickenpox, varicella zoster virus (VZV) infection

Primary maternal infection in pregnancy is uncommon as more than 90% of mothers are immune.

Early in pregnancy

• Intrauterine infection is rare (2% risk).
• Can lead to eye and CNS damage, skin scarring (Fig. 11.9) and limb hypoplasia.
• 1% risk of herpes zoster (shingles) in infancy.

Late in pregnancy

Infants born to mothers who develop chickenpox between 5 days before or 5 days after delivery should be given varicella zoster immune globulin (VZIG). This reduces but does not eliminate the risk of neonatal varicella zoster virus (VZV).

They should be closely monitored, and should be started on aciclovir (intravenous) if any signs of infection develop.

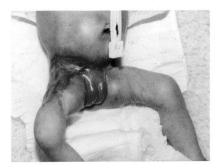

Fig. 11.9 Skin scarring from maternal VZV infection early in pregnancy. This is rare.

Parvovirus B19

• 50% of pregnant women are susceptible to infection.
• Transmission rate is 20–30%.
• In most cases there is a normal outcome of pregnancy but rarely infection in pregnancy leads to severe fetal anemia (aplastic anemia), causing hydrops fetalis (edema and ascites from heart failure). Anemia is associated with an abnormally elevated middle cerebral artery velocity on Doppler ultrasound. Can lead to intrauterine death, but if identified and treated by intrauterine transfusion prognosis is usually good.

12 Adaptation to extrauterine life

The transition from intrauterine to extrauterine life involves a complex sequence of physiologic changes that begin before birth. Remarkably, although infants experience some degree of intermittent hypoxemia during labor, most undergo this transition smoothly and uneventfully. If not, cardiorespiratory depression requires prompt and appropriate resuscitation.

Physiologic changes in fetal–neonatal transition

• Before birth, the lungs are filled with fluid. Oxygen is supplied by the placenta. On reaching the right atrium, some of the oxygenated blood from the placenta flows directly to the left atrium via the patent foramen ovale, bypassing the lungs. This ensures that the most oxygenated blood goes to the heart and brain. In addition, the blood vessels that supply and drain the lungs are constricted (providing high pulmonary vascular resistance), so most blood from the right side of the heart bypasses the lungs and flows through the ductus arteriosus into the lower aorta (Fig. 12.1a).
• Shortly before and during labor, lung liquid production is reduced.
• During descent through the birth canal, the infant's chest is squeezed and some lung liquid exudes from the trachea.
• Multiple stimuli (thermal, chemical, tactile) initiate breathing. Serum cortisol, ADH (antidiuretic hormone), TSH (thyroid-stimulating hormone) and catecholamines dramatically increase.
• The first gasp is usually within a few seconds of birth. A negative intrathoracic pressure is generated to achieve this. Most lung liquid is absorbed into the bloodstream or lymphatics within the first few minutes of birth.
• Aeration of the lungs is accompanied by increased arterial oxygen tension; the pulmonary artery blood flow increases and the pulmonary vascular resistance falls.
• Contraction of the umbilical arteries restricts access to the low resistance placental circulation. This results in increased peripheral vascular resistance and an increase in systemic blood pressure.

• The fall in pulmonary vascular resistance and the rise in systemic vascular resistance result in near equalization of pressures across the duct and virtual cessation of ductal flow and also closure of the foramen ovale (Fig. 12.1b).

Abnormal transition from fetal to extrauterine life

The transition may be altered by a variety of antepartum or intrapartum events, resulting in cardiorespiratory depression, asphyxia or both (Table 12.1).

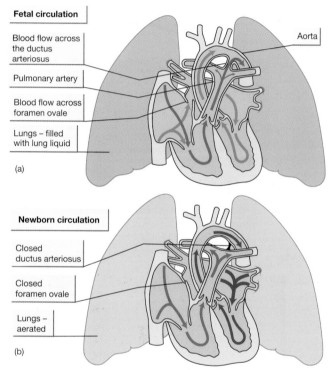

Fig. 12.1 Changes in the circulation at birth. (a) Fetal circulation. (b) Newborn circulation.

Table 12.1 Conditions assciated with abnormal neonatal adaptation to extrauterine life.

Fetal	Maternal	Placental
Preterm/post-dates	General anesthetic	Chorioamnionitis
Multiple birth	Maternal drug therapy, e.g. narcotics, magnesium sulfate	Placenta previa
Forceps or vacuum-assisted delivery	Pregnancy-induced hypertension	Placental abruption
Breech or abnormal presentation	Chronic hypertension	Cord prolapse
Shoulder dystocia	Maternal infection	
Emergency cesarean section	Maternal diabetes mellitus	
Intrauterine growth restriction (IUGR)	Polyhydramnios	
Meconium-stained amniotic fluid	Oligohydramnios	
Abnormal fetal heart rate trace		
Congenital malformations		
Anemia, infection		

Neonatology at a Glance, Third Edition. Edited by Tom Lissauer, Avroy A. Fanaroff, Lawrence Miall and Jonathan Fanaroff.
© 2016 John Wiley & Sons, Ltd. Published 2016 by John Wiley & Sons, Ltd.

The Apgar score

The Apgar score, named after Virginia Apgar, an anesthesiologist, is used to describe an infant's condition during the first few minutes of life (Table 12.2). It is assigned at 1 and 5 minutes of life. If the score is still below 7 or the infant is requiring resuscitation, it is continued every 5 minutes until normal or 20 minutes of age. Although often assigned, few babies truly attain a score of 10, because it is uncommon for the baby to be pink all over. The Apgar score is useful as a shorthand record of the newborn infant's condition after birth.

Table 12.2 Apgar score.

	Apgar score		
	0	**1**	**2**
Heart rate	Absent	<100 beats/min	>100 beats/min
Respiration	Absent	Slow, irregular	Good, crying
Muscle tone	Limp	Some flexion of extremities	Active motion
Reflex irritability (response to stimulation)	No response	Grimace	Cough, sneeze, cry
Color	Blue or pale	Body pink, blue extremities	Pink

Questions

Does resuscitation alter how the Apgar score is assigned?

No. The Apgar score is assigned according to the infant's condition irrespective of whether or not resuscitation is being performed.

Can one determine Apgar scores in preterm infants?

Yes. However, the extremely preterm infant's maximum score is reduced by poor muscle tone and weaker response to stimulation than term infants.

Question

What is the long-term significance of a low Apgar score (3 or less)?

An infant with a low Apgar score at 1 minute but responding rapidly to resuscitation has an excellent prognosis.
An infant with a low Apgar score beyond 10 minutes of age in spite of adequate resuscitation is at markedly increased risk of neurologic damage resulting in cerebral palsy; the longer the score remains low, the greater the risk.

Key point

The Apgar score is not used to determine the need for resuscitation.
Evaluation for resuscitation is made second by second and is based on breathing, heart rate and tone.

Asphyxia

Sustained, severe asphyxia (Fig. 12.2) *in utero* or during labor or postnatally results in the infant making increased respiratory effort, followed by a period of apnea (primary apnea). During primary apnea the heart rate falls to about half its normal rate but the blood pressure is initially maintained.

With continuing asphyxia, the infant starts to gasp, the heart rate slowly falls, as does the blood pressure. After several minutes, after a last gasp, there is secondary apnea. Anaerobic metabolism produces lactic acidosis and cardiac function deteriorates. To recover, positive pressure ventilation, if necessary accompanied by cardiac compressions, is required.

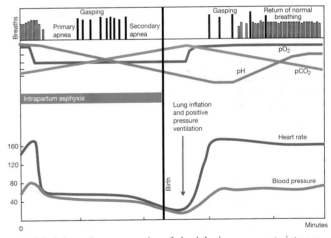

Fig. 12.2 Schematic representation of physiologic responses to intrapartum asphyxia and neonatal resuscitation. (Adapted from Resuscitation Council UK Newborn Life Support.)

Relatively few infants require resuscitation at birth. The aim of resuscitation is to optimize the airway, breathing and circulation as quickly as possible. Most infants respond to lung inflation. Very few require chest compressions or medications. As the need for resuscitation has become uncommon, there is increasing emphasis on simulation and teamwork training to ensure proficient resuscitation when it is required.

Preparation

The presence of antenatal or intrapartum risk factors often allows anticipation that resuscitation may be required. This enables those skilled in neonatal resuscitation to be present. However, the need for resuscitation cannot always be predicted. There should always be at least one health professional skilled in basic resuscitation readily available at every delivery. Staff skilled in advanced resuscitation should attend high risk deliveries and be readily available at all times (**see video: Basic newborn resuscitation**).

Before delivery

- Introduce yourself to parents and explain why you are present.
- Review maternal history and obstetric records.
- Turn on the radiant warmer.
- Wash hands and put on gloves.
- Check equipment is present and functional:
  - several warm towels (and plastic wrap or bag for preterm infants)
  - clock
  - stethoscope
  - suction equipment
  - gas supply and pressure-limited T-piece circuit (e.g. Neopuff®) or self-inflating bag and mask
  - oropharyngeal (Guedel) airway
  - laryngoscope, tracheal tubes and introducers
  - exhaled CO_2 detector
  - pulse oximeter
  - venous access equipment and drugs.

Specific questions to consider

- Will you need help? If so, call for it early.
- Is neonatal transport going to be needed?

Cord clamping

Delay in cord clamping of at least 1 minute from complete delivery of the infant is recommended for uncompromised infants. For the compromised infant, resuscitation is the priority and a plan of action should be agreed with the obstetric team. Resuscitation tables that can be placed directly adjacent to the mother to allow resuscitation with intact cord have been developed; studies are currently determining their impact on outcomes.

Temperature control

Thermoregulation is critical as hypothermia contributes to hypoglycemia, acidosis and even mortality, especially in extremely preterm infants (**see video: Resuscitation of preterm**).

Action

- Resuscitation area should be warm and draft free.
- Perform resuscitation under radiant warmer.
- Dry infant, remove wet towel, then wrap in dry towel.
- For preterm infants (<30 weeks), place wet infant directly in plastic wrap (bag) with only face exposed. Cover head with hat. An exothermic mattress may also be used.

Key point

Thermoregulation is critical. The vigorous term infant can be dried then placed against the mother's chest and covered with a warm towel.

If resuscitation is required – rapidly dry and place under radiant warmer. Preterm babies should be placed (wet) in plastic wrapping under a radiant heater with head covered. If neonatal admission temperature is >36.5 °C (97.8 °F), time on mechanical ventilation, length of stay and mortality are reduced.

After prolonged resuscitation in term infants, passive cooling should be started pending a decision about therapeutic hypothermia. Hyperthermia can worsen the outcome and should be avoided

Initial assessment at birth

Start the clock or note the time.
  Is the baby:
- term gestation?
- crying or breathing vigorously?
- good muscle tone?
  If this is the case, the baby should dried, placed skin-to-skin with the mother if desired and covered with dry linen to maintain temperature.
  If not, assess breathing (rate, depth and symmetry), heart rate (stethoscope on apex), color and tone and initiate resuscitation as required. Drying often produces enough stimulation to induce breathing.

A – Airway

If gasping or not breathing – open airway:
- Position – optimize head position, avoiding head overextension or flexion, using a towel beneath the shoulders if desired.
- Suction – only if obvious obstruction (e.g. blood, meconium) and unable to achieve chest rise. Suction should be under direct vision with a wide-bore suction device (bulb syringe or Yankauer).

Neonatology at a Glance, Third Edition. Edited by Tom Lissauer, Avroy A. Fanaroff, Lawrence Miall and Jonathan Fanaroff.
© 2016 John Wiley & Sons, Ltd. Published 2016 by John Wiley & Sons, Ltd.

Tracheal suctioning of meconium-stained fluid is only indicated for depressed, hypotonic babies. Care is required as pharyngeal suctioning may cause laryngeal spasm and vagal bradycardia. Suctioning meconium from the oropharynx at the perineum, routinely practiced for many years, does not improve outcome.
• For congenital airway abnormalities – choanal atresia, severe micrognathia (small jaw) or macroglossia (large tongue) – consider using an oral airway or laryngeal mask airway.

B – Breathing

Assessment

• Look for chest movement – check if inadequate or absent or if heart rate is <100 beats/min.
• Attach oxygen saturation monitor to right hand if resuscitation is anticipated, if baby remains cyanotic or if positive-pressure ventilation or supplementary oxygen required. Oxygen saturation monitors provide continuous reading of heart rate and oxygen saturation but take time to apply and may not function if poor perfusion. In healthy term infants following vaginal birth, it takes about 10 minutes for preductal oxygen saturation to reach levels >90%.

Action

If inadequate respiratory effort, gasping or not breathing or heart rate is <100 beats/min, the priority is to inflate the lungs with mask ventilation (Fig. 13.1), using a T-piece pressure device or self-inflating bag (Fig. 13.2).

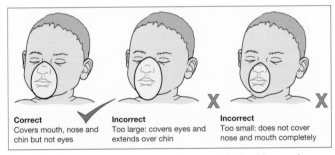

Correct
Covers mouth, nose and chin but not eyes

Incorrect
Too large: covers eyes and extends over chin

Incorrect
Too small: does not cover nose and mouth completely

Fig. 13.1 Correct size and position of face mask. It should cover the mouth, nose and chin.

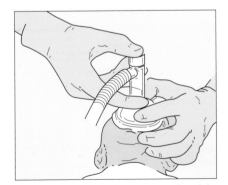

Fig. 13.2 Mask ventilation via a T-piece connected to air/oxygen blender from a pressure-limited circuit.

Mask ventilation

Most infants will respond to lung inflation.
• Term infants – start with air. Titrate additional oxygen according to oxygen saturation level.
• Preterm infants – as above but use air/oxygen blender and pulse oximetry. Use minimum oxygen required, according to preductal saturation targets in first 10 minutes of life. Avoid oxygen saturation above target range 91–95% as hyperoxemia can be damaging to eyes, lungs and brain.

Achieving lung inflation

The aim is good chest rise using the lowest pressure.
   Assess regularly, observing for:
• Increasing heart rate to >100 beats/min.
• Improving color (or saturations).
• Spontaneous breathing.
   If lung inflation is not achieved and the heart rate is not responding, further airway maneuvers may be required. Recheck the airway position and consider suction (if obstruction seen), increased peak pressure and inspiratory time, airway adjuncts (Guedel airway or laryngeal mask airway) or endotracheal intubation.

Key point

The Golden Minute:
   Initial assessment, dry the baby, observe breathing, check heart rate and start positive-pressure ventilation if required – all should be done in first minute after birth.

Endotracheal intubation (see Chapter 74)

Indications

• If *effective* mask ventilation is not sustaining adequate ventilation (but only when all the basic measures described above have been checked).
• Consider in all babies who require cardiac compressions to maintain the airway.
• If prolonged ventilation is needed.
• Congenital diaphragmatic hernia and some congenital upper airway abnormalities.
• If direct tracheal suction is needed for thick meconium or other obstruction in depressed, hypotonic infant.
   However:
• Should only be attempted by those with advanced airway skills.
• Limit each attempt to <30 seconds.
• Confirm tube in trachea with symmetrical air entry and end-tidal CO_2 detector.
• Provide effective mask ventilation between attempts if necessary.
If no response to intubation consider **DOPE**:
• **D**isplaced tube:
   – Is it in oesophagus? (no chest movement, air entry over stomach greater than chest, no CO_2 detected)
   – Is it in one (usually right) main bronchus?- asymmetrical chest rise or air entry, CO_2 may still be detected.

- **O**bstructed tracheal tube (especially meconium) – aspirate or replace tube, or tube too small for baby
- **P**atient:
  – Lung disorders i.e. lung immaturity, surfactant deficiency, pneumothorax, diaphragmatic hernia, lung hypoplasia, pleural effusion
  – Shock from blood loss, anemia
  – Neonatal encephalopathy – perinatal asphyxia, head trauma, CNS hemorrhage or abnormality
- **E**quipment failure-exhausted or disconnected gas supply.

C – Circulation

- Assess heart rate regularly with stethoscope or feel pulse at base of the umbilical cord (or observe heart rate on saturation monitor, if connected).
- Start chest compressions (Fig. 13.3) if heart rate <60 beats/min despite adequate ventilation.
- Call for help – if not already available.

There should be a 3:1 ratio of compressions to breaths (approximately 90 compressions and 30 breaths/minute) to maximize ventilation at an achievable rate. Compressions and ventilations should be coordinated to avoid simultaneous delivery.

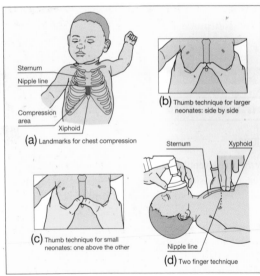

Fig. 13.3 (a) Apply pressure to lower third of sternum, just below an imaginary line joining the nipples. Avoid the xiphoid. Depress to reduce anteroposterior diameter of the chest by one-third with no bounce. The thumb technique (b and c) is more effective than the two-finger technique and is recommended, but the two-finger technique (d) is easier if you are alone.

Key points

- Before starting chest compressions, ensure the lungs are inflated, i.e. good chest movement. If not, chest compressions are unlikely to be effective.
- Call for help – giving chest compressions is easier with two people.

Drugs (Table 13.1)

Table 13.1 Resuscitation drugs

Medication	Concentration	Dosage/route	Indications
Epinephrine (adrenaline)	1 in 10000 (0.1 mg/mL)	IV: 0.1 to 0.3 ml/kg Endotracheal: 0.5–1 ml/kg	No response in spite of visible lung inflation and cardiac compressions
Volume expander	Normal saline Whole blood	10 mL/kg IV over 5–10 min	Suspected acute blood loss and/ or signs of hypovolemia
Sodium bicarbonate	0.5 mEq/mL (0.5 mmol/mL)	1–2 mEq/kg (1–2 mmol/kg) (2–4 mL/kg of 4.2% solution)	Consider only after prolonged arrest in spite of effective ventilation
Glucose	10%	2–2.5 mL/kg (250mg/kg) IV	For documented hypoglycemia

Drugs are rarely indicated; only use if no response in spite of:
- visible lung inflation
- cardiac compressions for at least 30 seconds.

Epinephrine (adrenaline) administered intravenously via umbilical venous catheter is recommended. Whilst intravenous access is obtained, administration in higher dose via endotracheal tube may be considered, but its efficacy has not been established.

Volume expansion with saline or blood may be indicated when blood loss is suspected e.g. pale infant, history of hemorrhage.

The role of sodium bicarbonate is controversial. It may be considered in prolonged resuscitation to correct metabolic acidosis, but may potentially be harmful as it may exacerbate intracellular acidosis if breathing is inadequate.

Prevention of hypoglycemia should be considered following prolonged resuscitation.

Drugs should be flushed with a bolus of saline.

Withholding and discontinuing resuscitation

Difficult decisions arise at the margins of viability and for infants with conditions that have unacceptably high morbidity or almost certain early mortality. Attitudes and practices vary widely between practitioners, institutions and countries. Whenever possible, decisions should be made with parental agreement.

Discontinuation of resuscitation should be considered if the heart rate is undetectable at birth and remains so for 10 minutes despite full resuscitation. If there is doubt, rather than hasty decisions in the delivery room, it is often best to transfer to the neonatal unit for detailed assessment.

Key point

In neonates, drugs are not indicated unless there is no response to effective ventilation (visible lung inflation) and optimally performed cardiac compressions.

Key point

The principles of neonatal resuscitation are agreed internationally and regularly updated [see ILCOR (International Liaison Committee on Resuscitation)]. As details differ between countries, the UK/European and US algorithms are shown.

Question

What are the guidelines used in the UK and Europe?

The UK/European Resuscitation guidelines are shown in Fig. 13.4.

Particular features are:
- **Airway** – neutral position (Fig. 13.5).

Suction airway only if obvious airway obstruction not corrected by appropriate airway positioning, and only under direct vision.

- **Breathing** – if not breathing or heart rate is not established, give five inflation breaths, preferably using air (pressure of $30\,cmH_2O$ for 2–3 s for term babies, 20–$25\,cmH_2O$ for preterm).

If heart rate increases but baby not breathing, provide regular ventilation breaths at 30–40 breaths/min.

If heart rate does not increase, check that chest is moving effectively. If not, check that baby's head is in neutral position, consider the need for jaw thrust, longer inflation time, a second person's help with the airway (Fig. 13.6), obstruction in the oropharynx or trachea, need for oropharyngeal (Guedel) airway.

If the heart rate remains at <60 breaths/min despite effective chest movement, start cardiac compression.

- **Cardiac compression** – ratio of 3 compressions to 1 inflation, rate of 90 compressions and 30 inflation breaths per minute.

- **Drugs** – rarely needed (<1 in 1000 births) if there is effective lung inflation and chest compression.

If epinephrine required, intravenous route is recommended. Tracheal route only if intravenous delivery not possible.

If blood loss suspected, give blood or 0.9% sodium chloride. Consider sodium bicarbonate and dextrose.

- **Meconium-stained liquor** – aspirating meconium from the nose and mouth before complete delivery is not recommended. If breathing is compromised and infant is hypotonic, inspect oral pharynx rapidly and aspirate obstructions to airway. Tracheal intubation may be helpful, if expertise is available (**see video: Resuscitation after meconium**).

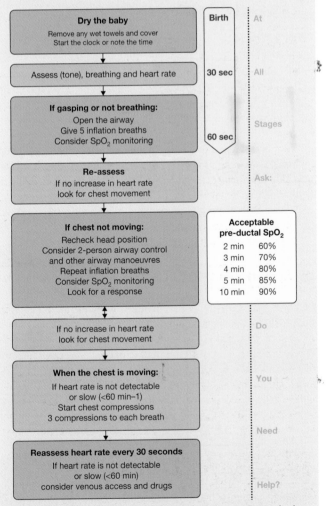

Fig. 13.4 Algorithm for newborn life support. (Source: Resuscitation Council UK, 2010.)

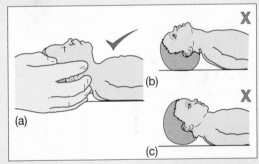

Fig. 13.5 Head position, the key to airway management. (a) Head in the correct neutral position. (b) Head overextended – incorrect. (c) Head flexed – incorrect.

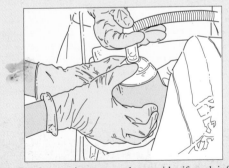

Fig. 13.6 Two-person airway control – consider if mask inflation ineffective. One person holds the head in the correct position, applies jaw thrust and holds the mask in place, the assistant operates the T-piece to provide lung inflation.

Question

What are the neonatal resuscitation guidelines used in the US?

The algorithm used is shown in Fig. 13.7.

Particular features are:
- **Airway** – place head in slightly extended 'sniffing position' to open airway. Clear airway if necessary with bulb syringe or suction catheter only if obvious obstruction to breathing or require positive pressure ventilation.
- **Breathing** – positive-pressure ventilation is started if the infants remains apneic or gasping or if heart rate remains at <100 beats/min.

Initial inflation pressure of 20 cmH$_2$O may be effective, but 30–40 cmH$_2$O may be required in some term babies. Ventilation should be delivered at 40–60 breaths/min to achieve promptly a heart rate >100 beats/min.

Endotracheal intubation may be indicated at any stage if there is inadequate response to mask ventilation.

- **Chest compression** – indicated for heart rate <60 beats/min despite adequate ventilation with supplementary oxygen for 30 s.

- **Drugs** –if heart rate remains at <60 beats/min despite adequate ventilation, usually with endotracheal intubation, with 100% oxygen and chest compressions.

Epinephrine (adrenaline) should be administered intravenously; endotracheal administration may be considered while access is obtained.

Volume expansion should be considered when blood loss is known or suspected.

Intravenous glucose should be considered as soon as practical after resuscitation in order to avoid hypoglycemia.

- **Meconium-stained liquor** – Endotracheal suctioning of meconium-stained amniotic fluid for non-vigorous babies. Monitor for subsequent respiratory distress and persistent pulmonary hypertension.

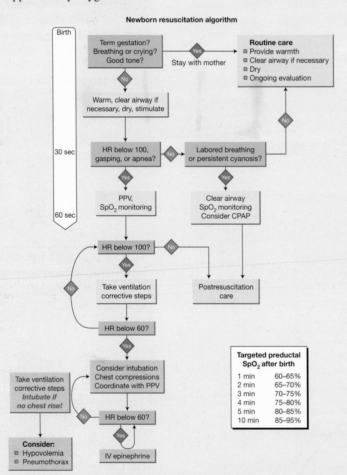

Fig. 13.7 Neonatal resuscitation algorithm. (Source: Kattwinkel J. *et al.* Neonatal Resuscitation: 2010 American Heart Association Guidelines for Cardiopulmonary Resuscitation and Emergency Cardiovascular Care. *Pediatrics* 2010; **126**; e1400–e1413. © American Heart Association, 2010; http://pediatrics.aappublications.org/content/126/5/e1400.full.html.)

Post-resuscitation care in the delivery room

Following resuscitation, stabilizing the extremely preterm or sick newborn infant starts in the delivery room before transfer to the neonatal unit (Fig. 13.8).

Airway and Breathing
Assess for respiratory distress
• Respiratory effort – both rate and pattern
• Chest retractions
• Nasal flare
• Grunting
• Cyanosis

If respiratory distress, provide respiratory support:
• CPAP/mechanical ventilation (see below)
• consider surfactant

Circulation
Examination:
Heart rate, pulses, capillary refill time, skin color
Immediate circulatory support if required

Thermoregulation:
Aim to maintain normal temperature 36.5–37.5°C by:
• Use of plastic wrap in preterm (<30 weeks) – apply prior to cord clamping (within sterile field at caesarian section); ensure wrap stays in place- make only small holes for oxygen saturation probe and umbilical catheter.
• Radiant heat and a hat. Exothermic mattresses may be useful.
• Monitor temperature regularly/continuously. Avoiding even moderate hypothermia reduces mortality, morbidity and length of stay in hospital.

Surfactant:
• Randomized trials have shown that routine prophylactic intubation and surfactant therapy is no longer indicated even in very preterm infants.
• Indicated in preterm infants who have significant respiratory distress ± oxygen requirement in spite of respiratory support.
• Requires tracheal instillation, followed by mechanical ventilation or non-invasive respiratory support.

Parents
Parents appreciate opportunity to touch their baby and understand what has been done. With support, fathers may be able watch delivery room stabilization and/or accompany baby to the NICU.

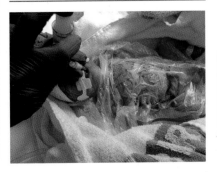

Investigations:
* Check blood glucose – if hypoglycemic, give glucose (Table 13.2); establish intravenous infusion to prevent hypoglycemia if indicated.
* Blood gas if indicated

Mechanical ventilation:
• Required prior to transfer in infants with significant respiratory distress and oxygen therapy in spite of non-invasive respiratory support and surfactant therapy.

Prophylactic CPAP:
• Extremely preterm infants are increasingly started on non-invasive respiratory support from birth instead of intubation and mechanical ventilation. CPAP soon after birth helps babies establish resting lung volume. Surfactant can be given later if sustained oxygen requirement develops.
• Given via face mask, binasal or single nasal prongs
• Use of CPAP ± surfactant in delivery room requires skill and experience.

Multi-disciplinary team
The team of health professionals, each with a clearly defined role, is required. If necessary, call for additional help.

Transport
Move to neonatal unit on resuscitation platform or in transport incubator. Using resuscitation table minimizes handling.

Oxygen saturation monitoring
Provides real-time measurements, also of heart rate. Apply probe to right hand for pre-ductal measurement. Titrate additional oxygen according to oxygen saturation, using range listed in algorithm. If preterm, keep oxygen saturation 91–95%.

Fig. 13.8 Post-resuscitation care in the delivery room.

14 Hypoxic–ischemic encephalopathy

Neonatal encephalopathy is a clinical description of generalized disordered neurologic function in the newborn. The most common cause is birth asphyxia. Asphyxia, from the Greek word meaning pulseless, is now used to mean a state in which gas exchange – placental or pulmonary – is compromised or ceases altogether, resulting in cardiorespiratory depression. Hypoxia, hypercarbia and metabolic acidosis follow. Compromised cardiac output diminishes tissue perfusion, causing hypoxic–ischemic injury to the brain and other organs. The origin may be antenatal, during labor and delivery or postnatal (Fig. 14.1).

Other causes of neonatal encephalopathy include transfer of maternal anesthetic agents, cerebral malformations, metabolic disorders (hypoglycemia, hypocalcemia, hyponatremia, inborn errors of metabolism), infection (septicemia and meningitis), hyperbilirubinemia, neonatal withdrawal (abstinence) syndrome and intracranial hemorrhage or infarction. The term "birth asphyxia" is best avoided because it is imprecise and implies that the baby's encephalopathy is a consequence of an asphyxial insult relating to birth, which may have medicolegal implications.

In hypoxic–ischemic encephalopathy (HIE), as opposed to other causes of encephalopathy, there is:
• a significant hypoxic or ischemic event immediately before or during labor or delivery or consistent fetal heart rate monitor pattern
• fetal umbilical artery acidemia (fetal umbilical artery pH < 7.0 or base deficit >/= 12 mmol/L, cord arterial pH < 7.20)
• Apgar score of < 5 at 5 and 10 minutes
• multisystem organ failure
• neuroimaging evidence of acute brain injury consistent with hypoxia-ischemia.

In developed countries, 0.5–1/1000 liveborn term infants develop HIE and 0.3/1000 have significant neurologic disability. HIE is more common in developing countries.

Pathogenic mechanisms

These include:
• failure of gas exchange across the placenta – excessive or prolonged uterine contractions, placental abruption, ruptured uterus
• interruption of umbilical blood flow – cord compression, cord prolapse, delayed delivery, e.g. shoulder dystocia
• inadequate maternal placental perfusion, maternal hypotension or hypertension – often with intrauterine growth restriction (IUGR)
• compromised fetus – anemia, IUGR
• failure of cardiorespiratory adaptation at birth – failure to breathe.

Compensatory mechanisms

These include:
• 'diving reflex' – redistribution of blood flow to vital organs (brain, heart and adrenals)
• sympathetic drive – increase in catecholamines, cortisol, antidiuretic hormone (ADH, vasopressin)
• utilization of lactate, pyruvate and ketones as an alternative energy source to glucose.

Primary and delayed injury

Following a severe ischemic insult, some brain cells die rapidly (primary cell death due to necrosis) and an excitotoxic cascade is triggered, including release of excitatory amino acids and free radicals. When circulation is re-established, there is a variable time delay before secondary energy failure and delayed cell death due to apoptosis. This offers a potential therapeutic window to ameliorate secondary damage (Fig. 14.2).

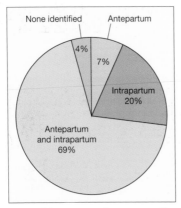

Fig. 14.1 Antepartum and intrapartum factors preceding neonatal hypoxic–ischemic encephalopathy. Data from Martinez-Biarge M. *et al.* Antepartum and intrapartum factors preceding neonatal hypoxic–ischemic encephalopathy. *Pediatrics* 2013; **132**; e952–e959.

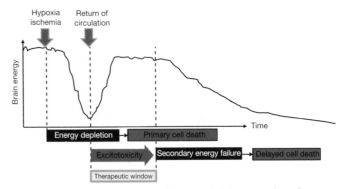

Fig. 14.2 Schematic diagram showing potential for prevention of secondary neuronal death.

Neonatology at a Glance, Third Edition. Edited by Tom Lissauer, Avroy A. Fanaroff, Lawrence Miall and Jonathan Fanaroff.
© 2016 John Wiley & Sons, Ltd. Published 2016 by John Wiley & Sons, Ltd.

Clinical manifestations

The clinical manifestations, investigations and management are summarized in Fig. 14.3.

Several large multicenter trials have demonstrated the benefit of therapeutic hypothermia in reducing death and disability and increasing survival with normal outcome at 18–24 months. The number needed to treat to prevent one death or disabled infant is seven. Selection criteria for cooling are gestation ≥36 weeks, need for prolonged resuscitation, clinical evidence of moderate or severe encephalopathy and severe metabolic acidosis within the first hour of life. aEEG or EEG are not required to initiate cooling, but may confirm the severity of the encephalopathy and determine if subclinical seizures are present (see Chapter 80). Cooling should be initiated within 6 h of birth. Core temperature is reduced to 33–34 °C and maintained for 72 h before slowly rewarming. Cooling is usually performed in a tertiary NICU but passive cooling (turning off radiant heaters and allowing the baby to lose heat naturally) may be commenced in the delivery room. Adjunct therapies to hypothermia that may further improve outcome are being evaluated, including xenon, melatonin and erythropoietin **(see video: Hypoxic–ischemic encephalopathy)**.

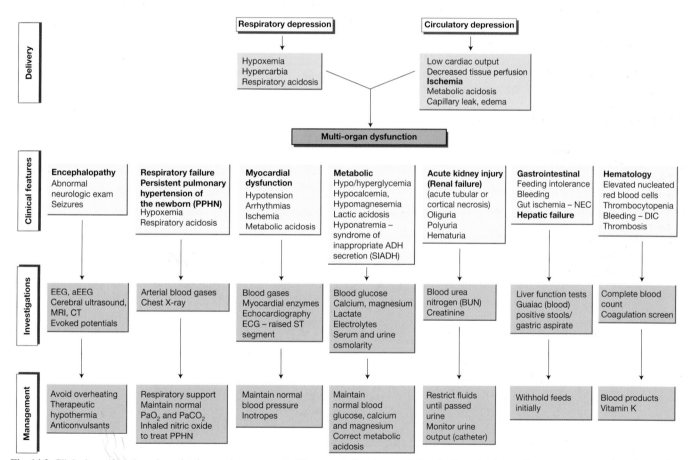

Fig. 14.3 Clinical manifestations, investigations and management of hypoxic–ischemic encephalopathy. Investigations and management are selected according to clinical features. (NEC – necrotizing enterocolitis; DIC – disseminated intravascular coagulation; EEG – electroencephalogram; aEEG – amplitude-integrated EEG, cerebral function monitor; CTG – cardiotochography.)

Key point

Avoid overheating – each degree above normal increases mortality and risk of brain injury.

Key point

Mild hypothermia (33–34 °C, within 6 h of birth for 72 h) has been shown to reduce morbidity and mortality of moderate and severe HIE (see Fig. 67.1).

Clinical staging of hypoxic–ischemic encephalopathy

Severity of brain injury can be systematically evaluated using a staging system which is performed sequentially and is of prognostic value. The most common is Sarnat (Table 14.1), although the simpler Thompson score is increasingly used.

Outcome

In general:
• A normal neurologic examination and feeding orally by 2 weeks of age suggest good prognosis.

• Mild HIE – usually good outcome.
• HIE without cooling:
– moderate HIE – increased risk for motor and cognitive abnormalities, including cerebral palsy (15–20%);
– severe HIE – 50–75% will either die or have severe disability in childhood (spastic quadriplegia, learning difficulties, visual and hearing impairment, and seizures).
• HIE with cooling:
– risk of death or disability is reduced by about 60%.
The postnatal markers of poor prognosis are shown in Table 14.3.

Table 14.1 Sarnat staging of hypoxic–ischemic encephalopathy.

	Grade 1 (mild)	Grade 2 (moderate)	Grade 3 (severe)
Level of consciousness	Irritable/hyperalert	Lethargy	Coma
Muscle tone	Normal or hypertonia	Hypotonia	Flaccid
Tendon reflexes	Increased	Increased	Depressed or absent
Myoclonus	Present	Present	Absent
Seizures	Absent	Frequent	Frequent
Complex reflexes			
Suck	Active	Weak	Absent
Moro	Exaggerated	Incomplete	Absent
Grasp	Normal to exaggerated	Exaggerated	Absent
Oculocephalic (doll's eye)	Normal	Overactive	Reduced or absent
Autonomic function			
Pupils	Dilated, reactive	Constricted, reactive	Variable or fixed
Respirations	Regular	Periodic	Ataxic, apneic
Heart rate	Normal or tachycardia	Bradycardia	Bradycardia
EEG	Normal	Low-voltage periodic or paroxysmal	Periodic or isoelectric
Prognosis	Good	Variable	High mortality and neurologic disability

Neuroimaging and functional studies (Table 14.2)

Table 14.2 Neuroimaging and functional studies and their indications and interpretation.

Procedure/test	Indication and interpretation
EEG or aEEG (amplitude-integrated EEG) (Fig. 14.4)	Best initiated as soon after birth as possible. Identifies encephalopathy, continuous seizure detection, monitoring background activity, and prognostic information. Good prognosis if normalizes in first 24 h.
Cranial ultrasound	Easy to perform at bedside. Useful for defining normal anatomy and for evidence of prenatal injury, congenital infection, intracranial hematoma or metabolic disorder. In HIE, may detect cerebral edema, hyperechogenic basal ganglia and/or abnormal blood flow velocity in middle and anterior cerebral arteries. Useful for following sequence and timing of any changes.
MRI scan	Imaging of choice for prognosis. Allows early recognition of injury to basal ganglia, internal capsule, white matter, brainstem and cortex, focal cerebral infarction, hemorrhage and malformations (Figs 14.5 and 14.6). Optimal between 7 and 21 days to determine the extent of cerebral injury. Diffusion-weighted imaging may detect abnormalities within the first week.

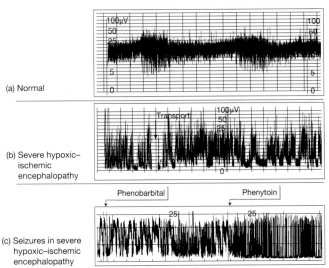

(a) Normal

(b) Severe hypoxic–
ischemic
encephalopathy

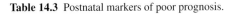

(c) Seizures in severe
hypoxic–ischemic
encephalopathy

Fig. 14.4 Amplitude-integrated EEG (aEEG) trace from cerebral function monitor showing (a) normal term newborn – normal baseline (>5 μV); (b) severe hypoxic–ischemic encephalopathy – low baseline amplitude; (c) seizures in severe hypoxic–ischemic encephalopathy unresponsive to phenobarbital but responsive to phenytoin, although the trace remains abnormal. (Courtesy of Professor Andrew Wilkinson.)

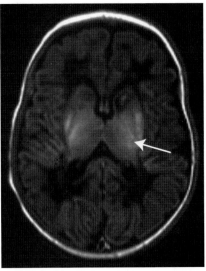

Fig. 14.5 Acute changes typically seen in the first week after perinatal asphyxia on MRI (axial T1W) at the level of the basal ganglia. There is an abnormal high signal in the posterolateral lentiform nuclei and thalami, loss of the normal high signal from myelin in the posterior limb of the internal capsule (arrow), abnormal signal in the head of the caudate nuclei and low signal throughout the white matter. (Courtesy of Dr Frances Cowan.)

Table 14.3 Postnatal markers of poor prognosis.

Abnormal EEG from birth or aEEG from 6 h with isoelectric pattern or burst suppression in non-cooled infants and later in cooled infants

Abnormal MRI (conventional or diffusion-weighted) – particularly basal ganglia/posterior limb of the internal capsule (PLIC) or marked brain atrophy or delayed myelination on later scan

Persistence of clinical seizures

Persistently abnormal neurologic exam after 1 week (reasonable sensitivity, poor specificity)

Not feeding orally by 2 weeks of age

Poor postnatal head growth

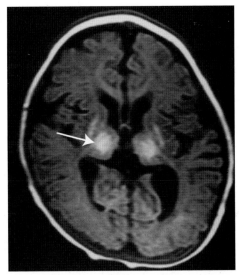

Fig. 14.6 Cerebral atrophy on MRI (axial T1W) developing several weeks after perinatal asphyxia. At the level of the basal ganglia there is severe atrophy of the basal ganglia (arrow), thalami and white matter with enlarged ventricles and extracerebral space. There is also plagiocephaly. (Courtesy of Dr Frances Cowan.)

15 Birth injuries

The incidence of severe birth injuries has fallen dramatically over the last 50 years. Prolonged, obstructed labor and difficult instrumental deliveries are usually avoided by cesarean section. However, birth injuries still occur, especially following instrumental deliveries, shoulder dystocia, malpresentation or preterm delivery. They are usually classified according to their anatomic location.

Common or important birth injuries

These are listed in Table 15.1. Scalp swellings can be differentiated by their position and relationship to the skull bones (Fig. 15.1).

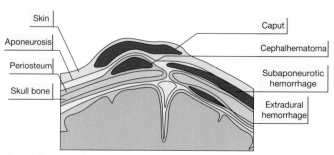

Fig. 15.1 Anatomic location of injuries to the head.

Table 15.1 Common or important birth injuries.

Lesion	Anatomic location	Comments	Clinical description and management
Injuries to the head			
Caput	Edema of the soft tissue of presenting part Crosses suture lines	Common and benign	Edema, bruising of scalp No treatment necessary; resolves in a few days, good prognosis
Chignon	Over site of vacuum extraction	Less common since soft, flexible cups introduced	Edema, sometimes bruising, skin damage Resolves over several days
Cephalhematoma	Subperiosteal Usually parietal Does not cross suture lines May be bilateral	Relatively common Associated with prolonged or instrumental labor	Hematoma maximal on second day May be associated with skull fracture May calcify Exacerbates jaundice Resolves in days to months
Subgaleal (subaponeurotic) hemorrhage	Between galea aponeurosis and periosteum (arrow)	Rare Risk factors: • prematurity • vacuum extraction May have underlying coagulopathy	Boggy appearance and pitting edema of scalp Anterior displacement of the ears Prompt recognition is crucial as may rapidly progress to hypovolemic shock Transfusion of blood, fresh frozen plasma, coagulation factors
Skull fractures	Usually parietal bone; occipital in breech deliveries	Uncommon Usually forceps delivery, but also normal delivery	Soft tissue edema and cephalhematoma Fractures may be linear or depressed Prognosis good
Minor injuries			
Forceps marks	From pressure of blades, especially rotational forceps	Less common as rotational forceps now seldom used	Bruising and/or skin abrasion Heals rapidly

Neonatology at a Glance, Third Edition. Edited by Tom Lissauer, Avroy A. Fanaroff, Lawrence Miall and Jonathan Fanaroff.
© 2016 John Wiley & Sons, Ltd. Published 2016 by John Wiley & Sons, Ltd.

Lesion		Anatomic location	Comments	Clinical description and management
Scalpel lacerations		Head or face	At caesarean section	May need tapes, suturing, plastic surgical referral

Injuries to the face

Lesion		Anatomic location	Comments	Clinical description and management
Facial palsy		Usually unilateral (right side in figure). If bilateral, suspect congenital cause	Pressure on maternal ischial spine or forceps delivery	Unilateral facial weakness on crying Eye on affected side remains open Resolves in 2–3 weeks If eye permanently open, use methylcellulose eye drops
Asymmetric crying facies		Unilateral absence of orbicularis oris muscle (left side in figure)	More common than facial palsy. Not a birth injury; needs to be differentiated from facial palsy	In contrast to facial palsy, eye can close; naso-labial crease is maintained

Injuries to the neck and shoulders

Lesion		Anatomic location	Comments	Clinical description and management
Fractured clavicle		Midclavicular area	Shoulder dystocia, breech Snap may be heard during delivery	Edema, bruising, crepitation at the site; decreased active movement of arm Clavicular lump from callus formation during healing phase. Confirm on x-ray Heals spontaneously
Brachial palsy Erb Nerves involved: C5, C6, ±C7			Shoulder dystocia, abnormal presentation, obstructed labor, macrosomia Phrenic nerve palsy – rare, diaphragm is elevated	Decreased shoulder abduction and external rotation, supination of wrist and finger extension (waiter's tip). Hand movement and grasp reflex are preserved 90% resolve by 4 months. Surgical referral if not recovered To avoid contractures, perform passive range of motion ± splints

Other injuries

Lesion		Anatomic location	Comments	Clinical description and management
Extremities – fractures		Fracture of the humerus/ femur	Breech, shoulder dystocia. May have underlying bone/ muscle disorder	Deformity, reduced movement of limb, pain on movement Orthopedic referral Splint to reduce pain. Rarely, hypovolemia from blood loss Bones rapidly remodel
Spinal cord		Cervical, thoracic, lumbar spine	Rare Instrumental delivery, may occur prenatally	Lack of movement below level of lesion Absent respiratory effort in high lesions Supportive care, steroids for spinal shock
Intra-abdominal organs		Ruptured liver, spleen	Macrosomia, breech, dystocia	Abdomen – distension, mass, discoloration, tenderness. Shock, pallor
		Renal injury Adrenal hemorrhage	Pre-existing hydronephrosis Prematurity, neuroblastoma	Hematuria Hypoglycemia, abdominal mass, coma, shock Intravascular volume support Abdominal ultrasound. Surgery unless bleed is contained (subcapsular hematoma)
Genitalia		Scrotum, labia majora	Breech	Bruising, hematoma. Resolves.

*Photograph of subgaleal hemorrhage reproduced with permission from Cheong, J.L.Y. *et al. Arch Dis Child Fetal Neonatal Ed* 2006; **91**: F202–F203.

16 Routine care of the newborn infant

Most term infants start to breathe several seconds after birth and become pink and active. If breathing normally, the baby can be dried and placed directly on the mother's front. This will allow direct skin-to-skin contact, the baby being kept warm with a towel. Alternatively, the baby can first be wrapped in warm towels. It is at this time that most babies are alert and are ready to begin to establish nursing at the breast.

After birth, the midwife or pediatrician will examine the baby briefly to check there are no abnormalities. A more detailed examination, the routine examination of the newborn, will be performed later, but within 24 hours of birth (see Chapter 17). Name tags will be attached to the baby and a record made to confirm that the baby passes urine and meconium within 24 hours of birth.

Routine care

Vitamin K
Vitamin K as prophylaxis against vitamin K deficient bleeding (hemorrhagic disease of the newborn) is recommended. It is most reliable if given as a single, large dose by intramuscular injection, but its disadvantage is that it is an injection. It can also be given orally, but this requires several doses to overcome its variable absorption, and protection is less reliable. Infants are at increased risk if they are breast-fed, as breast milk is low in vitamin K, if they have liver disease and if their mother is on anticonvulsant therapy.

Eye prophylaxis
In the US, most newborn infants are given erythromycin eye drops as prophylaxis against gonococcal and chlamydia eye infection. Silver nitrate eye drops have also been used, but can cause chemical conjunctivitis and do not prevent chlamydial infection.

In the UK, eye prophylaxis is not practiced, but gonococcal or chlamydia eye infection is rare.

Circumcision
This is widely performed in the US, but only for religious reasons in the UK. (see Chapter 52).

Breast-feeding
Mothers may need assistance and support to establish breast-feeding.

Umbilical cord care
Always wash hands before handling.
Keep dry and exposed to air.
Clean with water; avoid alcohol as it delays cord separation.
Fold diaper (nappy) below umbilicus.
In developing countries, application of chlorhexidine is recommended.

Meeting the family
Visiting by siblings, grandparents and other close family should be facilitated in order to be introduced to the new member of the family.

Emotions
Some mothers are emotionally labile during the first few days after birth. Even minor problems can cause considerable upset. Explanation and reassurance are required.

Mothers who develop postnatal depression or who are unable to care for their baby or have no suitable accommodation may be identified during this postnatal period. Liaison with mental health or social services, voluntary services or health visitors and other community health professionals may be required.

Infants with disabilities or complex medical needs may require a multidisciplinary planning meeting before discharge. This is considered further in Chapter 71.

Screening

The use of a screening test depends on:
- prevalence of the disease
- ease with which the test can be performed
- false-positive and-false negative screening rates
- whether it significantly improves the prognosis
- cost.

The availability of screening tests varies with judgment as to whether these criteria are satisfied.

Biochemical screening (Newborn bloodspot)

This is performed on all infants. Blood spots, usually from a heel prick, are placed on a card that is sent to a reference laboratory.

In most centers in the US, tandem mass spectrometry is used to screen a wide range of disorders (particular disorders vary by state), but all States screen for are least 29 disorders including:
- phenylketonuria
- hypothyroidism
- sickle cell disease
- thalassemia
- MCADD (medium-chain acyl-CoA dehydrogenase deficiency)
- Maple syrup urine disease (MSUD)
- Isovaleric aciduria (IVA)
- Glutaric aciduria type I (GA1)
- Homocysteinuria (HCU).

Cystic fibrosis screening is performed by measuring serum immuno-reactive trypsin (IRT) and DNA analysis for mutations in CFTR (cystic fibrosis transmembrane regulator gene). The trypsin level is raised

---

Neonatology at a Glance, Third Edition. Edited by Tom Lissauer, Avroy A. Fanaroff, Lawrence Miall and Jonathan Fanaroff.
© 2016 John Wiley & Sons, Ltd. Published 2016 by John Wiley & Sons, Ltd.

because of obstruction of the pancreatic ducts. It has a high false-positive rate, which can be reduced by combining it with DNA analysis.

In the UK, screening is confined to the disorders listed above, but an expanded program of tandem mass spectrometry is being assessed in some areas.

Audiology (see Chapter 62)

Neonatal hearing screening is universal for infants in the UK and in most States in the US.

Transcutaneous bilirubin

Used to identify infants at increased risk of developing hyperbilirubinemia and requiring more frequent monitoring (see Chapter 41).

Other possible screening tests

Pulse oximetry
Increasingly introduced in the US and UK to detect critical congenital heart disease in all infants (see Chapter 49).

Ultrasound for DDH (developmental dysplasia of the hips)
Used selectively in the UK and US, e.g. breech position, family history, but in all babies in some countries in Europe (see Chapter 17).

Routine hematocrit for polycythemia
Not recommended as not proven that treatment improves prognosis.

Health promotion

Parents should be provided with verbal and written advice about:
- feeding
- jaundice
- the importance of immunizations
- safe sleep practices to reduce the risk of SIDS (sudden infant death syndrome) (Fig. 16.1)

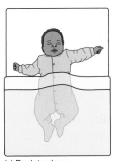
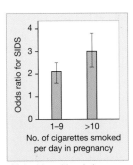

(a) Back to sleep
Always put babies to sleep on their back (not prone or side)

(b) Avoid smoking during pregnancy and in your baby's presence

Fig. 16.1 Advice for parents to reduce the risk of SIDS. (a) Back to sleep. (b) Odds ratio for SIDS and number of cigarettes smoked per day in pregnancy. A more detailed list of advice for parents is listed above in the Key points. (Adapted from Reduce the Risk of SIDS, Department of Health, UK, 2009 and American Academy of Pediatrics, 20011. Data from MacDorman M.F. *et al.* Sudden infant death syndrome and smoking in the United States and Sweden *Am J Epidemiol* 1997; **146**: 249–257.)

Key points

In order to reduce the risk of SIDS:
- Back to sleep (Fig. 16.1a)
- Avoid exposure to cigarette smoke (Fig. 16.1b)
- Avoid overheating:
  - No more than 1 more layer of clothing than an adult would wear.
  - Head and face uncovered.
- Safe sleep environment:
  - Sleep in own crib (cot) in parents' bedroom, but not in their bed.
  - Never sleep with baby on a sofa or armchair.
  - Infant should sleep on a firm surface, with no pillows or toys.
- Breast feed
- Consider pacifier at nap and bedtimes.

- the need for a car seat to take the baby home and whenever traveling in a car
- when to seek medical attention.

Discharge

Before discharge, check that:
- feeding is being established successfully
- the nursing staff do not have concerns about the mother's handling of the baby
- the baby is well and not significantly jaundiced
- timely follow-up arrangements are in place.

Question

Which immunizations should be given routinely in the immediate newborn period?

US:
- Hepatitis B: initial dose recommended as part of universal immunization program and given before discharge.

UK:
- BCG for TB: increasingly offered if living in high-risk area or for certain ethnic communities. Requires intradermal injection.
- Hepatitis B: given if mother is positive for hepatitis B surface antigen.

Key point

Every effort should be made to ensure successful breast feeding. Human milk provides not only optimal nutrients, but also provides hormones and enhances the immune system and gut microbiome.

17 Routine examination of the newborn infant

All babies are examined shortly after birth to check that transition to extrauterine life has proceeded smoothly and there are no major abnormalities. A comprehensive medical examination within 24 hours of birth, the 'routine examination of the newborn infant', should be performed.

The purpose is to:
• detect any abnormalities – a significant congenital anomaly is present at birth in 10–20 per 1000 live births
• confirm and plan the further management of any abnormalities detected antenatally
• consider potential problems related to maternal pregnancy history or familial disorders
• allow the parents to ask any questions and raise any concerns about their baby
• determine whether there is concern by caregivers about the care of the baby following discharge.
• provide health promotion, especially prevention of sudden infant death syndrome (SIDS) (see Chapter 16).

Preparation

Maternal charts (records):
• Check maternal antenatal, labor and delivery charts.

Equipment:
• Tape measure.
• Stethoscope.
• Ophthalmoscope.
Environment:
• Warm room free from drafts.
• Privacy, suitably lit.
• Examine on firm mattress in crib (cot).
• Both parents present if possible.
• Always wash hands and clean stethoscope before each examination.

The infant

• The baby must be completely undressed during the course of the examination so that all the body is observed.
• Need a content, settled infant for successful examination.
• Examination is performed opportunistically, i.e. eyes when open, heart when quiet, hips left until last. However, the examination must be complete.

Routine examination of newborn infants

(Table 17.1, Figs 17.2 and 17.3) **(see video: Newborn examination)**

Developmental dysplasia of the hip, DDH (congenital dislocation of the hip, CDH)

Clinical examination:
• Performed on all infants – part of routine neonatal examination.
• Infant must be relaxed – if crying or kicking there is tightening of the muscles around the hip.
• There may be asymmetry of skin folds around an affected hip and shortening of the affected leg.
• Fully abduct both hips; full abduction may not be possible if the hip is dislocated. Pelvis is stabilized with one hand; with the other, the examiner's middle finger is placed round the greater trochanter and the thumb around the distal medial femur.
• Check if dislocatable posteriorly (Barlow maneuver) (Fig. 17.1a).
• Check if hip is dislocated and can be relocated into acetabulum (Ortolani maneuver) (Fig. 17.1b) Minimal force is required.
Risk increased:
• in female infants (9:1)
• if positive family history (20% of affected infants)
• if breech presentation (30% of affected infants)
• in infants with a neuromuscular disorder.

If abnormal or questionable clinical examination, arrange consultation with experienced orthopedic surgeon. If normal examination but breech presentation or, in some centers, positive family history, arrange hip ultrasound at 4–6 weeks of age. Ultrasound screening of all infants can identify some missed on clinical examination and some with shallow acetabular shelf not detectable on clinical examination, but has appreciable false-positive rate (7%). Not recommended for all infants in US or UK.

For management see Chapter 61.

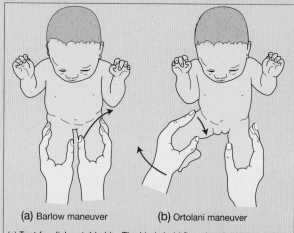

(a) Barlow maneuver   (b) Ortolani maneuver

(a) Test for dislocatable hip. The hip is held flexed and adducted. The femoral head is pushed downwards. If dislocatable, the femoral head will be pushed posteriorly out of the acetabulum with a palpable clunk

(b) Test for dislocated hip. Abduct hip with upward leverage of femur. A dislocated hip will return with a palpable clunk into the acetabulum

Fig. 17.1 Barlow and Ortolani maneuvers.

Neonatology at a Glance, Third Edition. Edited by Tom Lissauer, Avroy A. Fanaroff, Lawrence Miall and Jonathan Fanaroff.
© 2016 John Wiley & Sons, Ltd. Published 2016 by John Wiley & Sons, Ltd.

Table 17.1 Significant congenital abnormalities which may be identified on routine examination.

Dysmorphic infant (see Chapter 9)
Cataracts (see Chapter 62)
Cleft lip and palate (see Chapter 40)
Congenital heart disease (see Chapter 49)
Urogenital – hypospadias, undescended testes (see Chapter 52)
DDH (developmental dysplasia of the hip)
Imperforate anus (see Chapter 48)
Spinal anomalies (see Chapter 59)

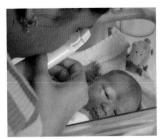

Fig. 17.2 Checking for red reflex. If absent, i.e. the pupil is white (cataracts, glaucoma, retinoblastoma), refer directly to an ophthalmologist. Also check eye looks normal, e.g. for a coloboma, a key-shaped defect in the iris. (see Chapter 62)

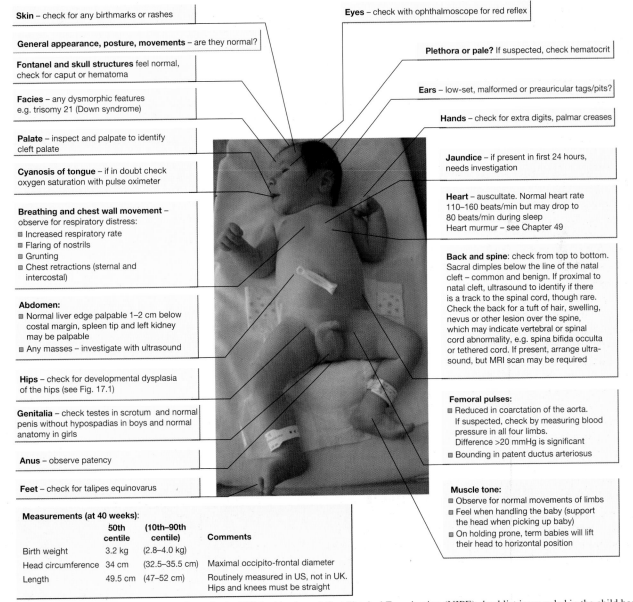

Skin – check for any birthmarks or rashes

General appearance, posture, movements – are they normal?

Fontanel and skull structures feel normal, check for caput or hematoma

Facies – any dysmorphic features e.g. trisomy 21 (Down syndrome)

Palate – inspect and palpate to identify cleft palate

Cyanosis of tongue – if in doubt check oxygen saturation with pulse oximeter

Breathing and chest wall movement – observe for respiratory distress:
- Increased respiratory rate
- Flaring of nostrils
- Grunting
- Chest retractions (sternal and intercostal)

Abdomen:
- Normal liver edge palpable 1–2 cm below costal margin, spleen tip and left kidney may be palpable
- Any masses – investigate with ultrasound

Hips – check for developmental dysplasia of the hips (see Fig. 17.1)

Genitalia – check testes in scrotum and normal penis without hypospadias in boys and normal anatomy in girls

Anus – observe patency

Feet – check for talipes equinovarus

Eyes – check with ophthalmoscope for red reflex

Plethora or pale? If suspected, check hematocrit

Ears – low-set, malformed or preauricular tags/pits?

Hands – check for extra digits, palmar creases

Jaundice – if present in first 24 hours, needs investigation

Heart – auscultate. Normal heart rate 110–160 beats/min but may drop to 80 beats/min during sleep Heart murmur – see Chapter 49

Back and spine: check from top to bottom. Sacral dimples below the line of the natal cleft – common and benign. If proximal to natal cleft, ultrasound to identify if there is a track to the spinal cord, though rare. Check the back for a tuft of hair, swelling, nevus or other lesion over the spine, which may indicate vertebral or spinal cord abnormality, e.g. spina bifida occulta or tethered cord. If present, arrange ultrasound, but MRI scan may be required

Femoral pulses:
- Reduced in coarctation of the aorta. If suspected, check by measuring blood pressure in all four limbs. Difference >20 mmHg is significant
- Bounding in patent ductus arteriosus

Muscle tone:
- Observe for normal movements of limbs
- Feel when handling the baby (support the head when picking up baby)
- On holding prone, term babies will lift their head to horizontal position

Measurements (at 40 weeks):

	50th centile	(10th–90th centile)	Comments
Birth weight	3.2 kg	(2.8–4.0 kg)	
Head circumference	34 cm	(32.5–35.5 cm)	Maximal occipito-frontal diameter
Length	49.5 cm	(47–52 cm)	Routinely measured in US, not in UK. Hips and knees must be straight

Fig. 17.3 Routine examination of newborn infants. In the UK the Newborn Infant Physical Examination (NIPE) checklist is recorded in the child health record and communicated to the family practitioner.

18 Neurologic examination

The newborn infant's neurologic development progresses markedly with gestational age. This needs to be taken into account when performing a neurologic examination, and accounts for many of the components of the neurologic examination used in the clinical assessment of gestational age (Ballard or Dubowitz score; see Chapter 83).

A detailed neurologic examination is performed if there are any concerns about neurologic abnormality. A normal neurologic exam is helpful prognostically, e.g. following hypoxic–ischemic encephalopathy, a normal neurologic examination and normal feeding by 2 weeks of age are associated with a good prognosis. Very low birthweight infants with a normal neurologic examination and intracranial ultrasound at 40 weeks are highly unlikely to develop significant motor disability and the predictive value of combined assessment is better than ultrasound alone.

The neurologic development described here is adapted from that described by Amiel-Tison, who has also devised a standardized examination with 10 components (**see video: Neurological examination**).

States of alertness

An infant's state of alertness can be classified (Prechtl scale):
- state 1: eyes closed, regular respiration, no movements
- state 2: eyes closed, irregular respiration, no gross movements
- state 3: eyes open, no gross movements
- state 4: eyes open, gross movements, no crying
- state 5: eyes open or closed, crying.

For satisfactory neurologic assessment infants need to be in state 3, when they are quiet but alert, i.e. able to fix and follow. However, the clinician may have to bring the baby to this state. Inability to do this may occur because the infant is abnormally lethargic or hyperexcitable (or deeply asleep or hungry!). An abnormal cry may also indicate abnormal neurology.

Visual fixing and following

A normal term infant should fix and follow a face or target of concentric black and white circles or a red ball moving from side to side. This starts at about 32 weeks' gestation. The infant should make eye-to-eye contact when held about 30 cm from the observer.

Hearing

Infants respond to noise with a facial grimace, turning of the head or startle.

Consolability

This is the response of the crying infant to a voice or soothing movements, such as rocking from side to side. It indicates communication between the infant and caregiver.

Head circumference

This is a surrogate measure of brain volume and subsequently of brain growth.

Face (cranial nerves)

There should be normal facial movements, blinking of the eyes and ability to suck strongly.

Posture and spontaneous motor activity

Posture

Posture at term is flexed (Fig. 18.1). Movements are smooth, symmetric and varied. The infant can move the fingers and can abduct the thumbs.

Passive tone in limbs and trunk

Develops from hypotonia at 24 weeks of gestation to strong flexor tone at 40 weeks, initially in the lower then upper limbs (Fig. 18.2).

Active tone in limbs and trunk

See Fig. 18.3.

32 weeks	40 weeks
Arms extended Some flexion of the legs	Full flexion of all four limbs

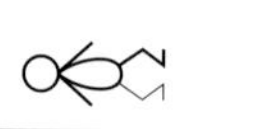

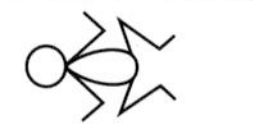

Fig. 18.1 Posture.

Popliteal angle		Foot dorsiflexion		Scarf sign	
With thigh beside abdomen, extend knee as far as possible		With knee flexed, ankle is dorsiflexed Measure angle between dorsum of foot and anterior of leg		Hand pulled across chest towards opposite shoulder Position of elbow noted	
32 weeks	Term	32 weeks	Term	32 weeks	Term
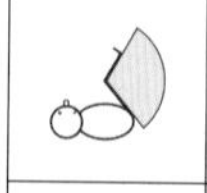	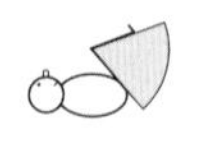	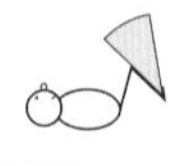	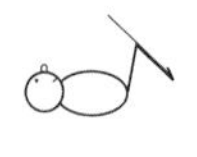	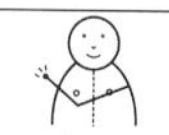 Largely passes midline	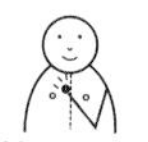 Very tight
120°–110°	90° or less	40°–30°	0°	Very weak resistance	Does not reach midline

Fig. 18.2 Passive tone in limbs and trunk.

Neonatology at a Glance, Third Edition. Edited by Tom Lissauer, Avroy A. Fanaroff, Lawrence Miall and Jonathan Fanaroff.
© 2016 John Wiley & Sons, Ltd. Published 2016 by John Wiley & Sons, Ltd.

Righting reaction		Neck flexor tone (raise to sit)		Ventral suspension	
Holding infant upright under axillae		Holding infant's shoulders, pull from lying to sitting			
32 weeks	40 weeks	32 weeks	40 weeks	32 weeks	40 weeks
Brief support of lower limbs only	Upright and takes weight for few secs	No movement of head forwards	Minimal head lag. Similarly for neck extensor tone (back to lying)	Some extension of head and back	Head extended above body, back extended and limbs fully flexed

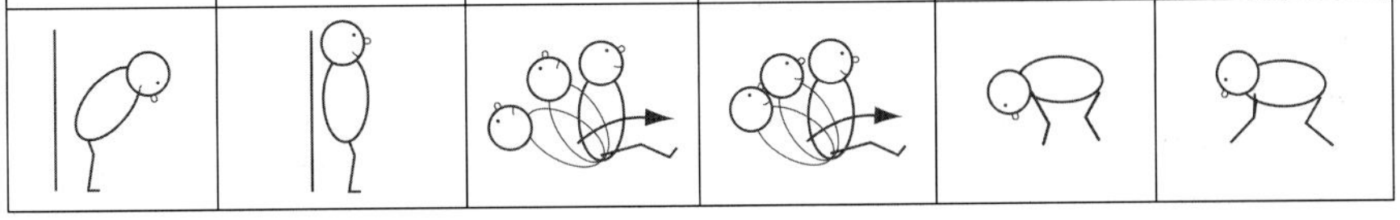

Fig. 18.3 Active tone in limbs and trunk.

Primary reflexes

Primary or primitive reflexes reflect brainstem activity (Fig. 18.4). They are a manifestation of central nervous system programming with later suppression by higher cortical function. If they cannot be elicited, suggests central nervous system depression. More important, their persistence suggests damage to upper cortical control (Table 18.1).

Key point

The hypertonic term infant – increased tone and tendon reflexes and head extension when held prone. Often hypotonic in neonatal period and hypertonia develops during infancy.
    The hypotonic term infant – see Chapter 60.

Table 18.1 Primary reflexes.

Reflex	Disappearance (corrected age)
Placing	3 months
Palmar grasp	3 months
Plantar grasp	3 months
Moro	4 months
Asymmetric tonic neck reflex (ATNR)	6 months

Deep tendon reflexes

May be depressed with lower motor neuron lesions, occasionally increased with upper motor neuron lesions. May reveal asymmetry. Ankle clonus is common and usually of no pathologic significance.

Plantar responses

Elicited by stroking the lateral part of the foot from heel to toe. Unhelpful at this age as normal response may be flexor (toe down) or extensor (toe up).

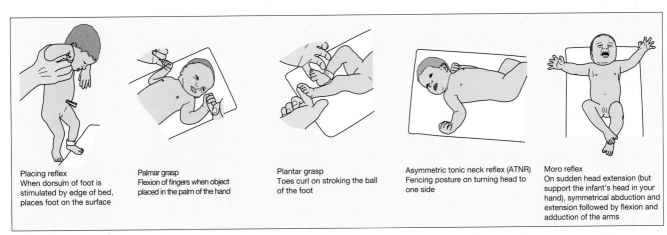

Placing reflex
When dorsum of foot is stimulated by edge of bed, places foot on the surface

Palmar grasp
Flexion of fingers when object placed in the palm of the hand

Plantar grasp
Toes curl on stroking the ball of the foot

Asymmetric tonic neck reflex (ATNR)
Fencing posture on turning head to one side

Moro reflex
On sudden head extension (but support the infant's head in your hand), symmetrical abduction and extension followed by flexion and adduction of the arms

Fig. 18.4 Primary reflexes.

19 Care and support for parents

The family must, of course, be included in the care of all newborn infants, whether well or critically ill. The birth of a healthy newborn infant is usually a joyous occasion fulfilling the dreams and hopes of the parents. If the baby is extremely premature, sick, has malformations or dies, these dreams will be shattered and the family will experience considerable distress. The family will need sensitive discussion and support. How this is done will influence their ability to cope and recover in the short and long term. Family centered care encourages parents to be partners in their infants' care and in decisions about treatment. The way parents see themselves as parents, respond to their baby and react to stressful situations is very individual and will be influenced by personal views and standards, family background and culture. Psychological support from an appropriately trained professional may be helpful for parents to deal with their distress and anxiety. This may also be needed to help with psychological problems that occur after the infant leaves hospital.

Attachment

What is maternal attachment?

It is the intense relationship which develops between a mother and her child, providing protection and nurturing for the child (Fig. 19.1).

In many animals, e.g. ducks or penguins, there is a critical, sensitive period for mother–infant bonding immediately after birth, when the mother and her offspring must be in direct contact. If this does not happen the mother fails to recognize that the newborn is hers. Attachment in humans does not necessarily happen instantly, but develops over time. Although touching and nursing the baby shortly after birth is helpful in promoting attachment, and should be encouraged, humans can still become attached to their infants where this does not occur, for example if the infant is admitted directly to the neonatal unit.

Fathers and other family members also develop attachment with the newborn baby. Attachment is the foundation of healthy emotional development. In childhood, secure attachment gives the child the confidence to explore and learn.

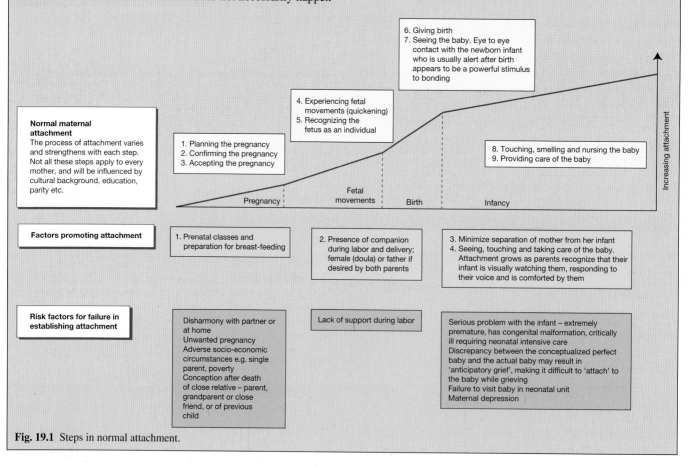

Fig. 19.1 Steps in normal attachment.

Neonatology at a Glance, Third Edition. Edited by Tom Lissauer, Avroy A. Fanaroff, Lawrence Miall and Jonathan Fanaroff.
© 2016 John Wiley & Sons, Ltd. Published 2016 by John Wiley & Sons, Ltd.

Communicating with parents

Parents and family want open communication about their baby. Professionals need to not only provide accurate and realistic information about the baby's problems but also listen to and address the family's anxieties and feelings. The needs of each of the family members should be elicited, as they may differ. Fathers, who may be at work much of the time, particularly value opportunities for communication.

Some specific circumstances regarding communicating with parents related to perinatal care are considered below.

Antenatal identification of fetal abnormality or potential abnormality

• Many problems, including major malformations and preterm delivery, are now identified before birth. The recognition of many minor malformations or the possibility of an abnormal finding in the fetus has become a common cause of additional anxiety for parents.
• The neonatal team should be involved and present a realistic picture. First discuss the positive aspects and present facts in a positive light – describe a glass as half full rather than half empty.

Facts should be disclosed but acknowledge uncertainty and do not overemphasize unsubstantiated fears.
• Problems should be anticipated and their consequences and management discussed with the family. If appropriate, a tour of the neonatal intensive care unit (NICU) before delivery should be conducted.

Admission of the infant to the neonatal unit

Parents of infants in the NICU are at increased risk of acute stress and post-traumatic stress disorder. See Chapter 22 for further details.

Infants with serious congenital malformations

The crisis of the birth of a child with a serious malformation can result in emotional turmoil, the parents mourning the loss of the normal child they expected whilst also needing to attach to their newborn. Doctors and other health professionals will need to explain the nature and implications of the disorder to the parents and family and may need to provide considerable emotional support to help families in this difficult situation (Table 19.1).

Table 19.1 How parents wish to be told about a serious problem or life-threatening illness. (Adapted from Wooley H. et al. Imparting the diagnosis of life-threatening illness in children. *BMJ* 1989; **298**: 1623–1626.)

Setting	**Explain long-term prognosis**
In private and comfort	If child is likely to die, listen to concerns about time, place and nature
Uninterrupted	of death
Unhurried	Outline the support/treatment available
Both parents present if possible	
If desired, also a trusted person who can help review the conversation afterwards.	**Address feelings**
Senior doctor	Be prepared to tolerate reactions of shock, especially anger or weeping
Nurse present	Acknowledge uncertainty
Translator if necessary	How is it likely to affect the family?
Some families find it helpful to have a tape recording of the interview or to take notes	What and how to tell other children, relatives and friends?
	Concluding the interview
Establish contact	Elicit what parents have understood
Find out what the family knows or suspects	Clarify and repeat, particularly highlighting immediate situation and next steps
Respect family's vulnerability	Acknowledge that it may be difficult for parents to absorb all the
Use the child's name and parents' names – do not call them mum and dad	information and they should not be afraid to ask questions over and over again
Do not avoid looking at them	Mention sources of support
Be direct, open, sympathetic	Give parents a contact telephone number or e-mail
	Give web-site or address of self-help group
Provide information	Check if there is anything else they would like to know
Flexibility is essential	
Pace rather than protect from bad news. Some families want a lot of information at once, others prefer shorter interviews more often	**Follow-up**
Name the illness or condition	Offer early follow-up and arrange date
Describe symptoms relevant to child's condition	Suggest to families that they write down questions before next appointment
Discuss etiology – parents will usually want to know	Ensure adequate communication of content of interview to other members
Anticipate and answer questions. Don't avoid difficult issues because parents have not thought to ask	of staff, family practitioner and health visitor and other professionals, e.g. a referring pediatrician

Human milk is recommended as the exclusive food for all term infants for the first 6 months of life. Human milk is also recommended for preterm infants but may need fortification. Donor breast milk is increasingly available for preterm infants to supplement maternal milk. All mothers should be encouraged and supported to breast-feed. Counseling should commence early in pregnancy and mothers should be assisted by nursing or lactation specialists.

The choice to breast- or bottle-feed is personal and formula feeding should not be criticized.

Nutritional characteristics of human milk compared with unmodified cow's milk

Protein

- Low protein content (whey: casein, 60:40) – more easily digestible.
- High free amino acids and urea; glutamine, the predominant amino acid, stimulates enterotropic hormones, enhancing feeding tolerance.

Fat

- Unsaturated.
- Contains long-chain polyunsaturated fatty acids (LCPUFAs) – needed for nervous system development (now incorporated into formula, as is arachidonic acid, ARA).

Carbohydrate

- High lactose.

Minerals

- Low renal solute load.
- Reduced phosphate:calcium ratio.

Vitamins

Supplementation required to breast milk to meet daily requirements.

Formula

Formula is humanized, i.e. manipulated to resemble human milk. However, there are still differences in amino acid and fatty acid composition and it does not contain the anti-infective properties of human milk. In developing countries, infection from reconstituting milk powder with contaminated water is a major health problem.

Unmodified cow's, goat's and sheep's milks are unsuitable for infants. Soy formula is sometimes used to prevent allergic disorders such as eczema and asthma, although evidence for this is lacking. About 10–30% of infants with cow's milk protein intolerance become sensitive to soy. Soy formula is not recommended for premature infants.

Steps to successful breast-feeding

- Place the infant on the breast either immediately or soon after birth.
- Provide quiet, supportive environment with comfortable positioning (Fig. 20.1).
- Demand feeding is preferable to a fixed schedule. This stimulates milk production and reduces feeling of fullness and discomfort. May be put to the breast 8–12 or more times per 24 hours.
- Put to both breasts at each feeding. Switch sides when baby pauses and lets go of breast. Allow unrestricted duration of feeds. Begin each feeding with the breast last nursed from.
- Emptying the breast adequately avoids engorgement.

- Initial milk is colostrum – low in volume, high in protein and immunoglobulin content. Takes 24–72 hours for breast milk to come in.
- Warn mothers that babies initially lose weight (up to 7–10% of birthweight) and only put on weight after day 4 of life. They should be back to birthweight by 10–14 days.
- Do not give supplementary water or formula unless medically indicated.
- Allow mothers and infants to stay together (rooming-in) 24 hours per day.
- Inform mothers of breast-feeding support groups.

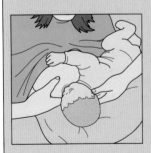 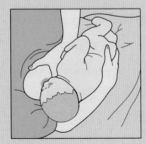 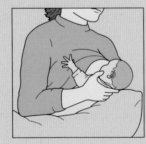

Fig. 20.1 Positioning for breast-feeding. (Adapted from UNICEF UK Baby Friendly Initiative.)

Neonatology at a Glance, Third Edition. Edited by Tom Lissauer, Avroy A. Fanaroff, Lawrence Miall and Jonathan Fanaroff.
© 2016 John Wiley & Sons, Ltd. Published 2016 by John Wiley & Sons, Ltd.

Breast-feeding

Advantages of breast-feeding for the infant

Immediate:
- Promotes mother–infant bonding.
- Ideal nutritional composition (see below).
- Contains immune factors (e.g. secretory IgA).
- Reduces gastroenteritis and respiratory infections.
- Less feeding intolerance.
- Reduces incidence of necrotizing enterocolitis in preterm infants.
- Promotes ketone production as an alternative energy substrate to glucose in first few days of life.
  Long term:
- Reduced risk of SIDS (sudden infant death syndrome).
- May decrease incidence and severity of eczema and asthma.
- Less obesity, insulin-dependent diabetes mellitus (type 1) and inflammatory bowel diseases (Crohn disease and ulcerative colitis).

Advantages of breast-feeding for the mother
- Enhances mother–infant bonding.
- More rapid postpartum weight loss.
- Decreased risk of osteoporosis.
- Decreased risk of breast and ovarian cancer.
- Increases time between pregnancies, which is important in developing countries.

Potential complications of breast-feeding for the infant
- Cannot tell how much milk the baby has taken. This is determined by monitoring baby's weight and urine output.
- Dehydration may occur if:
  - inadequate milk supply/poor feeding technique
  - hot weather.
- Jaundice associated with breast milk:
  - common
  - exacerbated by dehydration
  - even if requiring phototherapy, breast-feeding should be continued
  - is prolonged (>2 weeks of age) in up to 15% – will require investigations to be performed.
- Multiple births:
  - twins can often be exclusively breast-fed (Fig. 20.2), but rarely higher-order births.
- Vitamin K:
  - low level in breast milk may predispose to hemorrhagic disease of the newborn
  - prophylaxis is required.

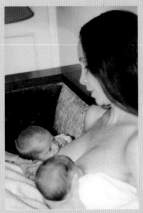

Fig. 20.2 Successful breast-feeding of twins.

Potential complications of breast-feeding for the mother
- Maternal feeling of inadequacy/upset if unsuccessful.
- Breast engorgement, cracked nipples – may be helped by manual expression or breast pump.
- Mastitis–requires maternal treatment and may disrupt feeding.

Contraindications to breast-feeding
- **Maternal HIV** – breast-feeding contraindicated in developed countries. In resource-poor environment, breast-feeding is advised unless formula feeds can be given safely. Under these circumstances, for Prevention of Mother-to-Child Transmission (PMCT), the World Health Organization now recommends lifelong combination antiretroviral therapy for all pregnant women, exclusive breast-feeding with antiretroviral therapy for the newborn for the first 6 months (or minimum of the first 6 weeks). Mixed formula and breast-feeding should be avoided (see Chapter 73, Global neonatology).
- **Maternal TB** infection (active).
- **Inborn errors of metabolism** – galactosemia, phenylketonuria.

Drugs in breast milk
- Most drugs are excreted in breast milk in such small quantities they do not affect the infant.
- Where possible, all drugs, including self-medication, should be avoided during breast-feeding. Most mothers who need medications can continue breast-feeding, but a few drugs preclude breast-feeding. Some examples are listed in Table 64.1.
  Check a formulary.

Key point

'Breast is best' for feeding newborn infants.

21 Minor abnormalities in the first few days

Distortion of the shape of the head from delivery (molding)
Caput succedaneum, cephalhematoma Chignon after vacuum extraction

Swollen eyelids but no discharge from the eye

Subconjunctival hemorrhages – from delivery

Traumatic cyanosis – skin discoloration and petechiae over the head and neck or presenting part from cord around the baby's neck or from a face or brow presentation. The tongue is pink

Small white cysts along the mid-line of the palate (Epstein pearls). Cysts of the gums (epulis) or floor of the mouth (ranula)

Peripheral cyanosis of the hands and feet (acrocyanosis). Present in most newborn infants on the first day

Breast enlargement may occur in newborn infants of either sex (Fig. 21.2). A small amount of milk may be discharged

Lanugo: fine, downy hair, starts to shed at 32–36 weeks' gestation

Umbilical hernia – more common in Black infants, usually resolves within 2–3 years

Vernix: greasy, yellow-white coating present at birth, a mixture of desquamating cells and sebum which protects fetus from maceration *in utero*

Vaginal discharge – small white discharge or withdrawal bleed in girls. A prolapse of a ring of vaginal mucosa may be present

Positional talipes (Fig 21.3). Feet adopt *in utero* position. If marked, parents can be shown passive exercises by physical therapist

Cracking and peeling of skin, particularly over hands and feet. Most pronounced in post-term infants. This scaling and desquamation is physiologic

Fig. 21.1 Minor abnormalities noted in the first few days of life.

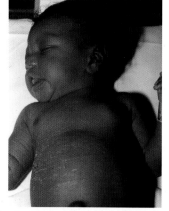

Fig. 21.2 Breast enlargement.

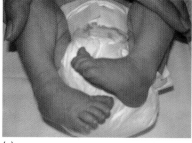
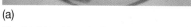
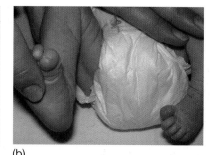

(a)   (b)

Fig. 21.3 Positional talipes. (a) Position of the feet. (b) The foot can be fully dorsiflexed to touch the front of the lower leg. In true talipes equinovarus this is not possible.

Neonatology at a Glance, Third Edition. Edited by Tom Lissauer, Avroy A. Fanaroff, Lawrence Miall and Jonathan Fanaroff.
© 2016 John Wiley & Sons, Ltd. Published 2016 by John Wiley & Sons, Ltd.

Skin lesions

Nevus flammeus (stork bites)
Pink macules on upper eyelids, mid-forehead (also called salmon patch) and nape of the neck (Fig. 21.4). Common. Dilated superficial capillaries. Those on the eyelids and forehead fade over the first year. Those on the neck persist but are covered with hair.

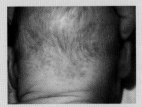

Fig. 21.4 Stork bite (nevus flammeus, salmon patch).

Milia
White, pinhead-sized pimples on the nose and cheeks and forehead. Resolve during first month of life. Are from retention of keratin and sebaceous material in the pilosebaceous follicles.

Miliaria
Pin-sized vesicles, particularly over the neck and chest. Usually develop at 2–3 weeks. Caused by sweat that is retained due to obstructed eccrine glands. Avoid excessive clothing and heating.

Erythema toxicum
Small, firm, white or yellow pustules on erythematous base (Fig. 21.5). It is the most common transient lesion, usually appears at 1–3 days but up to 2 weeks of age; primarily on trunk, extremities and perineum. Moves to different sites within hours. Contains eosinophils. May be present at birth.

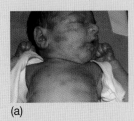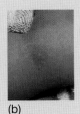

(a)   (b)

Fig. 21.5 (a) Erythema toxicum showing patchy pustules on erythematous base. (Courtesy of Dr Nim Subhedar.) (b) Close-up of skin lesion.

Mongolian spots
Blue–black macular discoloration at base of the spine and on the buttocks (Fig. 21.6). Usually but not invariably in Black or Asian infants. Sometimes also on the legs and other parts of the body. Fade slowly over the first few years. Of no significance unless misdiagnosed as bruises.

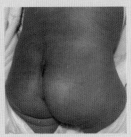

Fig. 21.6 Mongolian spot.

Transient pustular melanosis (transient neonatal pustulosis)
Resembles miliaria, but present at birth and may continue to appear for several weeks. Superficial vesiculo-pustular lesions rupture within 48 hours to leave small pigmented macules with white surround. More common in Black infants, in whom the lesions are often hyperpigmented.

Harlequin color change
Sharply demarcated blanching down one half of the body – one side of the body red while the other is pale. Lasts a few minutes. Thought to be due to vasomotor instability. It is benign.

Sucking blisters
Vesicles on hand, fingers or lips, from vigorous sucking *in utero*.

Other minor abnormalities (Figs 21.7–21.9)

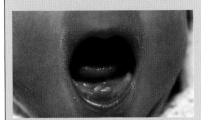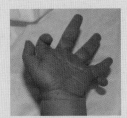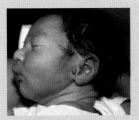

Fig. 21.7 Natal teeth. Front lower incisors present at birth. Remove if loose to avoid the risk of aspiration.

Fig. 21.8 Extra digits. Usually connected by a skin tag but may contain bone. Common anomaly – often hereditary. Cosmetic outcome is better if removed surgically rather than tying off with silk thread, which may leave residual neuroma.

Fig. 21.9 Ear tags. Consult plastic surgeon. Check that the ear and hearing is normal. If there is an ear anomaly, some centers ultrasound the kidneys as slight increased risk of renal abnormalities.

22 Common problems of term infants

Anticipation

Many neonatal problems can be anticipated or prevented by awareness of conditions that are detected antenatally (Tables 22.1 and 22.2) or which develop during labor or delivery (Table 22.3). This necessitates close liaison between the health professionals caring for the mother and fetus and pediatricians. Some common examples of problems and management plans which may occur in the neonatal period are listed below. They are described in more detail in the relevant chapters.

Maternal or antenatal conditions (Table 22.1)

Table 22.1 Neonatal problems associated with maternal conditions.

Maternal medical condition	Neonatal problem
Diabetes mellitus	Neonatal hypoglycemia Polycythemia Jaundice Congenital malformations
Maternal hyperthyroidism	Neonatal hyperthyroidism or hypothyroidism from maternal drug treatment
Autoimmune thrombocytopenia	Neonatal thrombocytopenia
SLE (systemic lupus erythematosus)	Heart block, rash
Red blood cell isoimmunization	
Rhesus and other red cell antibodies. ABO incompatibility (mother group O, infant A or B)	Jaundice, anemia
Hepatitis B positive	Immunization ± prophylaxis
HIV infection	Preventative therapy, advice about breast-feeding
Syphilis serology positive	Treatment if necessary
Chlamydia screening (in US)	
Chlamydia trachomatis identified	Check for conjunctivitis
Maternal drugs	
Drug abuse	Neonatal drug withdrawal
Alcohol	Fetal alcohol syndrome
Prolonged rupture of membranes	Neonatal infection
Chorioamnionitis	Neonatal infection
Maternal fever >38°C	Neonatal infection
Maternal group B streptococcal bacteriuria or colonization	Neonatal infection

Fetal conditions (Table 22.2)

Table 22.2 Neonatal problems associated with fetal conditions.

Fetal condition	Neonatal problem
Abnormal ultrasound	
Renal (commonest), e.g. hydronephrosis	May need prophylactic antibiotics, ultrasound and VCUG (vesicocystourethrogram)
Cardiac	May need repeat echocardiography – liaise with pediatric cardiologist
Other abnormalities	Management as planned antenatally
Intrauterine growth restriction (IUGR) or large for gestational age	Hypoglycemia Polycythemia
Multiple births	Anemia/polycythemia Twin–twin transfusion syndrome Congenital malformations Intrauterine growth restriction (IUGR)

Labor and delivery (Table 22.3)

Table 22.3 Neonatal problems associated with abnormal labor and delivery.

Labor and delivery	Neonatal problem
Antepartum hemorrhage	Hypoxic–ischemic encephalopathy, anemia
Markedly abnormal fetal heart trace	Hypoxic–ischemic encephalopathy
Cesarean section	TTNB (transient tachypnea of the newborn)
Vacuum extraction	Chignon, jaundice Subgaleal (subaponeurotic) hemorrhage – anemia, shock
Forceps	Localized bruising Facial palsy
Breech position	DDH (developmental dysplasia of the hip) Birth injuries Hypoxic–ischemic encephalopathy
Shoulder dystocia	Hypoxic–ischemic encephalopathy Erb palsy Fractured clavicle or humerus
Meconium	Meconium aspiration
Need for prolonged resuscitation at delivery	Hypoxic–ischemic encephalopathy

Neonatology at a Glance, Third Edition. Edited by Tom Lissauer, Avroy A. Fanaroff, Lawrence Miall and Jonathan Fanaroff.
© 2016 John Wiley & Sons, Ltd. Published 2016 by John Wiley & Sons, Ltd.

Overview of common medical problems

Most newborn infants are healthy, but may develop some of the clinical problems described below. Differentiating the clinically significant from the transient and benign can be difficult. An approach to these problems is given in Fig. 22.1. For details see specific chapters.

Conjunctivitis
Sticky eyes – common
Clean with sterile water
If conjunctivitis purulent or eyelids red and swollen, exclude bacterial cause including gonococcus and chlamydia

Vomiting
Babies often vomit milk. If persistent or bile stained may be from intestinal obstruction. If it contains blood, malrotation must be excluded, but is usually sallowed maternal blood from maternal cracked nipple or delivery
Abdominal distension may be from lower intestinal obstruction

Poor feeding
Usually related to problems in establishing breast-feeding
However, can be presentation of:
▫ Infection
▫ Hypoglycemia
▫ Electrolyte disturbance
▫ Inborn error of metabolism

Cyanotic/dusky spells
Normal infants sometimes become dusky or cyanosed around the mouth, often during feeds, in the first few days.
Conditions which need to be excluded are:
▫ Cyanotic congenital heart disease
▫ Polycythemia
▫ Infection

Mucus
Many babies produce a considerable amount of mucus on the first day. This needs to be differentiated from the infant with esophageal atresia who is unable to swallow saliva, which pools in the mouth

Jaundice
Check bilirubin on blood sample if:
▫ Jaundice at <24 hours of age
▫ Significant level on transcutaneous monitor

Skin lesions
Erythema toxicum or milia – common and harmless
Septic lesions – contain pus
Bullous impetigo – serious (staphylococcal or streptococcal) infection. Sacs of serous fluid; their roof is easily broken leaving denuded skin (Fig. 43.4)

Pallor/plethora
▫ Check hematocrit for anemia or polycythemia
▫ Check breathing and circulation

Jitteriness/seizures/lethargy
Jittery movements are common. They stop on holding the limb, in contrast to seizures. If pronounced check blood glucose and consider other causes, e.g. drug withdrawal
Seizures can be subtle, but are rhythmic jerky movements of the limbs
Seizures require prompt treatment and investigation – admit to the neonatal unit
Lethargy may be a sign of sepsis, hypoglycemia or inborn error of metabolism

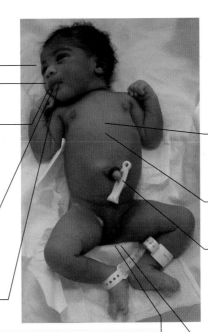

Delay in passing meconium (>48 hours)
Check for intestinal obstruction

Delay in voiding urine (>24 hours)
Voiding may be unobserved – often void immediately after birth
Consider urinary outflow obstruction (palpable bladder, ultrasound) or renal impairment (serum creatinine, ultrasound)

Weight loss
Babies initially lose weight (1–2% of birth weight per day up to 7–10% of birth weight). They may take up to 10–14 days to regain their birth weight

Collapse (rare but important)
Maintain Airway, Breathing, Circulation
Causes:
▫ Sepsis – bacterial or viral
▫ Duct-dependent heart disease – closure of ductus arteriosus
▫ Inborn error of metabolism

Hypoglycemia
Monitor if preterm, small or large for gestational age, maternal diabetes or ill infant.
Clinical features include:
• Jitteriness/irritability/high-pitched cry
• Depressed consciousness/lethargy/hypotonia
• Apnea
• Seizures.

Respiratory distress
Most common cause – TTNB (transient tachypnea of the newborn), but need to exclude infection and other causes
Check Airway, Breathing, Circulation, Oxygen saturation
Give oxygen, respiratory and circulatory support as required
Admit to neonatal unit
Check – complete blood count, blood culture, C-reactive protein and chest X-ray
Start antibiotics

Apneic attacks
The pauses in normal periodic breathing are sometimes misinterpreted as apnea by parents
True apnea with desaturation is uncommon in term infants and is a serious symptom; infection must be excluded

Umbilical cord
Red flare in skin around umbilicus – usually staphylococcal or streptococcal. Give intravenous antibiotics

Sepsis
A combination of some of these clinical features:
▫ Apnea and bradycardia
▫ Slow feeding or vomiting or abdominal distension
▫ Fever, hypothermia or temperature instability
▫ Respiratory distress
▫ Irritability, lethargy or seizures
▫ Jaundice
▫ Petechiae or bruising
▫ Reduced limb movement (bone or joint infection)
▫ Collapse or shock
▫ Hypoglycemia
In meningitis (late signs):
▫ Tense or bulging fontanel
▫ Head retraction (opisthotonus)
Management:
    Admit to neonatal unit
    Check – complete blood count, blood and other cultures, C-reactive protein/procalcitonin and chest X-ray
    Consider lumbar puncture
    Start antibiotics
    Provide supportive care

Fig. 22.1 Common medical problems of term infants in the first few days of life.

23 Admission to the neonatal unit

Newborn infants should not be separated from their mothers unless it is essential for their well-being. Additional nursing and medical care can be provided on postpartum (postnatal) wards or by providing continuing (transitional) care facilities beside their mother. However, 6–10% of newborn infants are admitted to a neonatal unit and 1–2% require intensive care.

Families often find neonatal units daunting and frightening. The environment is unfamiliar and their small and fragile baby is surrounded by high-tech equipment. There are large numbers of highly skilled nurses, doctors and other health professionals caring for their baby, and parents and families often feel superfluous as they are unable to help and care for their baby. Much can be done for parents and families to avoid these difficulties or help them cope with them.

If premature delivery or other reason for admission is anticipated, arrangements should be made for the parents to visit the neonatal unit and meet the neonatal team before the birth.

Welcoming parents and families

• Parents and families should always be made welcome by staff (however busy they are).
• Parents should be shown around to make sure they know what facilities are available for them, e.g. where they can rest, prepare food and drink, make phone calls, use the internet.
• Ask them how they would like to be addressed and call them by name.
• Always make sure you use the correct gender and name when talking about the baby.

Open access

• Open visiting policy for parents (Fig. 23.1) and ability to exchange information 24 hours per day. Mothers should be transported to be near their baby.
• Visits by grandparents (Fig. 23.2) and close family members who are part of the parents' support network, as well as supervised sibling visits (Fig. 23.3) should be encouraged.

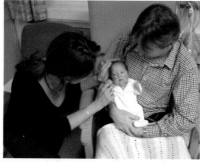

Fig. 23.1 Encourage parents to visit at any time.

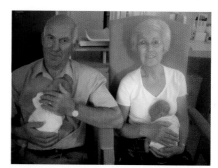

Fig. 23.2 Grandparents on the neonatal unit visiting the latest additions to their family.

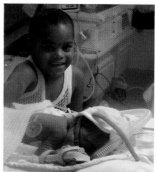

Fig. 23.3 Supervised sibling visits should be encouraged.

Explanation and facilitating communication

• Explain the infant's medical condition and equipment. Provide written information.
• Check with parents how they think their baby is doing and determine their level of understanding about their infant's condition and care. Correct misconceptions. Listen to the parents. Use interpreters if necessary.
• Arrange privacy for more detailed discussions. Parents appreciate respect for personal values and being involved in decision-making as appropriate.
• Assist the family to experience their new baby as a little person by visualizing the infant beyond the tubes and devices.
• Utilize other professionals, e.g. counselors, social workers. They may also provide helpful liaison between the neonatal intensive care unit (NICU) team and family as they may be perceived by the family as being less threatening than health-care professionals.
• The primary nurse, who is responsible for that baby, can facilitate identification of areas of concern and organize discharge.
• Arrange care conferences with the family, including all subspecialists involved in the care of infants with complex problems. These meetings are invaluable in keeping the family up-to-date and planning for discharge and subsequent care.
• Make sure that fathers do not miss out on communications.
• Listen and acknowledge parents when they express concerns about changes in their baby's behavior.

Neonatology at a Glance, Third Edition. Edited by Tom Lissauer, Avroy A. Fanaroff, Lawrence Miall and Jonathan Fanaroff.
© 2016 John Wiley & Sons, Ltd. Published 2016 by John Wiley & Sons, Ltd.

Assisting attachment

• Give the mother the opportunity to touch and hold her baby in delivery room, if at all possible.

• Explain the value of breast milk and encourage the mother to express breast milk if the baby cannot be nursed at the breast. This enables her to make a unique contribution to her baby's care. Success depends on support and encouragement by staff.

• Encourage parents to touch their baby (Fig. 23.4); even if on a ventilator the parents can soothe their baby. Like all new parents, the parents of premature infants need time to watch their baby to learn their ways of responding.

• Encourage parents to actively participate in their infant's care (Fig. 23.5). From the beginning parents can provide comfort and begin to take part in caregiving, e.g. with mouth care and tube feeds. When the baby is stable enough, parents may hold their baby during feeding (Fig. 23.6) and provide kangaroo care (Fig. 23.7a and b). Individualized nursing plans address the baby's behavioral and environmental needs and may reduce morbidity and length of stay (see Chapter 24).

• Encourage parents to keep a diary or journal and to collect mementos. Refer to the baby by name. Ensure the family has or is provided with good quality photos of their baby. Enable parents to personalize the incubator or crib (cot) with family pictures, religious texts etc. (Fig. 23.8).

Providing a family-friendly environment

• Make appearance of the unit as family-friendly as possible.

• Provide space and facilities for parents and families to have some privacy with their baby.

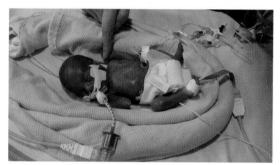

Fig. 23.4 Mother touching her baby after the baby was stabilized in the neonatal unit.

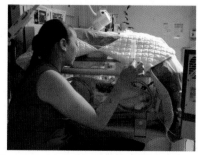

Fig. 23.5 Mother gavage (tube) feeding her ill baby. Parents also need to feel comfortable to watch their baby for as long as they like.

• Try to create a quiet calm environment with soft lighting

• Provide facilities for families to relax near but separate from the bedside, with play area for siblings.

• Provide rooms for parents to stay overnight. This is particularly important if their infant is critically ill or prior to discharge.

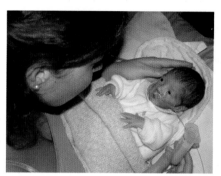

Fig. 23.6 Mother gavage (tube) feeding her baby. One of many activities that give mother and baby an opportunity to get to know each other.

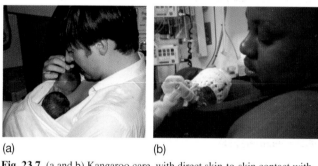

(a)   (b)

Fig. 23.7 (a and b) Kangaroo care, with direct skin-to-skin contact with parent. In many developing countries, continuous kangaroo mother care is used for stable preterm babies instead of incubator care; mortality is lower than with incubator care and it promotes breast-feeding and attachment.

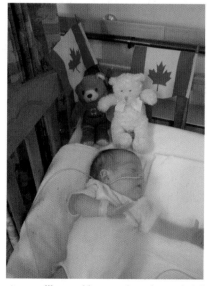

Fig. 23.8 Parents may like to add personal touches to their baby's bed, with toys and in this case flags to represent the baby's home country.

24 Developmental care

Developmental care complements high-tech medical and nursing care with strategies that reduce stress and promote the development of infants in NICU. Some of these strategies are of general benefit to all infants, e.g. adapting the nursery environment, and require understanding and commitment rather than skill. Others are individualized to suit the condition, stage of development and characteristics of the infant; these depend on professionals and parents understanding infant behavioral cues.

Observing newborn behavior

Babies tell us how they are coping by their behavioral cues. These include physiological signs (e.g. color changes, breathing pattern, heart rate and blood oxygen); motor signs (e.g. muscle tone, smoothness of movements, pattern of movement and posture); signs of state organization (e.g. level of arousal, quality of sleep and alertness); and capacity to pay attention. There are many different behavioral patterns that are helpful in understanding when a baby is comfortable and ready to interact (approach cues), or uncomfortable and needing rest or support (avoidance cues) (Table 24.1).

Table 24.1 Behavioral observation.

	Approach behavior	Avoidance behavior
Autonomic	Regular, gentle breathing	Breathing irregular, fast, labored
	Healthy pink coloring	Pale, dusky, flushed or mottled
	Comfortable digestion	Straining, gagging, vomiting
Motor	Smooth varied movement	Jerky, disorganized movement
	Softly flexed posture	Extended (Fig. 24.1b) or flat posture
	Modulated muscle tone	Flaccid or stiff tone
State	Restful sleep	Restless sleep
Attention	Sustained, focused alertness (Fig. 24.1a)	Glazed, strained, hyperalert look
Self-regulation	Self-calming	Inconsolable
	Socially responsive	Shut down

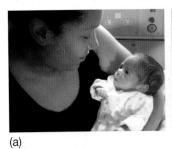 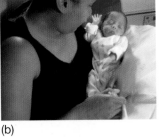

(a)   (b)

Fig. 24.1 (a) This baby's controlled posture and focused expression show successful self-regulation and readiness for interaction, i.e. approach behavior. (b) Extended limbs and turning away suggest avoidance behavior.

These observations take into account the context in which patterns of behavior occur, helping us to adjust the infant's experience and challenges to fit current developmental needs.

Parent participation

Developmental care can help parents to tune into their baby's behavior, laying the foundations for a secure attachment relationship, the basis of healthy emotional and social development. Parents are the baby's most consistent and dedicated carers and even in intensive care they can be involved, e.g. by placing a finger in the palm of the baby's hand or comforting their baby by cradling with still hands, Wherever possible plan the baby's day with parents to make opportunities to participate (Fig. 24.2). Share with parents observations about how their baby reacts to sounds, touch and movement, to build up a picture of each infant's individual characteristics and preferences (Fig. 24.3). Close physical contact, including skin to skin 'kangaroo care', helps parents to enjoy loving contact with their baby and grow in confidence.

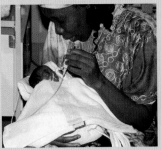 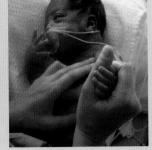

Fig. 24.2 Promotion of parental attachment by involvement with their baby's care.

Fig. 24.3 Promotion of parental attachment through touch.

The nursery environment

Preterm infants are not ready to deal with bright light, loud mechanical noises, hard surfaces, drafts, being moved through space and frequent sleep disruption. These experiences can be modified, e.g. ambient lighting can often be safely reduced and shade can be provided with incubator covers and crib (cot) canopies (Fig. 24.4); noise can be reduced with acoustic engineering, by lowering the volume of alarms and encouraging staff to work and talk quietly; nesting and soft bedding can be used to support the baby in a comfortable position (Fig. 24.5).

Adapting care

All caregiving activities and procedures can be adapted to make them go smoothly and provide opportunities for communication (Fig. 24.6). Infants in intensive care are frequently disturbed for

Neonatology at a Glance, Third Edition. Edited by Tom Lissauer, Avroy A. Fanaroff, Lawrence Miall and Jonathan Fanaroff.
© 2016 John Wiley & Sons, Ltd. Published 2016 by John Wiley & Sons, Ltd.

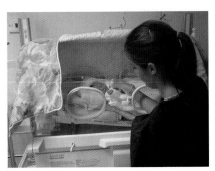

Fig. 24.4 Incubator covered to shade the baby. A flap always folded back so that the baby can be observed.

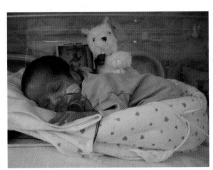

Fig. 24.5 Soft bedding with supportive nesting can contain disorganized movement and provide the baby with comforting boundaries.

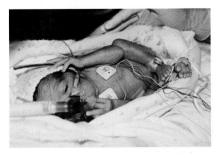

Fig. 24.6 Many activities can be done with the baby lying on one side to give more control of movement – lying quietly and calmly with legs folded in, one hand holding onto his head and the other grasping the pacifier which he is sucking.

nursing observations, examinations, diaper (nappy) changes, blood and other tests, giving medications, etc. Procedures can often be performed together to minimize disturbing a sleeping baby, even if this means being flexible about timing routine observations and care, or when to perform tests and therapy. Very sensitive babies may find this too challenging and will need periods of rest between procedures. A soft spoken greeting with gentle touch helps the baby to adjust at the start. Timing and pacing of procedures can be

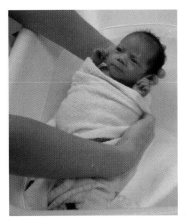

Fig. 24.7 Help sensitive infants to find bathing pleasurable by loosely wrapping in a towel.

adjusted according to the behavioral cues that show when the baby needs time out to rest and recover. Ask parents or a colleague to soothe a sensitive or agitated baby. Wrap the baby when moving through space, e.g. for weighing or bathing (Fig. 24.7). Try positioning the baby on the side for procedures and diaper (nappy) change. Give the baby opportunities to steady him or herself by grasping your finger, sucking a pacifier or pressing feet against the nest wall.

Questions

What is the Newborn Behavioral Assessment Scale (NBAS)?

A neurobehavioral assessment suitable for infants from term to 2 months. It reveals infant maturity and individuality with a series of maneuvers designed to test habituation, orientation to visual and auditory stimuli, state regulation, motor maturity and reflex responses. The baby's reactions to increasingly demanding activities are noted. The examiner must be skillful in eliciting the baby's best response as well as in scoring the assessment. It enables parents and professionals to enhance the parent–infant relationship and promote the baby's capacity for self-regulation. The Assessment of Preterm Infant Behaviour (APIB) is an adaptation of the NBAS to give a detailed description of preterm infant development. The Newborn Behavioral Observation (NBO) is a recent shorter version.

What is NIDCAP®?

This is the Newborn Individualized Developmental Care and Assessment Program. Promotes preterm and newborn development using strategies based on systematic behavioral observation and understanding of fetal, preterm and newborn neurodevelopment. These strategies are individualized to fit each infant's current needs and to support family participation.

25 Stabilizing the sick newborn infant

Seriously ill newborn or extremely preterm infants need to be stabilized following resuscitation in the delivery room (Fig. 25.1).

Airway, Breathing
Assess for respiratory distress:
◻ Tachypnea (>60 breaths/min)
◻ Chest retractions
◻ Expiratory grunting, nasal flaring
◻ Cyanosis
Respiratory support, as required:
◻ Clear the airway/oxygen/CPAP/high-flow nasal therapy/mechanical ventilation

Surfactant
Given to preterm infants with respiratory distress syndrome needing respiratory support or as prophylaxis in extremely preterm infants, according to unit policy

Circulation
Examination:
◻ Heart rate, pulses, capillary refill time, skin color and temperature
◻ Blood pressure
Treat shock—see facing page

Multidisciplinary team
Team of health professionals, each with clearly defined roles, is required

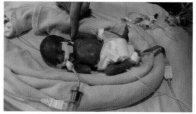

Temperature control
To keep the infant warm, stabilization is performed under a radiant warmer or in an incubator
Exothermic mattress may be helpful
Aim for 36.5–37.5°C

Venous and arterial lines
Peripheral intravenous line:
◻ Required for intravenous fluids, glucose, antibiotics, other drugs and parenteral nutrition
Umbilical venous catheter:
◻ Sometimes used for immediate intravenous access or for CVP (central venous pressure) monitoring or obtaining blood samples or administration of fluid or medications. Some centers use multilumen catheters to avoid the need for peripheral IV lines
Arterial line:
◻ Inserted if frequent blood gas analysis, blood tests and continuous blood pressure monitoring is required. Usually umbilical artery catheter (UAC), sometimes peripheral cannula if for short period or no umbilical artery catheter possible
Central venous line for parenteral nutrition:
◻ Inserted peripherally when infant is stable

Central nervous system
Examination:
◻ Response to handling
◻ Posture
◻ Movements
◻ Tone
◻ Reflexes

Monitoring
◻ Oxygen saturation
◻ Heart rate
◻ Respiratory rate
◻ Apnea >20 seconds
◻ Temperature – peripheral and central if ill
◻ Blood pressure
◻ Blood glucose
◻ Blood gases
◻ Weight
◻ Transcutaneous O_2 and CO_2—used in some centers

Antibiotics
Usually given before results of cultures and other investigations are available (although most infants are not septic)

Pain/sedation
Analgesia and sedation given according to assessment of need, e.g. painful procedures, artificial ventilation

Vitamin K
Routine prophylaxis against vitamin K deficiency bleeding (hemorrhagic disease of the newborn) if not already given

Parents
Time needs to be found to explain to parents and immediate relatives what is happening. If the mother cannot see the baby, e.g. following cesarean section or severe hypertension, photographs or videos are reassuring
Advise mother of benefits of early breast milk expression and ensure given practical advice and support

Investigations
◻ Hemoglobin/hematocrit
◻ Neutrophil count
◻ Platelets
◻ Blood urea nitrogen (urea), creatinine
◻ Electrolytes
◻ Culture—blood, CSF, urine if indicated
◻ Blood glucose
◻ CRP/acute phase reactant
◻ Surface cultures if indicated
◻ Coagulation screen if indicated

X-rays
Chest X-ray +/– abdominal X-ray assist in identifying cause of respiratory distress, position of tracheal tube and central lines
Ensure gavage (nasogastric) tube is placed prior to CXR to rule out esophageal atresia.

Fig. 25.1 Stabilization in the neonatal unit.

Heart rate

What information can be obtained by monitoring heart rate?
(Table 25.1)

Interpreting the heart rate is best done in conjunction with respiratory rate and oxygen saturation. Episodes of apparent desaturation are mostly transient. They may be caused by movement artifact, but if more severe and prolonged will be accompanied by bradycardia and require prompt attention.

Circulation

How is the need for circulatory support determined?

Difficult, but features of circulatory impairment are:
• Heart rate – usually tachycardia; bradycardia is a late sign.

Table 25.1 Some causes of isolated changes in heart rate.

Increased heart rate (>160 beats/min)	Decreased heart rate (<100 beats/min)
Movement/crying	Apnea, hypoxia
Respiratory distress	Seizures
Hypovolemia	Shock (uncompensated)
Fever, infection	Heart block, arrhythmia
Pain	Raised intracranial pressure
Fluid overload, e.g. heart failure, patent ductus arteriosus	Hypothermia (therapeutic or environmental)
Supraventricular tachycardia or other tachyarrhythmias	Artifact
Anemia	
Thyrotoxicosis	
Inotropes	
Iatrogenic hyperthermia	
Artifact	

Neonatology at a Glance, Third Edition. Edited by Tom Lissauer, Avroy A. Fanaroff, Lawrence Miall and Jonathan Fanaroff.
© 2016 John Wiley & Sons, Ltd. Published 2016 by John Wiley & Sons, Ltd.

- Central – peripheral ('toe–core') temperature difference >2 °C. (Can also be caused by a cold environment.)
- Capillary refill time – prolonged if >3 seconds.
- Metabolic acidosis (increased lactate levels).
- Oliguria.
- Echocardiography – used to help identify low cardiac output secondary to cardiac underfilling suggesting hypovolemia and/or poor contractility from myocardial dysfunction (see Chapter 82, Echocardiography for the neonatologist).
- Chest X-ray – cardiovascular function may be compromised by overinflation of lungs or high mean airway pressure on mechanical ventilation (especially high frequency) obstructing venous return to both the right and left atrium.

- Blood pressure, ideally invasive. After 1 hour of age, hypotension often defined by mean blood pressure (mmHg) persistently below the baby's gestational age (completed weeks). However, a large PDA (patent ductus arteriosus) can lead to a low mean blood pressure due to low diastolic pressure.

Management of shock is directed at the underlying cause wherever possible (Fig. 25.2).

Fluid resuscitation with or without inotropic support may be needed (Fig. 25.3 and Table 25.2).

Treatment thresholds and management of hypotension or circulatory impairment without shock are uncertain.

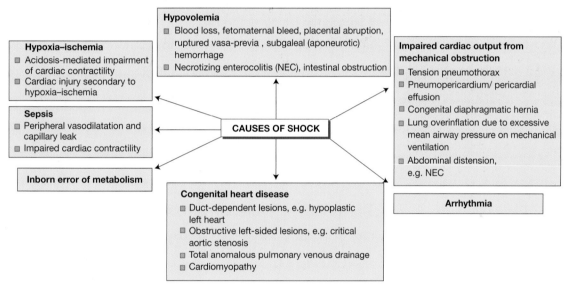

Fig. 25.2 Causes of shock.

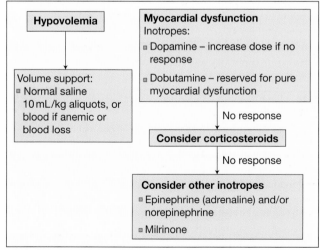

Fig. 25.3 Circulatory support. This differs between centers.

Table 25.2 Inotropes.

Inotrope	Pharmacology	Main effect
Dopamine	D1, D2, β_1, β_2 agonist	Increases contractility and SVR. Increases BP but may not increase cardiac output
Dobutamine	β_1 agonist	Increases heart rate and contractility without affecting SVR. May improve cardiac output
Norepinephrine (noradrenaline)	α_1, α_2, β_1 agonist	Mainly increases SVR by vasoconstriction
Epinephrine	α_1, α_2, $\beta_{1,2,3}$ agonist	Mainly increases SVR by vasoconstriction
Milrinone	Phosphodiesterase-III inhibitor- increases cAMP	Increased contractility and vasodilatation reduces afterload. Little research
Hydrocortisone	Unknown mechanism	Proven inotrope and vasopressor sparing effect

SVR – Systemic vascular resistance.

26 Respiratory support

Forms of respiratory support

Respiratory support includes:
- supplemental oxygen
- CPAP – continuous positive airway pressure
- high-flow nasal therapy (HFNT)/high-flow nasal cannulae (HFNC)
- non-invasive mechanical ventilation (NIMV/NIPPV)
- positive-pressure ventilation (PPV)
- HFOV – high-frequency oscillatory ventilation
- iNO – inhaled nitric oxide
- ECMO – extracorporeal membrane oxygenation.

The approach to respiratory support is continually evolving and new strategies and modes of support are being introduced. Whilst aiming to maintain adequate gas exchange, there is an emphasis on minimizing the risk of ventilator-induced lung injury. Hyperinflation from high pressures (volutrauma) and repeated opening and closing of alveoli (atelectotrauma) may cause lung damage. Non-invasive respiratory support, which includes CPAP, high-flow nasal therapy and non-invasive mechanical ventilation with or without surfactant therapy in preterm infants, are used increasingly either as the primary mode of support or following extubation to avoid reintubation (Fig 26.1). Positive-pressure ventilation is required for infants with significant respiratory distress that cannot be managed with non-invasive respiratory support; some of the newer approaches are described in this chapter.

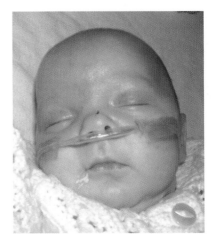
Fig. 26.2 Oxygen delivered via nasal cannula.

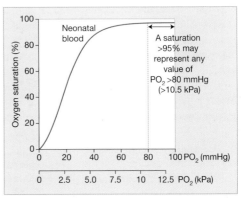
Fig. 26.3 Saturation measurements above 95% in preterm infants receiving supplemental oxygen may represent dangerously high oxygen tensions.

Supplemental oxygen therapy

Oxygen is given to prevent hypoxia (Fig. 26.2), which may cause ischemic damage to the brain and other organs, apnea and pulmonary hypertension. Hyperoxia should also be avoided as elevated levels of oxygen in the blood may cause tissue damage due to the release of oxygen free radicals and retinopathy of prematurity in preterm infants.

The optimal values for arterial oxygen tension and saturation have not been established, but in practice:
- In preterm infants, arterial oxygen tension (PaO_2) is maintained at 45–80 mmHg (6.0–10.5 kPa) and oxygen saturation at 91–95%. Lower saturations are associated with less retinopathy of prematurity but increased mortality. Saturation above 95% in infants receiving supplemental oxygen may represent dangerously high oxygen tensions (Fig. 26.3).
- Term infants – maintain oxygen saturation at 95–99% and PaO_2 between 60–80 mmHg (8–10.5 kPa).

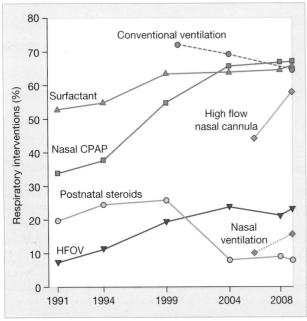
Fig. 26.1 Changes in use of respiratory interventions in VLBW (very low birthweight) infants with time. (Vermont–Oxford Network; data from Soll R.F. et al. Obstetric and neonatal care practices for infants 501–1500 g from 2000 to 2009. *Pediatrics* 2013; **132**: 222–228 and Dr Jeff Horbar.)

Neonatology at a Glance, Third Edition. Edited by Tom Lissauer, Avroy A. Fanaroff, Lawrence Miall and Jonathan Fanaroff.
© 2016 John Wiley & Sons, Ltd. Published 2016 by John Wiley & Sons, Ltd.

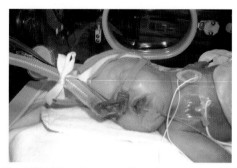

Fig. 26.4 Nasal CPAP (continuous positive airway pressure) with flow driver that maintains a constant pressure by changing the direction of gas flow during expiration (fluidic flip).

Continuous positive airway pressure (CPAP)

Distending pressure is usually applied via nasal prongs (Fig. 26.4) in the nasal airway or by a close-fitting nasal mask. CPAP aims to prevent alveolar collapse at end expiration, stabilize the chest wall and reduce the work of breathing. It also allows supplemental oxygen to be delivered continuously. It is used for infants with moderate respiratory distress and for recurrent apnea. There is increasing use of early CPAP as respiratory support immediately after birth even for very preterm infants, with mechanical ventilation used only as rescue. CPAP may also facilitate weaning from mechanical ventilation. Larger infants may not tolerate CPAP well.

CPAP may be delivered as:
• bubble CPAP – the pressure is determined using a water manometer
• flow-driver CPAP – the flow driver provides a constant stream of air/oxygen; special nasal prongs maintain a constant pressure throughout the infant's respiratory cycle by changing the direction of gas flow during expiration (fluidic flip).

A pressure of $6-8\,cmH_2O$ is used and there needs to be minimal air leak around the nasal prongs or mask.

Complications of CPAP are:
• pneumothorax
• feeding difficulties due to gaseous distension of the stomach
• nasal trauma causing nasal septum breakdown or erosion and nasal deformity; minimized by correct size and fixation of prongs or mask.

If respiratory failure develops, mechanical ventilation is required. CPAP can be stopped abruptly or weaned by gradually reducing the PEEP or increasing the period of time off CPAP. The limited evidence suggests that gradually weaning pressure is superior and reduces length of stay. If weaned too quickly, there may respiratory deterioration or poor growth.

Some infants with bronchopulmonary dysplasia require nasal CPAP for many weeks.

High-flow nasal therapy

Increasingly used as an alternative for CPAP or to wean off ventilators or CPAP. Warmed, humidified oxygen/air is delivered at a high flow rate (>2 L/min) via nasal cannulae. It probably generates some distending pressure to the lungs but works mainly by

flushing CO_2 from the nasopharynx. Babies, especially when more mature, tolerate it better than CPAP. In contrast to CPAP, there is leakage of gases around loose- fitting cannulae. Its efficacy as a mode of support compared with CPAP is being evaluated; for weaning infants off mechanical ventilation it appears to have similar efficacy to CPAP with less nasal trauma.

Non-Invasive Mechanical Ventilation (NIMV)

The terms NIMV (non-invasive mechanical ventilation or nasal intermittent mandatory ventilation) and NIPPV (nasal intermittent positive pressure ventilation) are used interchangeably for positive-pressure respiratory support without the use of a tracheal tube. It is gaining popularity as a primary means of respiratory support and also after extubation to prevent reintubation.

Whereas CPAP provides only continuous positive airway pressure, NIMV also delivers intermittent peak inspiratory pressure, either mandatory or triggered, via rigid nasal prongs. This is postulated to provide better oxygenation and CO_2 removal than CPAP. There is currently no convincing evidence that it is better than CPAP in preventing reintubation or bronchopulmonary dysplasia in preterm infants.

Positive-pressure ventilation (PPV)

Indications

• Increasing oxygen requirement or work of breathing or increasing $PaCO_2$ while on nasal CPAP/HFNT.
• Respiratory failure – inadequate oxygenation (hypoxia) and/or CO_2 elimination (hypercarbia).
• Apnea – prolonged/recurrent.
• Upper airway obstruction or vocal cord paralysis.
• Congenital diaphragmatic hernia.
• Perioperative respiratory support for anesthesia.
• Circulatory failure.

Intermittent positive-pressure ventilation (IPPV)

Respiratory support is administered using a mechanical ventilator through a tracheal tube. With conventional ventilation, intermittent positive-pressure ventilator breaths are given on a background of continuous distending pressure (positive end-expiratory pressure, PEEP) (Fig. 26.5). Alveolar ventilation (CO_2 clearance) is determined by the difference between peak inspiratory pressure (PIP) and PEEP and the respiratory rate. Oxygenation is determined by the mean airway pressure (area under the curve) and administered oxygen concentration (FiO2).

Conventional ventilation is pressure limited and time cycled. Peak inspiratory pressure is set by the operator and tidal volume varies from breath to breath depending upon lung compliance and airway resistance. This may increase the risk of volutrauma and atelectotrauma.

Volume-limited or targeted ventilation is increasingly used. In volume-limited ventilation, instead of setting the desired peak inspiratory pressure, a maximum tidal volume is set (limited) by the

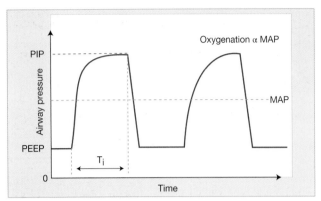

Fig. 26.5 Intermittent positive-pressure ventilation (IPPV). Diagram of change in airway pressure with time. (PIP – peak inspiratory pressure; PEEP – positive end-expiratory pressure; Ti – inspiratory time; MAP – mean airway pressure.)

volume. Tidal volumes are usually 4–6 mL/kg, the normal tidal volume of neonates, but higher volumes may be required by infants with bronchopulmonary dysplasia and lower volumes with lung hypoplasia. This mode of ventilation is particularly useful when lung compliance is changing rapidly, e.g. rapid improvement of compliance after surfactant administration, when the ventilator will be able to deliver the desired tidal volume using lower pressures, reducing the risk of an air leak. It is less useful if there is a large leak around the tracheal tube (>40%). Advances in ventilator technology allow the measurement and delivery of small tidal volumes, which was not previously possible. Studies suggest that there may be a decreased risk of pneumothorax and bronchopulmonary dysplasia compared with pressure-limited ventilation.

operator so that the peak inspiratory pressure generated will only rise to meet the desired volume. In volume-targeted ventilation, a desired tidal volume is set (targeted) and the peak inspiratory pressure will automatically adjust to achieve the desired tidal

Key points

In the presence of marked chest retractions, provide respiratory support, including mechanical ventilation if necessary, even if the blood gases are normal. Evidence of respiratory failure on blood gases is a late feature.

Question

How are the settings of conventional ventilators adjusted?

Monitoring
Continuous oxygen saturation, vital signs, regular blood gases, transcutaneous PaO_2 and $PaCO_2$ (if available) – to identify acute changes in infant's condition.

Target arterial blood gases
- PaO_2: 45–80 mmHg (6–10.5 kPa)
- $PaCO_2$: 40–65 mmHg (5–8.5 kPa)
- pH: 7.20–7.4.

Abnormal blood gases
Check:
- Infant – for satisfactory chest wall movement, bilateral air entry, exclude pneumothorax (transilluminate chest if necessary), check airway patency and ventilator functioning correctly.
- Breathing and circulation – adjust ventilator settings if necessary. Consider rechecking blood gases 30–60 minutes after changing settings or if there has been a change in the infant's condition.

Oxygen
To increase oxygenation, options are:
- increase inspired oxygen concentration
- increase mean airway pressure – increase PIP, PEEP, or inspiratory time, or flow (Fig. 26.5).
Consider surfactant therapy or HFOV (high-frequency oscillation).

Carbon dioxide
- Keep $PaCO_2$ in normal range during first 72 h in preterms – to keep cerebral blood flow stable during time of maximum risk of

intraventricular hemorrhage. Thereafter, allow somewhat higher levels of $PaCO_2$ (permissive hypercapnia) to minimize ventilator-induced lung injury, but keep pH above 7.20.
- Avoid low $PaCO_2$ (<40 mmHg, 5 kPa) as this lowers cerebral blood flow and is associated with ischemic brain injury (periventricular leukomalacia).
To reduce $PaCO_2$:
- increase ventilator rate (but allow sufficient expiratory time for carbon dioxide removal)
- increase breath size – increase PIP, or reduce PEEP.
Consider if tracheal tube is blocked (suction or replace if necessary), or if excessive dead space in circuit.

Metabolic acidosis
In extremely preterm infants this may be due to:
- circulatory hypoperfusion
- hypoxemia
- urinary loss of bicarbonate (alkaline urine)
- anemia
- parenteral nutrition
- acute kidney injury (renal failure)

Ventilation strategy
When adjusting ventilator, aim to minimize ventilator-induced lung injury (inflammation, air leaks) by:
- using lowest PIP to reduce volutrauma and adequate PEEP to reduce atelectotrauma. Aim to synchronize ventilator with the infant's breathing – can use patient-triggered ventilation (PTV) or synchronous intermittent mandatory ventilation (SIMV), sedation, analgesia and occasionally muscle relaxants.

Question

How do ventilator graphics assist ventilator management?

Increasingly, ventilators display breath-by-breath measurements of pressure, flow and volume that can help to monitor lung physiology and individualize mechanical support.

Pressure–volume loop (Fig. 26.6)

Recognizing problems:
- As airway resistance increases, the loop widens, e.g. blocked ETT.
- As compliance decreases, the loop gradient flattens, e.g. RDS.
- In overdistension, the curve flattens or 'beaks' at the end of expiration.
- If the expiratory part of the loop does not return to baseline, it suggests there is a leak.

Pressure-time waveform – pressure modes (Fig. 26.7)

- Pressure increases rapidly from the level of PEEP until it reaches the level of PIP, then remains constant for the inspiratory time.
- Expiration is a passive process and pressure decreases gradually until it reaches the level of PEEP before the next breath.

- The waveform is not affected by changes in resistance or compliance.
- The area under the curve represents the mean airway pressure (MAP).
- There is a negative deflection just before the inspiratory part of the waveform with patient-triggered breaths.
- The higher the flow rate the squarer is the waveform (increases MAP).

Pressure–time waveform – volume modes (Fig. 26.8)

The waveform is affected by changes in resistance and compliance because pressure is variable. At the beginning of inspiration the ventilator generates pressure (P_{res}) to overcome airway resistance and no volume is delivered. Then pressure increases until the PIP is reached and the gradient depends on compliance. When the set tidal volume is delivered, the pressure quickly falls to a plateau pressure before passive expiration.

Recognizing problems:
- Increased resistance leads to higher P_{res}.
- Decreased compliance leads to increased PIP.

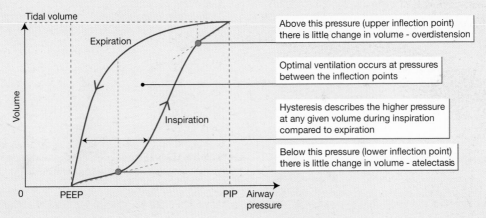

Fig. 26.6 Pressure–volume loop.

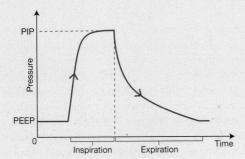

Fig. 26.7 Pressure–time waveform with pressure mode.

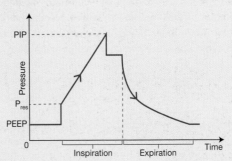

Fig. 26.8 Pressure–time waveform with volume modes.

Flow–time waveform

- The area underneath the flow curve represents the transferred volume.
- In pressure modes, the waveform is a slope because flow decreases when PIP is reached (Fig. 26.9).
- In volume modes the waveform is square because flow remains constant during inspiration (Fig. 26.10).
- If the waveform does not return to baseline before the next breath, there may be a leak or air trapping.

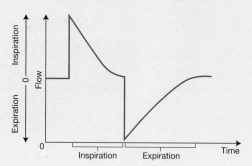

Fig. 26.9 Flow-time waveform in pressure mode.

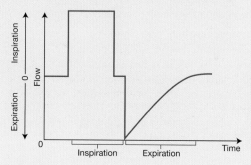

Fig. 26.10 Flow-time waveform in volume mode.

Question

What are the causes of deterioration of a ventilated infant?

Sudden deterioration (acronym DOPE):

- **D**isplaced tracheal tube.
- **O**bstructed tracheal tube, e.g. secretions, blood.
- **P**neumothorax or pneumomediastinum (air leaks).
- **E**quipment failure, e.g. ventilator circuit disconnected.

Slow deterioration:

- Increased lung secretions.
- Infection.
- Patent ductus arteriosus.
- Anemia.
- Developing bronchopulmonary dysplasia.

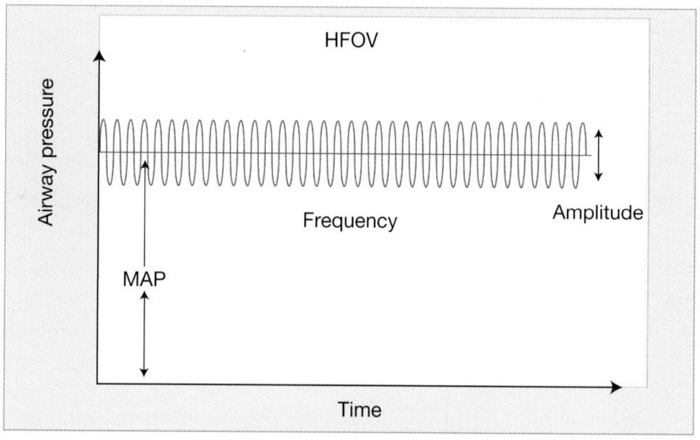

Patient-triggered ventilation (PTV) and synchronous intermittent mandatory ventilation (SIMV)

Two forms of synchronized mechanical ventilation are available to promote synchrony between the ventilator and an infant's own respiratory efforts – patient-triggered ventilation (PTV) and synchronous intermittent mandatory ventilation (SIMV). Both methods use the infant's own spontaneous respiration to trigger the ventilator to deliver a breath, usually from the change in airway pressure or flow measured in the ventilator circuit, or from a recording of the infant's respiration. In patient-triggered ventilation, also called assist control (AC) or spontaneous intermittent positive-pressure ventilation (SIPPV), each breath is supported by the ventilator; in SIMV, only a preset number of breaths in a given time is supported by the ventilator and other breaths are unsupported. In both, there is a backup ventilation rate if the infant does not breathe.

Fig. 26.11 High - frequency oscillatory ventilation (HFOV). Diagram showing changes in airway pressure with time. (MAP – mean airway pressure.)

High-frequency oscillatory ventilation (HFOV)

High-frequency ventilators operate at frequencies approximately 10 times greater than conventional ventilators and can achieve good gas exchange despite using tidal volumes smaller than dead space (Fig. 26.11). The rationale for using high-frequency ventilation is to recruit collapsed alveoli ('open' the lung) and minimize ventilator-induced lung damage. The mechanism of gas exchange is unclear but may include facilitated diffusion and turbulence. Rescue treatment with high-frequency ventilation in term and preterm infants with severe respiratory failure is associated with short-term improvement in gas exchange, especially when used in combination with inhaled nitric oxide. Some units choose to ventilate all their extremely preterm infants by HFOV to minimize barotrauma. Studies have failed to show a decrease in duration of

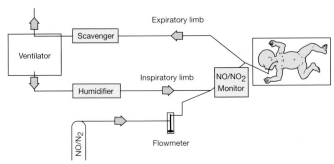

Fig. 26.12 Components in delivery of inhaled nitric oxide. There is a scavenger for removing nitric oxide released into the atmosphere. The blood concentration of methemoglobin, a potentially toxic by-product, is checked periodically. Inspired nitrogen dioxide (NO_2) levels (a by-product of mixing nitric oxide and oxygen) are monitored continuously.

ventilation, incidence of bronchopulmonary dysplasia, mortality or need for extracorporeal membrane oxygenation (ECMO) compared with conventional ventilation.

Inhaled nitric oxide (iNO)

Inhaled nitric oxide causes selective pulmonary vasodilation. It is used in infants with hypoxemic respiratory failure with or without persistent pulmonary hypertension of the newborn (PPHN) to improve oxygenation (Fig. 26.12). It reduces the need for ECMO in term and near-term infants with severe respiratory failure. There is increasing evidence that sildenafil is as effective with reduced expense and complexity, but is not currently approved in the US for this purpose. The efficacy of inhaled nitric oxide in preterm infants remains to be established.

Respiratory failure

The severity of hypoxemic respiratory failure can be assessed by calculating the oxygenation index (OI):

$$OI = \frac{\text{mean airway pressure (cmH}_2\text{O)} \times FiO_2 \times 100}{PaO_2\,\text{(mmHg)}}$$

In term infants, OI ≥40 is associated with a 40% risk of mortality.

In preterm infants, OI ≥20 is associated with a 50% risk of mortality.

Therapeutic options for respiratory failure if on conventional mechanical ventilation with high pressures and in high concentration of oxygen are:
- extra rescue doses of surfactant
- high-frequency ventilation
- nitric oxide or sildenafil therapy (although sildenafil is not currently approved in the US for this purpose)
- ECMO for infants of ≥34 weeks' gestation.

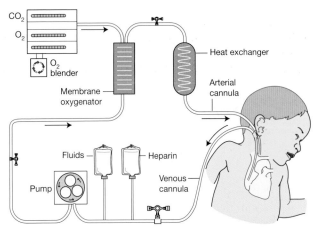

Fig. 26.13 ECMO (extracorporeal membrane oxygenation) circuit. The infant's venous blood is pumped through a membrane oxygenator (an artificial lung), which extracts carbon dioxide and adds oxygen. The blood is returned to the baby into the right carotid artery (veno-arterial ECMO, as shown in the diagram). In veno-venous ECMO, blood is removed and returned into the right atrium through a double-lumen catheter. The lungs continue to be ventilated but at a low resting level.

Table 26.1 Conditions that may require ECMO.

- congenital diaphragmatic hernia
- meconium aspiration syndrome
- persistent pulmonary hypertension of the newborn (PPHN)
- sepsis
- respiratory distress syndrome (RDS)
- severe airway obstruction/malformation
- heart disease – congenital or cardiomyopathy

Extracorporeal membrane oxygenation (ECMO)

Infants are placed on heart–lung bypass for up to 2–3 weeks to allow the lungs to recover (Figs 26.13 and 3.3). Blood is removed from the circulation, oxygenated and then returned to the circulation. It is performed in relatively few specialized centers. Because of the need for anticoagulation and large surgical catheters, there is a risk of intraventricular hemorrhage in preterm infants and it is therefore reserved for infants of ≥34 weeks' gestation and birthweight >=2 kg. Conditions that cause recoverable respiratory failure which may respond to ECMO are listed in Table 26.1. Indication is an oxygenation index of ≥40 in spite of optimal mechanical ventilation and circulatory support. Other requirements are <10–14 days' mechanical ventilation, no lethal congenital abnormalities and no significant intracranial hemorrhage. The need for ECMO has declined markedly since the introduction of inhaled nitric oxide, surfactant and HFOV. The most common indication is now congenital diaphragmatic hernia.

27 Preterm infants and their complications

The preterm infant differs markedly from the term infant in size, appearance and development. Some of these differences are shown schematically in Figs 27.1–27.4.

Gestation	23–25 weeks	29–31 weeks	37–42 weeks (term)
Birthweight (50th centile)	At 24 weeks – Female: 620 g; Male: 700 g	At 30 weeks – Female: 1.4 kg; Male: 1.5 kg	At 40 weeks – Female: 3.4 kg; Male: 3.55 kg
Skin	Very thin, gelatinous. Dark red all over body	Medium thickness. Pink	Thick skin with cracking on hands and feet. Pale pink: pink all over ears, lips, palms and soles
Ears	Pinna soft, no recoil	Cartilage to edge of pinna in places, recoils readily	Firm pinna cartilage to edge of pinna, recoils immediately
Breast	No breast tissue palpable	One or both breast nodules 0.5–1.0 cm	One or both nodules >1.0 cm
Genitalia	Male: scrotum smooth, testes impalpable. Female: prominent clitoris. Labia majora widely separated, labia minora protruding	Male: scrotum – few rugae, testes – in inguinal canal. Female: labia minora and clitoris partially covered	Male: scrotum – rugae, testes in scrotum. Female: labia minora and clitoris covered
Posture	Extended, jerky, uncoordinated	Some flexion of legs	Flexed, smooth limb movements
Vision	Eyelids may be fused or partially open. Absent or infrequent eye movements	Pupils react to light	Looks at faces. Follows faces, curvy lines and light/dark contrast in all directions
Hearing	Startles to loud noise		Turns head and eyes to sound. Prefers speech and mother's voice
Breathing	Needs respiratory support. Apnea common	Sometimes needs respiratory support. Apnea common	Need for respiratory support uncommon. Apnea rare
Sucking and swallowing	No coordinated sucking	Coordinated at 32–34 weeks' gestation	
Feeding	Usually need PN (parenteral nutrition)	Gavage (nasogastric) feeds. Sometimes need PN (parenteral nutrition)	At term, cries when hungry. Takes full feeds on demand Coordinates breathing, sucking and swallowing
Taste		Reacts to bitter taste	Differentiates between sweet, sour, bitter. Prefers sweet
Interaction	Seldom available for interaction. Easily overloaded by sensory stimulation		Makes eye contact and alert wakefulness
Cry	Very faint		Loud
Sleep/wake cycle	Intermediate sleep state		Clearly defined sleeping and waking states

Fig. 27.1 Maturational changes in appearance, posture and development with age.

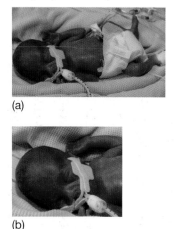

(a)

(b)

Fig. 27.2 Preterm infant at 23 weeks' gestation, showing thin, gelatinous skin and fused eyelids Legs flexed as nested. Tracheal and gavage (nasogastric) tubes.

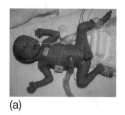

(a)

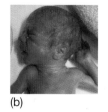

(b)

Fig. 27.3 Preterm infant at 30 weeks' gestation, showing medium-thickness skin and ear with cartilage to edge of pinna.

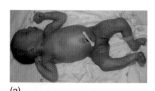

(a)

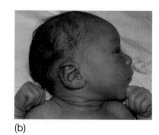

(b)

Fig. 27.4 Term infant showing flexed posture and thick skin, and well-formed ear.

Neonatology at a Glance, Third Edition. Edited by Tom Lissauer, Avroy A. Fanaroff, Lawrence Miall and Jonathan Fanaroff.
© 2016 John Wiley & Sons, Ltd. Published 2016 by John Wiley & Sons, Ltd.

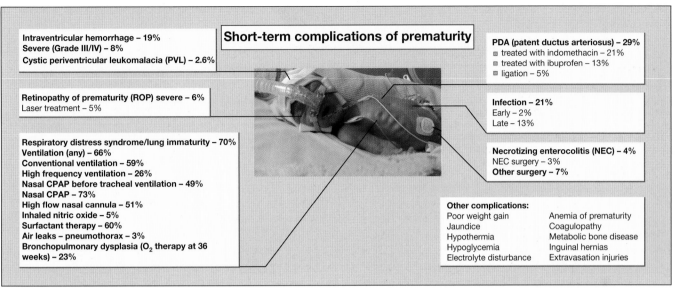

Short-term complications of prematurity

Intraventricular hemorrhage – 19%
Severe (Grade III/IV) – 8%
Cystic periventricular leukomalacia (PVL) – 2.6%

PDA (patent ductus arteriosus) – 29%
- treated with indomethacin – 21%
- treated with ibuprofen – 13%
- ligation – 5%

Retinopathy of prematurity (ROP) severe – 6%
Laser treatment – 5%

Infection – 21%
Early – 2%
Late – 13%

Respiratory distress syndrome/lung immaturity – 70%
Ventilation (any) – 66%
Conventional ventilation – 59%
High frequency ventilation – 26%
Nasal CPAP before tracheal ventilation – 49%
Nasal CPAP – 73%
High flow nasal cannula – 51%
Inhaled nitric oxide – 5%
Surfactant therapy – 60%
Air leaks – pneumothorax – 3%
Bronchopulmonary dysplasia (O$_2$ therapy at 36 weeks) – 23%

Necrotizing enterocolitis (NEC) – 4%
NEC surgery – 3%
Other surgery – 7%

Other complications:
Poor weight gain	Anemia of prematurity
Jaundice	Coagulopathy
Hypothermia	Metabolic bone disease
Hypoglycemia	Inguinal hernias
Electrolyte disturbance	Extravasation injuries

Fig. 27.5 Short-term complications of very low birthweight (<1.5 kg) infants. (Percentages are based on Vermont–Oxford Network data for 2013.)

Morbidity

Being born preterm has many disadvantages, including stress for the parents and family, prolonged hospitalization and being extremely expensive. After 30 weeks of gestation, most preterm infants in developed countries survive without neurologic or other impairment. However, at lower gestational age there is a considerable complication rate (Fig. 27.5). The rate is highly dependent on gestational age.

Mortality

Mortality is mainly determined by gestational age (Fig. 27.6) and birthweight (Fig. 27.7). They interact with each other as well as with other risk factors:
- gender (males have higher mortality)
- ethnicity
- multiple birth (increases mortality).

There has been a marked improvement in survival in infants born at the limit of viability, i.e. 23–25 weeks of gestational age. However, mortality, morbidity and adverse neurodevelopmental outcome are highest in these infants. This is considered further in Chapters 8 and 72.

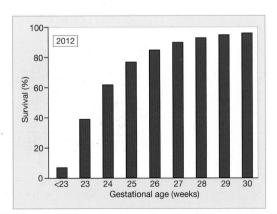

Fig. 27.6 Survival by gestational age of very low birthweight (VLBW) infants. Data from over 900 neonatal units from throughout the world. (Vermont–Oxford Network, 2012.)

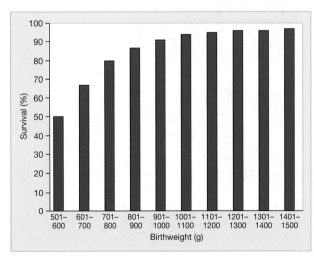

Fig. 27.7 Survival by birthweight of very low birthweight (VLBW) infants. Overall survival 88%. (Vermont–Oxford Network 2012.)

28 Lung development and surfactant

Structural development

The fetal lung passes through five main stages of lung development during gestation (Fig. 28.1).

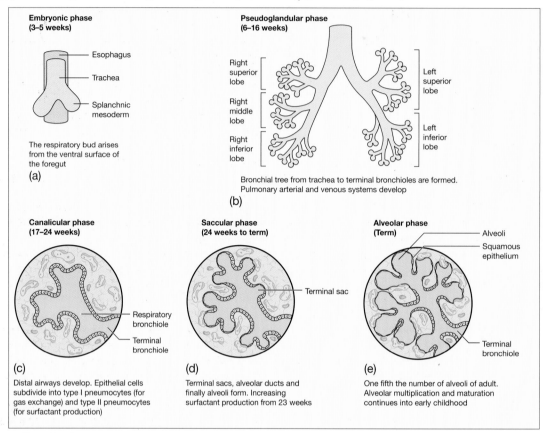

Fig. 28.1 Phases of lung development.

Physiology and composition of surfactant (Figs 28.2–28.4)

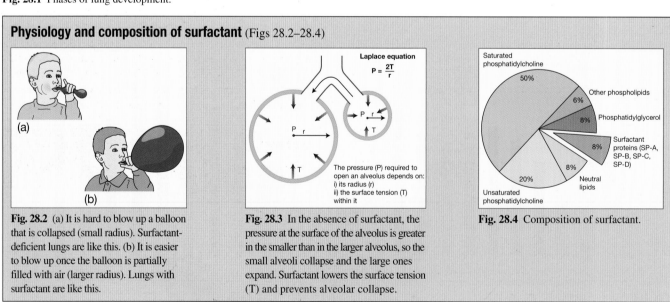

Fig. 28.2 (a) It is hard to blow up a balloon that is collapsed (small radius). Surfactant-deficient lungs are like this. (b) It is easier to blow up once the balloon is partially filled with air (larger radius). Lungs with surfactant are like this.

Fig. 28.3 In the absence of surfactant, the pressure at the surface of the alveolus is greater in the smaller than in the larger alveolus, so the small alveoli collapse and the large ones expand. Surfactant lowers the surface tension (T) and prevents alveolar collapse.

Fig. 28.4 Composition of surfactant.

Neonatology at a Glance, Third Edition. Edited by Tom Lissauer, Avroy A. Fanaroff, Lawrence Miall and Jonathan Fanaroff.
© 2016 John Wiley & Sons, Ltd. Published 2016 by John Wiley & Sons, Ltd.

Surfactant

Surfactant:
- Is a naturally occurring substance containing lipids (90%) and proteins (10%).
- Is synthesized in type II pneumocytes in the lung and released onto the alveolar surface.
- Lowers surface tension at the air–water interface in the alveolus through the action of its lipid components (mainly dipalmitoylphosphatidylcholine, DPPC).
- Production starts late in the second trimester and early third trimester.
- Deficiency causes respiratory distress syndrome (RDS).

Clinical implications of surfactant deficiency

In surfactant deficiency, the lung has low compliance (i.e. is stiff), so the change in lung volume for a given change in airway pressure is much less than in the normal healthy newborn lung (Fig. 28.5). The pressure required to initiate lung inflation ('opening pressure') is also higher. Without surfactant, the lung alveoli collapse during expiration and the next breath starts from a low lung volume. These changes result in increased work of breathing and hypoxemia (Fig. 28.6).

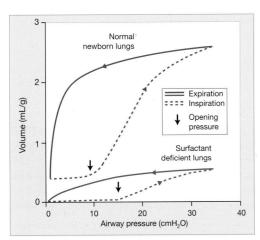

Fig. 28.5 Difference in lung volume for a given airway pressure between normal and surfactant-deficient lungs. If surfactant is present there is a lower opening pressure, a larger change in volume for a given change in pressure and the lungs do not collapse on expiration.

Antenatal corticosteroids

Corticosteroids promote surfactant synthesis and lung maturation. Recommended for preterm labor at 24–34 weeks, and to be considered at earlier gestations (see Chapter 67).

Surfactant therapy

Surfactant therapy is administered directly into the lungs.

There are two types of surfactant:
- natural surfactants – made from animal lung extracts: porcine – poractant alfa (Curosurf®), calf – beractant (Survanta®).
- synthetic surfactants – available, but not widely used. Aerosolized surfactant development is at an advanced stage.

Preterm infants are given surfactant to either prevent or treat RDS. The strategies used are:
- prophylactic surfactant – elective intubation and surfactant given in the first few minutes after birth irrespective of the presence or absence of respiratory distress.
- rescue surfactant therapy – once the baby develops significant RDS.

Once surfactant has been administered, it becomes incorporated into an endogenous pool that is recycled within the pneumocytes. Occasionally a second dose is needed 6–12 hours later, but after that endogenous surfactant production takes over.

Although early systematic reviews showed prophylactic therapy to be more effective than rescue treatment, many centers have switched to rescue therapy, commencing with CPAP in the delivery room and administering surfactant only if CPAP alone is ineffective, aiming to avoid positive-pressure ventilation. This approach is adopted even in very low birthweight infants; only 60% of them now receive surfactant therapy. Surfactant can be administered in these circumstances by the INSURE (intubation, surfactant, extubation) technique, or instilled through a catheter into the trachea, called 'minimal invasive surfactant treatment' (MIST). Otherwise, in infants on mechanical ventilation, it is administered down the tracheal tube either as prophylaxis or rescue treatment. Surfactant therapy may also be beneficial in term infants with severe meconium aspiration, pulmonary hemorrhage or pneumonia who develop secondary surfactant deficiency (**see video: INSURE technique**).

Key point

- Surfactant therapy has been a major advance in neonatal care.

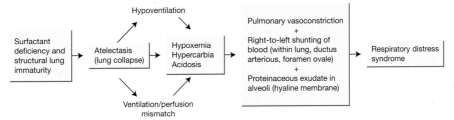

Fig. 28.6 Effect of surfactant deficiency and lung immaturity in preterm infants.

29 Respiratory distress syndrome

Respiratory distress syndrome (RDS) is:
- also called hyaline membrane disease (HMD) or surfactant deficient lung disease (SDLD)
- the commonest respiratory disorder affecting preterm infants (see Table 29.1)
- a major cause of morbidity and mortality in preterm infants, although this has decreased markedly in recent years.

Risk factors

The predominant risk factor is:
- prematurity (Fig. 29.1), as surfactant is only produced towards the end of the second trimester and early third trimester.

Other risk factors are:
- maternal diabetes mellitus
- sepsis
- hypoxemia and acidemia
- hypothermia.

Pathology

Characteristic histopathologic features include:
- collapsed terminal air saccules
- overdistended terminal airways
- influx of inflammatory cells into the airway lumen
- interstitial edema and protein leak onto the surface of the airways and air saccules
- hyaline membrane formation in distal and terminal airways (Fig. 29.2)
- necrotic damage to airway epithelial cells.

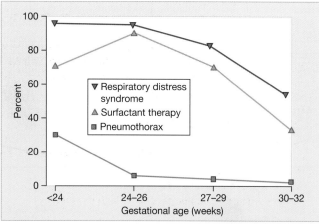

Fig. 29.1 Decline in incidence of RDS with gestation in very low birthweight infants. The use of surfactant and incidence of pneumothorax is also shown. (Vermont–Oxford Network data for 2012.)

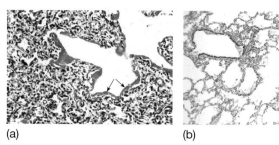

(a)   (b)

Fig. 29.2 Histology showing (a) characteristic features of RDS. The hyaline membrane is shown (arrows). (b) Normal preterm lung for comparison.

Pathogenesis

Caused by a deficiency in surfactant production or function. This results in alveolar collapse, which in turn leads to poor lung compliance (stiff lungs) and impaired gas exchange. Immature lung architecture may also contribute.

Clinical features

Onset within 4 hours of birth of respiratory distress:
- tachypnea (>60 breaths/min)
- chest retractions (sternal and intercostal retractions) (Fig. 29.3)
- nasal flaring
- expiratory grunting
- cyanosis (if severe).

Diagnosis is based on history, physical signs, characteristic chest X-ray (Fig. 29.4) and clinical course.

Causes of respiratory distress in preterm infants are listed in Table 29.1.

Natural course

The natural course is for the illness to become worse over the first 24–72 hours and then improve over the next few days. There is initially tissue edema from transudation of fluid into alveoli and subcutaneous tissues, which resolves with improvement of lung disease leading to diuresis. These features are ameliorated by antenatal corticosteroids and postnatal surfactant therapy (**see video**).

Management

This includes:
- reduced morbidity and mortality with antenatal corticosteroids
- surfactant therapy – prophylaxis/rescue (see Chapter 28)
- oxygen therapy
- prevention of alveolar collapse – by applying CPAP (continuous positive airway pressure), high flow nasal therapy or PEEP (positive end-expiratory pressure) on a mechanical ventilator
- lung expansion – by applying a peak inspiratory pressure with a mechanical ventilator, if necessary
- provision of intensive care (see Chapter 25).

Neonatology at a Glance, Third Edition. Edited by Tom Lissauer, Avroy A. Fanaroff, Lawrence Miall and Jonathan Fanaroff.
© 2016 John Wiley & Sons, Ltd. Published 2016 by John Wiley & Sons, Ltd.

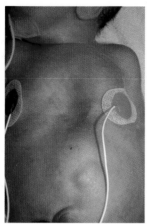

Fig. 29.3 Chest retraction in a preterm infant with respiratory distress.

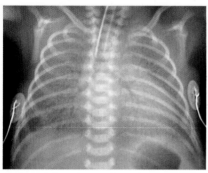

Fig. 29.4 Chest X-ray (after 4 hours of age) in RDS showing:
• diffuse, uniform granular (ground glass) appearance of the lungs from atelectasis
• air bronchogram – outline of air-filled large airways against opaque lungs
• reduced lung volume
• indistinct heart border as the lung fields are opaque ('white-out').
A tracheal tube is in place.

Table 29.1 Causes of respiratory distress in preterm infants.

Common
Respiratory distress syndrome (surfactant deficiency)
Pneumonia/sepsis
Transient tachypnea of the newborn
Uncommon
Pulmonary hypoplasia
Pneumothorax
Congenital heart disease
Rare
Diaphragmatic hernia
Non-respiratory – anemia, hypothermia, metabolic acidosis
Other causes
These are listed in Chapter 39

Complications

The main complications are:
• infection/lung collapse
• air leaks
• patent ductus arteriosus
• pulmonary hemorrhage
• intraventricular hemorrhage
• bronchopulmonary dysplasia.

Air leaks

Pulmonary interstitial emphysema (PIE)
There is tracking of air from the overdistended terminal airways into the interstitium. Increases risk of pneumothorax and bronchopulmonary dysplasia.

Pneumothorax
Occurs in 5–10% of infants ventilated for RDS. Presents with:
• increased oxygen requirement
• reduced breath sounds and chest movement on affected side
• hypoxemia, hypercarbia and acidosis on blood gases
• shock.
Confirmed by transillumination or chest X-ray (see Chapter 26).

A tension pneumothorax is treated by urgent aspiration and insertion of a chest tube.

Pneumothorax may occur spontaneously, but is less likely if the ventilator is well synchronized with the baby's breathing and high pressures are avoided.

Pulmonary hemorrhage

This is hemorrhagic pulmonary edema. In preterm infants it is usually associated with left heart failure from a patent ductus arteriosus (left-to-right shunting) and respiratory distress syndrome requiring mechanical ventilation.

Causes blood staining of tracheal aspirate with or without shock.

Occurs in about 3% of infants with respiratory distress syndrome requiring mechanical ventilation. Most of these infants will have received surfactant, but this is no longer considered to be a risk factor. Coagulation may be deranged.

Treatment:
• increase ventilation, especially PEEP.
• surfactant
• if necessary, administer blood/volume and clotting factors, but avoid fluid overload
• close patent ductus arteriosus.
Massive pulmonary hemorrhage has a high mortality.

30 Temperature control

Hypothermia

Temperature regulation is fundamental to neonatal care.

Hypothermia can cause:
- increased oxygen and energy consumption, resulting in hypoxia, metabolic acidosis and hypoglycemia
- apnea
- neonatal cold injury – redness of the skin from dissociation of hemoglobin
- coagulopathy
- poor weight gain
- increased mortality.

Newborn babies are particularly liable to hypothermia as:
- they have a large surface area relative to their mass, so there is an imbalance between heat generation (related to mass) and heat loss (surface area)
- their skin is thin and permeable to heat
- they have little subcutaneous fat for insulation
- they have a limited capacity to generate heat as they mainly rely on non-shivering thermogenesis using a special form of adipose tissue, brown fat, which is distributed in the neck, between the scapulae and surrounding the kidneys and adrenals
- their ability to produce heat from sympathetic responses is poor – shivering occurs only at an ambient temperature of <16 °C in term infants and does not occur in preterm infants until 2 weeks of age
- preterm infants are unable to curl up to reduce skin exposure. There is only one scenario where hypothermia is beneficial – for brain protection in term babies with perinatal asphyxia (see therapeutic hypothermia, Chapter 14).

Evaporative heat loss in preterm infants

Transepidermal water loss:
- is markedly increased in very premature infants (Fig. 30.2a)
- is increased by radiant warmers, phototherapy (if not using LED lights) and if the skin is denuded
- declines with increasing postnatal age, as the skin thickens
- is reduced by humidity (Fig. 30.2b).

How newborn infants lose heat

Convection (Fig. 30.1a)
Determined by:
- temperature difference between skin and air
- area of skin exposed to the air
- movement of surrounding air.

Is an important cause of heat loss, minimized by:
- clothing the infant
- raising temperature of ambient air
- avoiding drafts.

Radiation (Fig. 30.1b)
Depends on temperature difference between skin and surrounding surfaces, i.e. walls of incubator or, if under radiant warmer, windows and walls of room; is independent of the air temperature.

Reduced in incubators by having a double wall.

Evaporation (Fig. 30.1c)
Important:
- at birth, when skin is wet
- in preterm infants, as their skin is very thin and water-permeable
- from the respiratory tree with artificial ventilation/nasal CPAP unless air/oxygen is heated and humidified.

Minimized at birth by drying the infant and wrapping in a warm towel; preterm infants (<30 weeks) placed directly in plastic wrapping with only the face exposed and head covered with a hat.

Conduction (Fig. 30.1d)
Loss is small as babies are on mattresses, which may be heated.

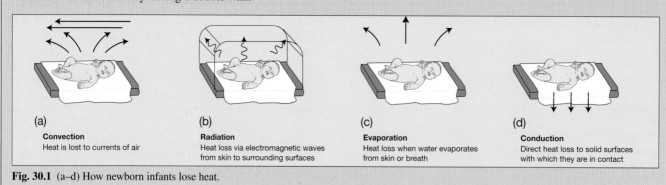

(a) **Convection**
Heat is lost to currents of air

(b) **Radiation**
Heat loss via electromagnetic waves from skin to surrounding surfaces

(c) **Evaporation**
Heat loss when water evaporates from skin or breath

(d) **Conduction**
Direct heat loss to solid surfaces with which they are in contact

Fig. 30.1 (a–d) How newborn infants lose heat.

Neonatology at a Glance, Third Edition. Edited by Tom Lissauer, Avroy A. Fanaroff, Lawrence Miall and Jonathan Fanaroff.
© 2016 John Wiley & Sons, Ltd. Published 2016 by John Wiley & Sons, Ltd.

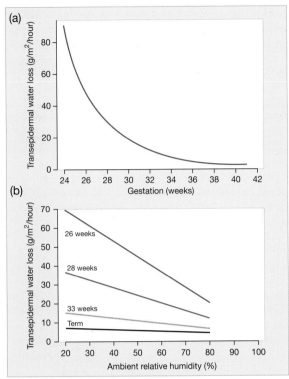

Fig. 30.2 (a) Transepidermal water loss increases with decreasing gestation. (b) Transepidermal water loss is reduced by humidity. (From Hammerlund *et al*. Transepidermal water loss in newborn infants. *Acta Paediatr Scand* 1983; **72**: 721–728.)

Keeping neonates warm

Infants should be nursed in their thermoneutral environment, with a core body temperature of 36.5–37.5 °C (Fig. 30.3). If the infant needs to be naked for observation/procedures:

- place under radiant warmer for resuscitation/stabilization or care of some term infants, incubator if preterm.
- ensure the NICU is warm and draft-free
- use warm, humidified ventilator gases
- cover the head with a hat (important as the surface area of babies' heads are large).

If premature but stable:

- clothe
- place in incubator or heated mattress in crib/cot
- wrap, keep in a warm, draft-free room
- can be kept warm with kangaroo mother care, even if gavage (nasogastric) feeding (See Chapter 73 Global Health).

Key point

At birth, preterm infants <30 weeks should be placed in a plastic wrap (bag), with a hat, and under a radiant heater until they are in a warm humidified incubator.

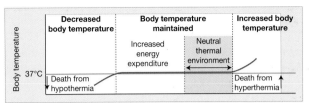

Fig. 30.3 The neutral thermal environment is the temperature range where heat production is at the minimum needed to maintain normal body temperature. It depends on birthweight, gestational and postnatal age and whether the infant is clothed or naked.

Key point

A normal core temperature does not mean a neutral thermal environment – it may be achieved by increased energy expenditure.

Incubators

Advantages

- Provide constant, warm environment, even when doors are open.
- Can minimize transepidermal water loss – with high relative humidity.
- Can reduce radiant heat loss if the baby is covered and the incubator has double walls.
- Allows continuous observation of infant's breathing and condition.

Disadvantages

- Reduced access for procedures, but improved in modern incubators
- May inhibit parental interaction.
- Noise from incubator's motor and doors.

Radiant warmers

Advantages

- Ease of access for resuscitation/stabilization and some practical procedures and care of term infants.
- Rapid increase in temperature.

Disadvantages

- High transepidermal water loss from radiant heat – makes fluid balance problematic in preterm infants, so best avoided.
- Difficult to provide extra humidity,
- High convective heat losses.

Combined incubators with inbuilt radiant warmers

Now widely used for infants requiring intensive care. Radiant heat is used only when access is required, e.g. for procedures.

Question

When are heated mattresses useful?

They may allow stable preterm infants to be nursed in a crib (cot) instead of an incubator. Also useful to warm infants who have become cold, or in the operating room, during imaging studies or transport.

31 Growth and nutrition

Growth

Between 24 and 36 weeks' gestation, a fetus growing along the 50th centile gains 15 g/kg/day. Infants who are fed enterally require 110–135 kcal/kg/day (85–95 kcal/kg/day if parenterally fed) to maintain this rate of growth. As these high energy requirements often cannot be met, the weight of extremely preterm infants is often initially static or may decline, and the infant may take up to 21 days to regain birthweight. Thereafter, their growth improves but is often suboptimal. The reason for this growth failure includes:
- the infant is unable to tolerate high volumes of nutrients
- fluids may be restricted, e.g. patent ductus arteriosus
- feeds restricted because of intercurrent illness, e.g. infection
- lower volume of milk given than protocol for fear that infant will not tolerate it or that it predisposes to necrotizing enterocolitis (NEC).

Nutrition

Which milk?

Breast milk
Is the milk of choice. Advantages over formula feeds (also see Chapter 20) are:
- better tolerated
- associated with a lower incidence of necrotizing enterocolitis and provides some protection against infection
- contains hormones and growth factors
- has better absorption of fats and improved bioavailability of trace minerals
- promotes mother–infant bonding
- it is associated with improved cognitive development later in childhood.

Disadvantages are:
- depends on the mother being able to express sufficient milk over a prolonged period; this can usually be achieved with support.

- growth of the preterm infant may be suboptimal. Breast milk may need to be enhanced with human milk fortifier to increase its energy, protein and mineral content. Human milk fortifiers contain cow's milk protein. Fortification is usually stopped once the infant is entirely breast-fed or weighs more than 2 kg.

Donor human milk
An increasing number of neonatal units give donor breast milk to extremely preterm infants or infants at increased risk of NEC (necrotizing enterocolitis) when maternal breast milk is not available, especially during the first few days of life. Donors are screened by questionnaire and serological testing for infection, the milk is pasteurized and screened for bacteria. Donor milk has been shown to have a lower incidence of feeding intolerance and necrotizing enterocolitis than preterm formula.

Low birthweight infant formulas
These have been developed to supply the increased energy (24 kcal/oz, 80 kcal/100 mL), protein, sodium, calcium and phosphate required by low birthweight infants (Table 31.1). They are increasingly further modified to be more like breast milk, with the addition of long-chain polyunsaturated fatty acids which are used as structural fats in nervous tissue, and oligosaccharides which act as prebiotics to encourage a more breast-fed-like gut bacterial flora.

Supplements

- **Iron** is given to preterm infants once they are on full enteral feeds and not receiving blood transfusions unless fully formula fed. Supplementation is for six months to one year.
- **Multivitamins** (A, B_{12}, C, D and E) are given routinely. Folic acid is given in some centers.
- **Vitamin K** is given to all infants, including the preterm, as prophylaxis against vitamin K deficient bleeding (hemorrhagic disease of the newborn).

Table 31.1 Composition of various milks.

	Mature term breast milk	Preterm breast milk	Fortified preterm breast milk	Low birthweight formula	Term formula
Energy (kcal/100 mL)	70	67	74	80	66
Carbohydrate (g/100 mL)	7	7.6	8	10–11	7.6
Fat (g/100 mL)	4.2	4	4	5	4.4
Protein (g/100 mL)	1.3	1.8–2.4	2.9	2.2–2.5	2.5
Na (mmol/L)	7	13	18	13–20	8
K (mmol/L)	15	15	17	18	17
Ca (mmol/L)	9	6	22	30	12–20
Phosphate (mmol/L)	5	5	18	21	12–18

(Source: ESPGHAN, 2010.) (MCT – medium chain triglyceride).

Question

What is the daily recommended nutritional requirement of a fully enterally fed very low birthweight infant?

It is (per kg/day):

Fluids	135–200 mL
Energy	110–135 kcal
Protein	3.5–4 g
Carbohydrate	11–13 g
Fat	4.8–6.6 g (<40% MCT)
Sodium	2–3 mmol
Potassium	2–3 mmol
Calcium	120–140 mg
Phosphate	60–90 mg

Neonatology at a Glance, Third Edition. Edited by Tom Lissauer, Avroy A. Fanaroff, Lawrence Miall and Jonathan Fanaroff.
© 2016 John Wiley & Sons, Ltd. Published 2016 by John Wiley & Sons, Ltd.

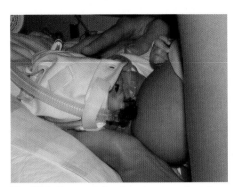

Fig. 31.1 Preterm infant learning to suck at the breast whilst still on continuous positive airway pressure (CPAP).

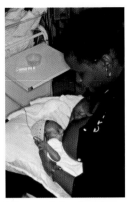

Fig. 31.2 Preterm infant learning to breast-feed whilst still receiving gavage (tube) feeds.

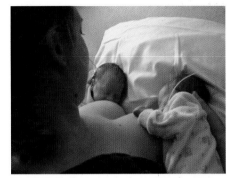

Fig. 31.3 Preterm twins successfully learning to feed at the breast.

Feeding

Whereas the healthy newborn term infant can be put to the breast shortly after birth, extremely preterm infants cannot feed for themselves as they:
• are unable to suck and swallow until about 32–34 weeks of gestation (Figs 31.1–31.3)
• are initially unable to tolerate milk in sufficient quantity to meet their nutritional requirements.

A number of strategies are adopted to overcome these problems.

Minimal enteral (non-nutritive) feeding

A small volume (e.g. 10–20 mL/kg/day), preferably with expressed breast milk, is given during the first few days to stimulate gut hormone production even when the infant is too unwell or unstable to tolerate the expected volume of feeds. This helps intestinal maturation, motility and gallbladder function, decreasing the time taken to establish full enteral feeding; it also lowers serum bilirubin concentrations. Feeding should be advanced cautiously in infants who are growth-restricted and have reversed end-diastolic blood flow velocity on antenatal Doppler ultrasound because of their increased risk of necrotizing enterocolitis.

Gavage (tube) feeding

Used when infants are too immature (<34 weeks' gestational age) or ill to feed for themselves but are able to tolerate enteral feeds. The volume of milk is gradually increased. Gastric residuals should not slow down advancement of feeding volumes unless bilious with abdominal distension, blood in the stool or other features suggesting necrotizing enterocolitis. Reduced gut motility in very low birthweight infants may necessitate suppositories for constipation.

The tube may be orogastric or nasogastric. As nasogastric tubes lie in the narrowest part of the upper airway, just behind the nose, a size 5 French gauge tube increases airway resistance by 30–50% in preterm infants. This increases the work of breathing and may increase the frequency of apnea. Some units avoid nasogastric tubes in extreme preterm infants, but orogastric tubes are more difficult to fix securely.

There is conflicting evidence regarding continuous versus bolus feeding in relation to weight gain and the incidence of apnea and bradycardia. The infant's oxygen tension falls with feeds in both preterm and term infants. It has been argued that continuous feeding is more physiologic for preterm infants because it is a closer approximation to the way a fetus is fed *in utero*. However, bolus feeds are preferred as the response of gut hormones is more physiologic.

Parenteral nutrition (PN)

A mixture of carbohydrate, protein, fat, vitamins and trace elements allows nutrition to be provided whilst oral feeding is established. It is usually given via a central venous line but may be given peripherally. It is associated with a number of complications:
• line-related infection
• conjugated hyperbilirubinemia
• electrolyte disorders
• hyperglycemia
• chemical burns from extravasation
• pleural or pericardial effusion – if tip of the central line lies in the heart and becomes displaced.

Volume of fluids

A guide to average total fluid intake is shown in Table 31.2. It is adjusted according to plasma electrolytes, creatinine, acid–base status and the infant's weight, all of which are measured regularly over the first few days. It is markedly affected by:
• gestational age
• thermal environment (radiant warmer or incubator)
• evaporative water loss (reduced by humidity, etc.).

Once the preterm infant is stable and on full enteral feeds, electrolytes, creatinine and phosphate, calcium and alkaline phosphatase can be checked weekly.

Table 31.2 Typical fluid intake according to postnatal age.

Postnatal age	Fluid intake (mL/kg/24 h)	
	<2.5 kg	>2.5 kg
Birth	60–100	60–80
Day 1	90–120	60–100
Day 2	120–150	90–120
Day 3	150	120–150
Days 4 and over	150–180	150

These are the most common causes of acquired brain injury in premature infants. Their incidence is inversely related to gestational age.

- **Hemorrhage** – occurs in about 20% of VLBW (very low birthweight) infants. Involves the germinal matrix, an immature capillary network, which overlies the head of the caudate nucleus. The hemorrhage may be confined to the germinal matrix (GMH–IVH), may extend into the ventricle (IVH) or involve the parenchyma. Parenchymal hemorrhages result from venous infarction. Hemorrhage usually occurs within 72 hours of birth. It is uncommon beyond 32 weeks' gestation by which time the germinal matrix has involuted.
- Cystic **periventricular leukomalacia (PVL)** – loss of periventricular white matter in watershed areas around the lateral ventricles from hypoxia–ischemia. Probably most occur before birth, but some postnatally. Periventricular flare or echodensity (PVE) may resolve or evolve into small cysts in fronto-parietal region or extensive periventricular or deep white matter cysts which are visible on ultrasound after 2–3 weeks in 3% of VLBW infants.

Diagnosis

This is by bedside cranial ultrasound (Table 32.2). In VLBW infants, it is performed shortly after birth to identify antenatal lesions, during the first week of life and after serious illness to identify hemorrhages, and repeated periodically to identify and monitor hydrocephalus and appearance of cystic periventricular leukomalacia (PVL). It is excellent for detecting hemorrhage and ventricular dilatation (see Chapter 79, Cranial ultrasound). It is relatively insensitive in detecting white matter damage; MRI when older is more sensitive (see Chapter 81, Perinatal neuroimaging).

Pathogenesis (Figs 32.1 and 32.2) and incidence (Table 32.1)

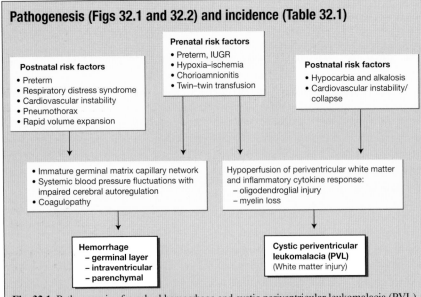

Fig. 32.1 Pathogenesis of cerebral hemorrhage and cystic periventricular leukomalacia (PVL).

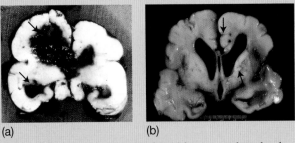

(a)   (b)

Fig. 32.2 Autopsy specimen showing (a) large parenchymal and intraventricular hemorrhage and (b) ventricular dilatation and cystic periventricular leukomalacia (PVL).

Question

What is meant by cerebral autoregulation?

It is the maintenance of normal cerebral blood flow over a wide range in blood pressure.

This blood pressure range is narrow in preterm infants; falls in blood pressure lead to cerebral hypoperfusion, leading to ischemic damage and hemorrhagic infarction.

Key point

There has been a marked reduction in the incidence of severe periventricular leukomalacia and post-hemorrhagic hydrocephalus requiring shunts.

Table 32.1 Incidence of severe intraventricular hemorrhage (IVH) and cystic periventricular leukomalacia (PVL) by gestational age (Vermont–Oxford Network data for 2012).

Gestational age (weeks)	Severe IVH (Grades III/IV) (%)	Cystic PVL (%)
<24	35	6.5
24–26	17	5
27–29	5	3
30–32	1.4	1

Neonatology at a Glance, Third Edition. Edited by Tom Lissauer, Avroy A. Fanaroff, Lawrence Miall and Jonathan Fanaroff.
© 2016 John Wiley & Sons, Ltd. Published 2016 by John Wiley & Sons, Ltd.

Table 32.2 A classification of lesions identified on intracranial ultrasound.

Hemorrhage
Grade I – isolated germinal matrix hemorrhage (GMH)
Grade II – intraventricular hemorrhage (GMH–IVH); <50% of
    ventricular area on parasagittal view
Grade III – intraventricular hemorrhage (GMH–IVH with dilatation); >50%
    of ventricular area on parasagittal view, usually distends lateral ventricle
Grade IV – hemorrhagic parenchymal infarct (parenchymal lesion)
Periventricular white matter echodensity (PVE) – echogenicity is
    comparable with that of choroid plexus
Cystic periventricular leukomalacia (PVL)
Porencephalic cyst – single, large cyst
Posthemorrhagic ventricular dilatation/hydrocephalus (PHVD)

Clinical features

Most infants are asymptomatic; more likely with large bleeds.
Clinical features of intraventricular hemorrhage include:
- increased ventilatory support
- abnormal neurologic signs, including seizures
- apnea and bradycardia
- shock.

Laboratory findings

Mostly not specific. For intraventricular hemorrhage may include:
- acute anemia
- hyperglycemia, hyperkalemia, electrolyte imbalance
- unexplained metabolic acidosis
- coagulation abnormalities.

Management

Optimize:
- airway and breathing – provide oxygenation/ventilation as
needed; avoid hypo- or hypercarbia, synchronize infant's breathing
and ventilator

- circulation – maintain adequate intravascular volume and blood
pressure
- comfort – avoid unnecessary or uncomfortable manipulation.
Treat seizures.
Correct significant coagulation abnormalities.
Monitor for complications (Fig. 32.3) – sequential head circumference measurements and serial head ultrasound for ventricular dilatation (see Chapter 79).

Prognosis

- Small germinal matrix or intraventricular hemorrhage – slightly increased risk of neurodevelopmental problems.
- Large parenchymal hemorrhage/large porencephalic cyst – may cause hemiplegic cerebral palsy and visual defect.
- Hydrocephalus needing shunt – appreciable mortality, high risk of neurodisability.
- Transient echodensities – normal.
- Widespread cysts – most have cerebral palsy, usually spastic diplegia or quadriplegia with or without learning difficulties and visual impairment.

Prevention

- Avoid delivery before 30 weeks of gestation unless essential.
- Give antenatal corticosteroids.
- Avoid perinatal hypoxia–ischemia when possible.
- Efficient resuscitation and stabilization at birth.
- Minimal handling
- Optimize intensive care – minimize hypotension and hypocarbia ($PCO_2 < 30$ mmHg, 4 kPa), which causes cerebral vasoconstriction.

    Prophylactic indomethacin reduces the incidence of severe hemorrhage but does not improve neurodevelopmental outcome.

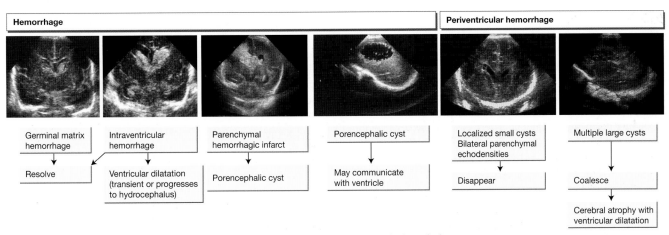

Fig. 32.3 Natural history and complications of cerebral hemorrhage and periventricular leukomalacia.

33 Patent ductus arteriosus (PDA)

The ductus arteriosus connects the pulmonary artery with the descending aorta (Fig. 33.1). *In utero*, patency of the arterial duct is maintained by a low PaO_2 and high concentrations of vasodilating prostaglandins (PGE_2 and PGI_2). In the fetus the ductus arteriosus allows 90% of the right cardiac output to bypass the lungs and helps deliver oxygenated blood form the placenta to the brain and other vital organs (see Chapter 12).

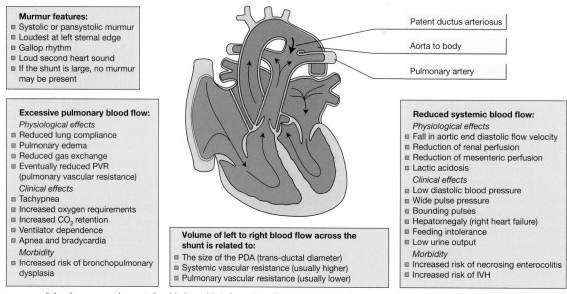

Murmur features:
- Systolic or pansystolic murmur
- Loudest at left sternal edge
- Gallop rhythm
- Loud second heart sound
- If the shunt is large, no murmur may be present

Excessive pulmonary blood flow:
Physiological effects
- Reduced lung compliance
- Pulmonary edema
- Reduced gas exchange
- Eventually reduced PVR (pulmonary vascular resistance)
Clinical effects
- Tachypnea
- Increased oxygen requirements
- Increased CO_2 retention
- Ventilator dependence
- Apnea and bradycardia
Morbidity
- Increased risk of bronchopulmonary dysplasia

Patent ductus arteriosus
Aorta to body
Pulmonary artery

Reduced systemic blood flow:
Physiological effects
- Fall in aortic end diastolic flow velocity
- Reduction of renal perfusion
- Reduction of mesenteric perfusion
- Lactic acidosis
Clinical effects
- Low diastolic blood pressure
- Wide pulse pressure
- Bounding pulses
- Hepatomegaly (right heart failure)
- Feeding intolerance
- Low urine output
Morbidity
- Increased risk of necrosing enterocolitis
- Increased risk of IVH

Volume of left to right blood flow across the shunt is related to:
- The size of the PDA (trans-ductal diameter)
- Systemic vascular resistance (usually higher)
- Pulmonary vascular resistance (usually lower)

Fig. 33.1 Anatomy of the ductus arteriosus (after birth), with left to right flow across it, and clinical/physiologic consequences.

Ductal closure

After birth, ductal constriction is promoted by:
- the rise in oxygen tension with the first breaths
- the fall in pulmonary vascular resistance and rise in systemic vascular resistance
- a fall in PGE_2 and PGI_2.

Ductal closure takes place in two stages:
- functional closure – 24–48 hours after birth
- anatomic closure – may take 2–3 weeks.

In preterm infants, there may be delay in anatomical closure. As pulmonary resistance falls, blood flows "left to right" across the patent ductus, from the higher systemic to the lower pulmonary vascular resistance. In severe respiratory distress syndrome, pulmonary artery pressure is increased and the shunt may be bidirectional. Eventually, the duct will close spontaneously, but intervention is sometimes required to achieve this. In contrast to preterm infants, in term infants, a patent ductus arteriosus is due to a permanent defect in the muscle wall of the duct and is unlikely to close spontaneously.

Ongoing patency of the ductus arteriosus may be beneficial in pulmonary hypertension or some forms of 'duct dependent' congenital heart disease as it augments systemic or pulmonary circulation (See Chapter 49 Cardiac disorders).

Risk factors

- prematurity – incidence increases with decreasing gestational age; most common in those less than 32 weeks' gestational age.
- respiratory distress syndrome
- fluid overload
- sepsis
- pulmonary hypertension.

Clinical features

A PDA becomes significant when the volume of left–right blood flow leads to hemodynamic compromise (Fig. 33.1). The clinical features are attributable to excessive pulmonary blood flow and reduced systemic perfusion from shunting of blood across the duct. The degree of shunting depends on the size of the duct and the difference between systemic and pulmonary vascular resistance.

Investigations

Chest X-ray (Fig. 33.2)

May show cardiomegaly and increased pulmonary vascularity or pulmonary edema.

Neonatology at a Glance, Third Edition. Edited by Tom Lissauer, Avroy A. Fanaroff, Lawrence Miall and Jonathan Fanaroff.
© 2016 John Wiley & Sons, Ltd. Published 2016 by John Wiley & Sons, Ltd.

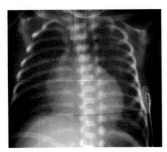

Fig. 33.2 Chest X-ray showing increased pulmonary vasculature markings and cardiomegaly. But often unhelpful diagnostically. (Courtesy of Dr Sheila Berlin.)

Echocardiography with pulsed color Doppler

- Confirms the diagnosis.
- Provides visualization of the size and direction of the shunt and its hemodynamic consequences (Fig. 33.3a and b). Significant if:
- Left atrial enlargement (left atrial:aortic root ratio >1.5:1).
- Left ventricular enlargement (cardiomegaly).
- High cardiac output (>350 mL/kg/min).
- Absent or retrograde diastolic flow in postductal aorta.
- Absent or retrograde diastolic flow in celiac, renal and middle cerebral arteries.

Management

Medical management

The aim is to eliminate the left to right shunt, thereby reducing pulmonary blood flow and restoring systemic blood flow. However, the duct often closes spontaneously and indications for medical or surgical closure remain uncertain.

- **Fluid management** – Fluid restriction is widely practiced to limit pulmonary edema and is appropriate during treatment with indomethacin or ibuprofen if oliguria/anuria and/or fluid retention ensue. However, prolonged fluid restriction may further worsen systemic hypoperfusion.
- **Shunt limitation strategies** – Through permissive hypercapnemia, elevated positive end-expiratory pressure and avoidance of excessive oxygen.
- **Diuretics** – Used only if in heart failure. Furosemide leads to increased renal production of prostaglandins, which may actually promote ductal patency. May also further compromise systemic blood flow. May be needed while awaiting surgery.
- **Prostaglandin synthase inhibitors**, also called cyclooxygenase inhibitors (COXi) – See Table 33.1. Indomethacin was used for many years. Prophylactic indomethacin will reduce the incidence of PDA and severe IVH but does not alter long-term neurodevelopmental outcome and risks intestinal

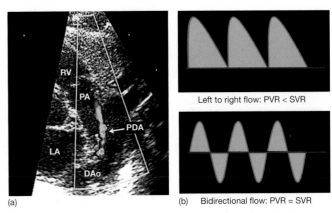

(a)   (b)   Bidirectional flow: PVR = SVR

Fig. 33.3 (a) Pulsed color Doppler showing shunting across the ductus arteriosus (arrow). (b) Different patterns of PDA flow. (PVR = pulmonary vascular resistance, SVR = systemic vascular resistance.)

Table 33.1 Indomethacin and ibuprofen.

Side effects	Contraindications
Decreased platelet aggregation, may worsen bleeding	Abnormal renal function with oliguria
Gastrointestinal bleeding	Gastrointestinal bleeding
Focal intestinal perforation	Thrombocytopenia
Fluid retention, leading to hyponatremia	Seldom effective if >4 weeks old

perforation. Ibuprofen has similar efficacy but less reduction in cerebral, renal and mesenteric blood flow. Usually given over 3 days. The duct closes in >60% after a single course; a second course may be required. Most effective in the first week of life. Paracetamol has recently been used if COXi are unsuccessful or contraindicated. Although it appears promising, its widespread use is not currently recommended owing to lack of safety data.

Surgical closure

Only if medical treatment fails. Thoracotomy usually to clip or ligate duct; minimally invasive gaining popularity.
Complications of surgery are:

- Postligation cardiac syndrome – hypotension and difficulty with oxygenation secondary to impaired left ventricular function. May benefit from prophylactic milrinone in immediate postoperative period.
- Recurrent laryngeal nerve damage – vocal cord paralysis.
- Chylothorax from damage to thoracic duct.
- Pneumothorax.
- Ligation of pulmonary artery by mistake.
- Adverse neurological outcome, mortality (<1%).

Infection

Infection is a major cause of morbidity and mortality in preterm infants. They are especially vulnerable because:
• they have reduced cellular and humoral immunity because IgG antibodies are transferred from mother to fetus mainly during the third trimester
• their skin is thin and readily denuded by skin electrodes, catheters and tape, providing a portal of entry and a site of colonization for organisms
• central venous catheters and tracheal tubes are a potential focus for infection, especially if left in place for prolonged periods
• cross-infection is readily spread from infant to infant in neonatal nurseries on the hands of staff and from contaminated equipment.

Early-onset infection (<72 hours)

Acquired before birth from chorioamnionitis or maternal bacteremia or from the birth canal.

The most common organisms are group B streptococci and Gram-negative bacteria.

Late-onset sepsis (>72 hours)

Mainly due to nosocomial (hospital-acquired) infection, rather than community-acquired infection. The most common cause is coagulase-negative staphylococcus (CONS). Other organisms are shown in Fig. 34.1.

There is marked variation in nosocomial infection rates among units. This results in wide variation in infection-related morbidity,

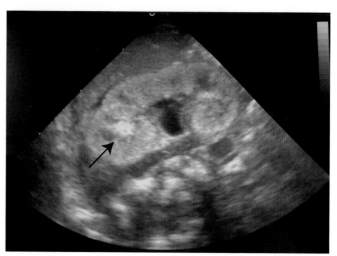

Fig. 34.2 Fungal ball (arrow) in the kidney from *Candida* sepsis on renal ultrasound.

duration of hospitalization, cost and mortality. Recent quality improvement initiatives with care bundles to reduce central line-associated bloodstream infection (CLABSI) have markedly reduced late-onset sepsis.

Fungal infections

In very low birthweight infants:
• incidence 1–10%
• mortality up to 35%.

Candida albicans is the most common organism (Fig. 34.2). The source of infection is colonization of the gastrointestinal tract. In some neonatal units, antifungal agents are given prophylactically to extremely low birthweight infants. However, this practice is not uniformly accepted. Broad-spectrum antibiotics, parenteral nutrition and central venous catheters are risk factors for fungal infection.

Treatment is with amphotericin B, fluconazole or flucytosine, depending on infection site and fungus species.

Presentation and management

These are described in Chapter 42.

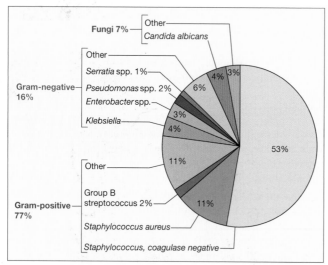

Fig. 34.1 Organisms causing late-onset sepsis in very low birthweight infants. (NICHD Neonatal Research Network. Boghossian N.S. *et al.* Late-onset sepsis in very low birth weight infants from singleton and multiple-gestation births. *J Pediatr* 2013; **162**: 1120–1124.)

Jaundice

Most preterm infants develop jaundice from unconjugated hyperbilirubinemia in the first week of life. The level of bilirubin that is potentially damaging is lower than in more mature infants. The bilirubin peaks at around day 5 of life and should be closely monitored.

Conjugated hyperbilirubinemia is mainly associated with parenteral nutrition (PN), necrotizing enterocolitis and congenital infection. Management is described in Chapter 41.

Neonatology at a Glance, Third Edition. Edited by Tom Lissauer, Avroy A. Fanaroff, Lawrence Miall and Jonathan Fanaroff.
© 2016 John Wiley & Sons, Ltd. Published 2016 by John Wiley & Sons, Ltd.

Anemia

Common in VLBW (very low birthweight) infants, mainly because of:
• blood loss from repeated blood sampling and the preterm infant's small blood volume of only about 90 mL/kg
• physiologic anemia of prematurity. This occurs at 1–3 months of age due to:
  – reduced red cell production
  – shortened red cell survival
  – markedly increased requirements from growth.

Treatment

Blood transfusions

Aim is to restore or maintain adequate tissue oxygen delivery, but as there are no reliable symptoms or signs to determine this, the indications in neonates are controversial and vary between centers (Table 34.1). Blood transfusions are kept to a minimum because of potential hazards. Splitting adult donor bags to allow several transfusions from the same donor is recommended to reduce potential risk of blood-borne pathogens by reducing number of donors.

Oral iron therapy

Given to prevent anemia of prematurity, unless the infant has received a recent blood transfusion or iron-fortified formula.

Oral folic acid

Given in some centers.

Table 34.1 An example of indications for blood transfusions in preterm infants (College of American Pathologists, 1998).

Acute blood loss with shock
Hb <12 g/dL – if in oxygen with mechanical ventilation, congenital heart disease with cyanosis or heart failure
Hb <10 g/dL – if moderate oxygen requirement via nasal cannula
Hb <8 g/dL – if apnea and bradycardia, sustained tachycardia, failure to gain weight, mild oxygen requirement
Hb <7 g/dL and reticulocyte count <100 000/mL – even if asymptomatic

Question

Is erythropoietin therapy helpful in newborn infants?

Recombinant human erythropoietin (EPO) could potentially reduce the need for red cell transfusions. However, it does not significantly reduce the transfusion requirements in the first 2 weeks of life, when sick neonates are most dependent on transfusion. It is therefore used selectively. It may be useful for treatment of chronic anemia when transfusion is declined (e.g. for religious or cultural reasons). It is not useful for treatment of acute anemia because of the lag of >1 week after starting treatment before the hemoglobin increases significantly.

Osteopenia of prematurity

Metabolic bone disease may occur at several weeks of age, causing:
• reduced bone mineralization with widening and cupping of the wrists, knees and ribs on X-ray, as with rickets (Fig. 34.3a and b)
• failure in linear growth
• pathologic fractures, particularly of ribs and long bones.
  Investigations show:
• calcium – normal or raised
• phosphate – low
• alkaline phosphatase (a marker of bone turnover) – markedly raised.
  Osteopenia of prematurity is due to phosphorus deficiency from urinary loss and increased requirements.

It can be prevented by providing additional phosphate in parenteral nutrition, by fortifying expressed breast milk or by giving oral phosphate to maintain age-appropriate plasma phosphate levels. It can be problematic to provide sufficient phosphate for infants requiring parenteral nutrition for a prolonged period.

Treatment is with sodium or potassium acid phosphate and vitamin D supplements.

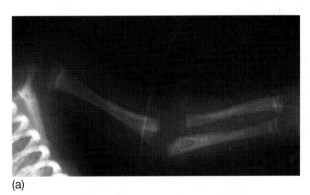

(a)

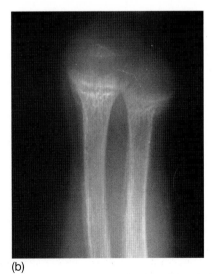

(b)

Fig. 34.3 Osteopenia of prematurity. (a) Reduced bone mineralization with some widening, fraying and cupping of the metaphyses. (b) Marked widening, fraying and cupping of the metaphyses of the wrist bones. (Courtesy of Dr Sheila Berlin.)

35 Apnea, bradycardia and desaturations, retinopathy of prematurity

Apnea, bradycardia and desaturations

Common in VLBW (very low birthweight) infants.

Definition (Fig. 35.1)

Interrelationship between apnea, bradycardia and desaturation is complex, so monitor not only respiration but also heart rate and oxygen saturation.

Hypoxemia with bradycardia is harmful if prolonged.

Classification

- **Central** – cessation of chest wall motion due to loss of respiratory neural output (no signal is sent to breathe).
- **Obstructive** – persistence of obstructed inspiratory efforts throughout the apnea with no airflow. May be associated with neck flexion. Presents with bradycardia with or without desaturation. May not be detected on standard clinical impedance respiratory monitor as they detect chest wall movement as a breath, although there is no airflow.
- **Mixed** – most common for prolonged apnea; a combination of both of above, with obstructed inspiratory efforts intermittently throughout the apnea.

Episodes of desaturation

- May accompany short (5–10 seconds) respiratory pauses, especially if baseline SaO₂ is low.
- During assisted ventilation they are secondary to hypoventilation.
- Variable relationship with bradycardia.

Causes

Usually due to prematurity – must consider or exclude:
- infection (most common)
- necrotizing enterocolitis
- heart failure – patent ductus arteriosus, etc.
- hypoglycemia, electrolyte abnormality
- inborn error of metabolism
- anemia
- seizures.

Treatment

Most apneic spells are brief and self-limiting.
If not:
- Check airway.
- Gentle tactile stimulation.
- Nasal CPAP (continuous positive airway pressure) – very effective, eliminates obstructive apnea. Non-invasive ventilation may also be used.
- Methylxanthines – caffeine or theophylline. Caffeine more widely used as fewer side-effects and drug level monitoring not needed.

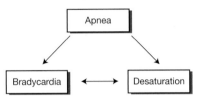

Fig. 35.1 Apnea is absence of breathing for more than 10–15 seconds and may result in bradycardia and/or desaturation.

Caffeine lowers the incidence of bronchopulmonary dysplasia (BPD) and improves neurodevelopmental outcome.
- Mechanical ventilation.

Prognosis

Apnea and bradycardia continue in some preterm infants beyond 36 weeks of gestational age, particularly in association with bronchopulmonary dysplasia (chronic lung disease), but rarely beyond 43–44 weeks. Continue to hospitalize if symptomatic apnea and bradycardia until absent for several days. Not a risk factor for later SIDS (sudden infant death syndrome).

Question

What is the relationship of apnea to feeding?

Hypoventilation, apnea and even cyanosis commonly accompany onset of oral (especially bottle) feeds.

These episodes of hypoventilation typically resolve rapidly without the need for further intervention.

Gastroesophageal reflux and apnea are both common in preterm infants, but rarely temporally related.

Pharmacologic treatment of reflux often fails to abolish apnea.

Retinopathy of prematurity (ROP)

Eye disease of prematurity. Highest incidence in extremely low birthweight infants.

Hyperoxia restricts retinal vascular growth by inhibiting vascular endothelial growth factor (VEGF). Subsequent hypoxia acts as a stimulus for inappropriate and excessive growth of retinal vessels, mediated by increased VEGF. Keeping preterm infants in inappropriately high oxygen concentrations results in a high incidence of ROP, causing blindness (see Chapter 67). However, in VLBW infants, even with oxygenation closely monitored (attempting to keep PaO₂ at 50–80 mmHg, i.e. 6.5–10.5 kPa, oxygen saturation 91–95%), about 30–40% develop ROP, which is severe in 6%, treatment is needed in 3% and 1% have severe visual impairment.

Visual outcome also depends on associated neurologic injury, myopia and squint.

Neonatology at a Glance, Third Edition. Edited by Tom Lissauer, Avroy A. Fanaroff, Lawrence Miall and Jonathan Fanaroff.
© 2016 John Wiley & Sons, Ltd. Published 2016 by John Wiley & Sons, Ltd.

ROP causes 3–10% of childhood visual impairment in developed countries. Visual impairment from ROP is also emerging as a problem in low and middle income countries in preterm infants >1500 g birthweight, from use of excessively high concentrations of oxygen.

Screening

Preterm infants are screened selectively (Table 35.1). Findings are classified according to the stage of advancement and the zone affected (Table 35.2 and Fig. 35.2).

Table 35.1 Screening guidelines for retinopathy of prematurity.

	US (2013)	UK (2008)
Who?	Birth: ≤1500 g or ≤30 weeks	Birth: <1501 g or <32 weeks
	Bigger/older infants who are particularly unstable	
When?	≤27 weeks gestational age at 31 weeks	<27 weeks gestational age at 30–31 weeks
	≥28 weeks at 4 weeks postnatal age	>27 weeks at 4–5 weeks postnatal age
Follow up?	Screen until retinopathy shows signs of regression or until fully vascularized	
	Post-discharge follow-up of visual development	

Table 35.2 International classification of retinopathy of prematurity (revised 2005).

Stage 1 – flat demarcation line between normally vascularized and non-vascularized retina (Fig. 35.3)

Stage 2 – demarcation line extends off the retina as a ridge

Stage 3 – new vessels behind the ridge with or without vitreous hemorrhage (extraretinal fibrovascular proliferation) (Fig. 35.4)

Stage 4 – partial retinal detachment

Stage 5 – total retinal detachment (Fig. 35.5)

Plus disease – abnormal dilatation and tortuosity of posterior pole vessels

Pre-plus disease – mild abnormal dilatation and tortuosity of posterior pole vessels

Aggressive posterior ROP – rapidly progressing, severe form

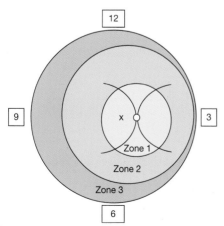

Fig. 35.2 Zones of retina. Numbers at the periphery indicate clock hour.

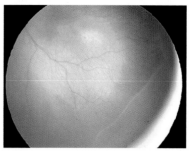

Fig. 35.3 Stage 1 retinopathy of prematurity. (Courtesy of Prof. Alistair Fielder.)

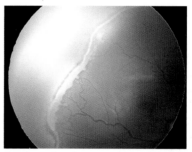

Fig. 35.4 Stage 3 retinopathy of prematurity in a Black infant. (Courtesy of Prof. Alistair Fielder.)

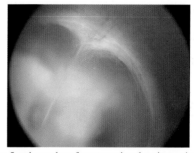

Fig. 35.5 Stage 5 retinopathy of prematurity showing retinal detachment.

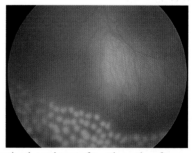

Fig. 35.6 Following laser therapy for retinopathy of prematurity.

Treatment

Stage 1 or 2 disease resolves spontaneously. Severe retinopathy requires treatment with laser therapy to ablate the peripheral avascular retina (Fig. 35.6). Intravitreal injections of VEGF blocking antibody fragments are under investigation as an alternative form of treatment.

36 Necrotizing enterocolitis

Necrotizing enterocolitis (NEC) is the most serious abdominal disorder of preterm infants. It occurs in 2–10% of VLBW (very low birthweight) infants and has a mortality of 15–25%.

The incidence increases with decreasing gestational age; it is rare in term infants. It is characterized by abdominal distension, bilious aspirates, bloody stools and intramural air (pneumatosis intestinalis) on abdominal X-ray.

There is inflammation of the bowel wall, which may progress to necrosis and perforation. It may involve a localized section of bowel (most often the terminal ileum) or be generalized.

It is usually sporadic but occasionally occurs in epidemics. In preterm babies the onset is usually at 1–2 weeks but may be up to several weeks of age. In term babies it occurs earlier, usually after an ischemic insult.

Risk factors

Pathogenesis is unknown, but several risk factors have been identified (Fig. 36.1). Exclusive feeding with human milk reduces the risk of NEC.

There is a change in the microbiome pattern in the gut preceding NEC (and late onset sepsis) revealing less diversity and changes in the community of gut microorganisms which become dominated by Proteobacteria and Firmicutes.

Clinical features

Onset is at 1–2 weeks but may be up to several weeks of age, with:
- bilious aspirates/vomiting
- feeding intolerance
- blood or mucus in stools
- abdomen – distension, distended veins, discoloration of the abdominal wall and tenderness (Fig. 36.2), which may progress to perforation (Table 36.1).
- features of sepsis – temperature instability, apnea and brady-cardia, jaundice, lethargy, hypoperfusion and shock.

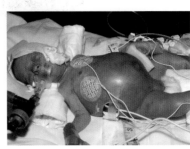

Fig. 36.2 Abdominal distension and shiny discolored, abdominal skin in severe necrotizing enterocolitis.

Table 36.1 Clinical signs of peritonitis/perforation.

Abdominal tenderness
Guarding
Tense, discolored abdominal wall
Abdominal wall edema
Absent bowel sounds
Abdominal mass

Laboratory findings

These include:
- raised acute-phase reactant (C-reactive protein (CRP), or procalcitonin)
- thrombocytopenia
- neutropenia, neutrophilia
- anemia
- blood culture positive
- coagulopathy
- metabolic acidosis
- hypoxia, hypercapnia
- hyponatremia, hyperkalemia
- increased BUN (blood urea nitrogen/urea)
- hyperbilirubinemia.

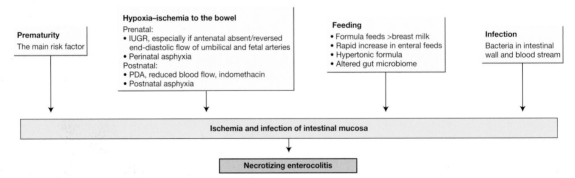

Fig. 36.1 Risk factors in the pathogenesis of necrotizing enterocolitis.

Neonatology at a Glance, Third Edition. Edited by Tom Lissauer, Avroy A. Fanaroff, Lawrence Miall and Jonathan Fanaroff.
© 2016 John Wiley & Sons, Ltd. Published 2016 by John Wiley & Sons, Ltd.

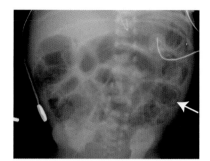

Fig. 36.3 Abdominal X-ray showing dilated loops of bowel and intramural air (arrow). (Courtesy of Dr Sheila Berlin.)

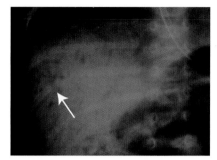

Fig. 36.4 Air in portal venous system (arrow). This is often a transient sign. (Courtesy of Dr Annemarie Jeanes.)

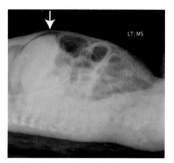

Fig. 36.5 Bowel perforation showing air under the diaphragm on lateral x-ray (arrow). (Courtesy of Dr Sheila Berlin.)

Radiologic abnormalities

- Dilated loops of bowel.
- Thickened intestinal wall.
- Inspissated stool (mottled appearance).
- Intramural air (*pneumatosis intestinalis*, pathognomonic sign) (Fig. 36.3).
- Air in portal venous system (Fig. 36.4).
- Bowel perforation:
  - gasless abdomen/ascites
  - pneumoperitoneum
  - air below diaphragm/around the falciform ligament (Fig. 36.5).

Management (Table 36.2)

Sequelae

- Complications of prolonged parenteral nutrition – infection, electrolyte derangement, conjugated hyperbilirubinemia, etc.
  Short bowel syndrome following bowel resection:
- Diarrhea (from loss of bowel mucosa and rapid gastrointestinal transit)
- Growth failure
- Vitamin B_{12} deficiency if terminal ileum resected
- Dependence on parenteral nutrition
- Stricture formation – causes intestinal obstruction and/or intestinal hemorrhage.

Prevention

- Use breast milk if possible.
- Avoid hyperosmolar feeds.
- Avoid rapid increase in feed volume in very immature infants, especially if intrauterine growth restriction with absent/reversed end-diastolic Doppler waveform antenatally.
- Probiotics with or without prebiotics and lactoferrin help maintain normal gut flora and may reduce risk of NEC.

Table 36.2 Management of necrotizing enterocolitis.

Management	Rationale/goals
Secure airway and support breathing	Abdominal distension may compromise breathing
	May require artificial ventilation
Circulation	
• establish vascular access	Infusion of fluids
• give intravascular volume replacement (saline, blood, fresh frozen plasma)	Treat hypoperfusion/hypovolemic shock
• correct metabolic acidosis	Improve organ and tissue perfusion
Place large-bore naso/orogastric tube	Intestinal decompression, bowel rest
NPO (nil by mouth) – start parenteral nutrition	Support nutritional demands for growth
Broad-spectrum antibiotics	Gram-positive, -negative and anaerobic coverage
	Consider antifungal agents
Treat coagulopathy (fresh frozen plasma, platelets, cryoprecipitate)	Avoid bleeding complications
Monitor regularly – clinical, radiographic and laboratory investigations	Necrotizing enterocolitis can worsen very quickly to bowel perforation
Surgery – options are:	Indications – bowel perforation or failure to resolve on medical treatment
• peritoneal drainage at bedside	
• laparotomy – resection of non-viable bowel and anastomosis or ileostomy or colostomy	However, peritoneal drainage alone is associated with worse neurodevelopmental outcome than laparotomy

Key point

NEC is often suspected before all the classic clinical features are present. Treatment may need to be started whilst awaiting investigation results and before the clinical course becomes evident. Surgical consultation should be initiated early.

37 Bronchopulmonary dysplasia

Bronchopulmonary dysplasia (BPD) develops in 20–30% of very low birthweight infants and is a major cause of morbidity and mortality. The incidence is highest in the extremely preterm (Fig. 37.1); it is uncommon in infants born after 32 weeks' gestational age.

Definition

A consensus conference recommended the following definitions:
• oxygen requirement at 28 days of age (used in many trials)
• oxygen requirement and characteristic chest X-ray at 28 days
• oxygen requirement confirmed by physiologic challenge at 36 weeks' postmenstraual age. This is ascertained by checking if oxygen saturation is maintained in spite of a stepwise reduction in supplemental oxygen until breathing room air. This is the most widely used definition as it identifies infants most likely to have long-term complications.

The conference also recommended that the term 'bronchopulmonary dysplasia' be used rather than 'chronic lung disease'.

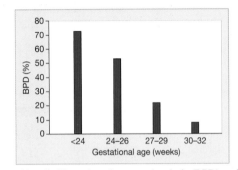

Fig. 37.1 Incidence of bronchopulmonary dysplasia (BPD), at 36 weeks by gestational age at birth in VLBW (very low birthweight infants). (Vermont–Oxford Network data for 2012.)

Predisposing factors

Bronchopulmonary dysplasia is a multifactorial disorder (Fig. 37.2).

It most often develops in extremely preterm infants with surfactant deficiency or immature lungs who require mechanical ventilation. Higher pressures (causing barotrauma), excessive tidal volumes (causing volutrauma), high oxygen concentration and longer time on mechanical ventilation all contribute to an increased risk of developing bronchopulmonary dysplasia. However, with current respiratory management of minimal ventilatory support, bronchopulmonary dysplasia is increasingly seen in extremely preterm infants with minimal lung disease during the first few days of life and whose lungs are subjected to minimal barotrauma and volutrauma. Developmental arrest or delay in pulmonary maturation is thought to be primarily responsible ('new' BPD), where the histology shows minimal airway lesions, pulmonary edema with little fibrosis but decreased alveolar divisions and vascular development. There may be a genetic predisposition. This contrasts with the postnatal insults causing structural lung injury which were the main causes of bronchopulmonary dysplasia in the past ('old' BPD), where there was emphysema and atelectasis, interstitial fibrosis, smooth muscle hyperplasia of the airways and pulmonary vessels and right ventricular hypertrophy.

Clinical features

In addition to the need for oxygen with or without respiratory support:
• skin pallor
• tachypnea
• hyperexpanded chest
• chest retractions

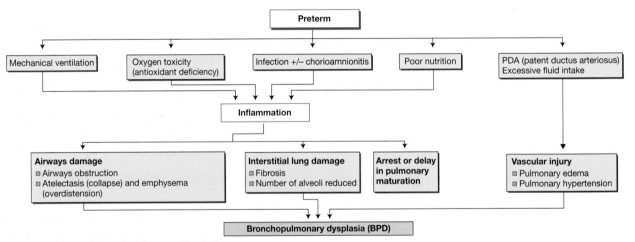

Fig. 37.2 Pathogenesis of bronchopulmonary dysplasia.

Neonatology at a Glance, Third Edition. Edited by Tom Lissauer, Avroy A. Fanaroff, Lawrence Miall and Jonathan Fanaroff.
© 2016 John Wiley & Sons, Ltd. Published 2016 by John Wiley & Sons, Ltd.

- auscultation – crackles and wheezes
- fluid retention, heart failure
- recurrent pneumonia
- growth failure.

Investigations

- chest X-ray (Fig. 37.3)
- overnight oxygen saturation monitoring.

Management

Management of BPD includes:
- Oxygen and respiratory support (low-flow nasal cannula, high-flow nasal therapy, CPAP or mechanical ventilation) but with oxygenation (SaO_2) targeted to 91–95%) (Fig. 37.4).
- Attention to nutritional problems of:
  - increased caloric requirements (130–150 kcal/kg) because of increased work of breathing
  - delay in establishing feeding
  - gastroesophageal reflux (may result in aspiration)
  - prevention of osteopenia of prematurity with phosphate supplements.
- Drug therapy may be considered:
  - inhaled bronchodilators (short-term benefit only)
  - diuretics (transient improvement only)
  - corticosteroid therapy (see below).
  - sildenafil if severe pulmonary hypertension.

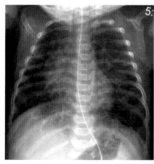

Fig. 37.3 Chest X-ray in bronchopulmonary dysplasia showing generalized, patchy opacification of lung fields, lung collapse, cystic changes and overdistension of the lungs. (Courtesy of Dr Sheila Berlin.)

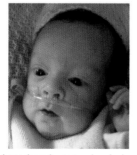

Fig. 37.4 Infant with bronchopulmonary dysplasia receiving low-flow nasal oxygen.

Long-term consequences of severe BPD

- Prolonged oxygen therapy and non-invasive or invasive respiratory support may be required for many months. May need to be provided at home.
- Feeding problems requiring prolonged nasogastric/gastrostomy feeding.
- Inguinal hernias (from raised intra-abdominal pressure and muscular weakness associated with suboptimal growth).
- Risk of RSV (respiratory syncytial virus) infection causing bronchiolitis (risk of hospitalization reduced by passive immunization with monoclonal antibody palivizumab).
- Rehospitalization because of respiratory infection.
- Increased risk of asthma and sleep-disordered breathing including obstructive sleep apnea.
- Increased risk of neurodevelopmental problems.
- Rarely, death from acute chest infection or cor pulmonale (pulmonary hypertension).

Strategies for prevention

These include:
- antenatal corticosteroids
- surfactant therapy
- minimizing exposure to mechanical ventilation
- non-invasive respiratory support (CPAP or high flow nasal therapy)
- avoidance of fluid overload
- closure of patent ductus arteriosus
- vitamin A (given in some centers)
- mesenchymal stem cells (via endotracheal tube) – encouraging results in initial therapeutic trials.

Question

What is the controversy about postnatal corticosteroid therapy?

In infants still requiring oxygen at several weeks of age, corticosteroid therapy was widely used as it dramatically reduces their oxygen requirement and allows weaning from mechanical ventilation. But high-dose corticosteroid therapy is associated with serious side-effects, especially if prolonged:
- short term – high blood pressure, hyperglycemia, increased risk of sepsis
- longer term – Cushingoid facies, hypertrophic cardiomyopathy, osteopenia, failure of growth in length and head circumference and increase in cerebral palsy.

As a result of the increased incidence of cerebral palsy and other side-effects, it is now used sparingly in ventilator-dependent infants, using only a low dose and as short a course as possible (see Fig. 26.1 showing reduction in use of postnatal corticosteroid therapy).

Survival in high-income countries of extremely preterm (<28 weeks) infants has increased dramatically, and many babies of 23–24 weeks of gestation now survive (Figs. 27.6 and 27.7). However, this increased survival has been achieved at the expense of high rates of neurodisability, although recent outcome data suggest that the neurodisability rates in early life are falling (Fig. 38.1).

The development of VLBW infants is monitored in a neonatal follow-up program (see Chapter 72) or in the community. Data from these programs can then be compared with other programs, but such comparisons may be misleading if based on an individual unit as the sample size will be small, with wide variations from year to year, and there may be differences in the demography of the mothers and referral patterns.

The most meaningful outcome data are regional or national, provided that the data collection is standardized and complete. A follow-up rate greater than 90% is desirable for all cohorts but difficult to achieve.

Growth

At discharge from hospital, over 90% of VLBW infants are below the 10th centile for weight, length and head circumference. Many show catch-up growth in the first 2–3 years, first of head circumference, then weight and then length. Growth is better if the infant is in good health. Catch-up growth may occur across childhood and adolescence, but may be less in infants with intrauterine growth restriction.

Medical complications

These include:
• bronchopulmonary dysplasia (BPD) – may require additional oxygen therapy for many months
• pneumonia/wheezing/asthma – more common with BPD
• bronchiolitis from RSV (respiratory syncytial virus) infection (hospitalization reduced by giving RSV monoclonal antibody, palivizumab)
• gastroesophageal reflux – especially with BPD

• complex nutritional and gastrointestinal disorders – following necrotizing enterocolitis or gastrointestinal surgery
• inguinal hernias – require surgical repair.

Rehospitalization rate is increased, mainly for respiratory disorders and surgical repair of inguinal hernias.

Disability and impairment

Neurodisability at 18 months to 2 years is usually classified (Table 38.1) as:
• severe – unable to walk, very low IQ, blind or profoundly deaf
• moderate – walk with support, IQ 55–70, hear with aids
• mild – less severe impairments, IQ 70–85.
Many studies combine the severe and moderate categories.

The risk of developing cerebral palsy rises steeply as gestational age falls (Fig. 38.2), but severe cerebral palsy with functional impairment has become relatively uncommon, comprising only 8% of babies at 23 weeks and 5–6% of babies at 24–25 weeks of gestation. 1–2% of extremely preterm infants have hearing impairment requiring amplification. 1% are blind in both eyes, but a much greater proportion have refraction errors requiring glasses and squints, probably related to resolved retinopathy of prematurity.

Cognitive impairment

By far the most common impairments following very preterm birth are learning difficulties, which become apparent when performance is compared with that of their peers at nursery, and become increasingly evident during school years (Fig. 38.3) The prevalence of cognitive impairment and of other associated difficulties increases with decreasing gestational age at birth (Fig. 38.4). In addition, children may have difficulties with:
• fine motor skills, e.g. threading beads
• concentration, with short attention span

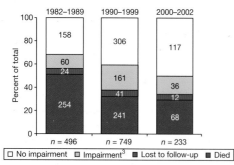

Fig. 38.1 Neurodevelopmental outcome for babies of <1000 g birthweight over 20 years in a tertiary perinatal center. The proportion with impairment has decreased. (Source: Wilson-Costello D. *et al. Pediatrics* 2007; **119**: 37–45.)

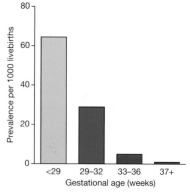

Fig. 38.2 Gestation-specific prevalence of cerebral palsy in 4 Child Register 1984–2003. (Data from Surman G. *et al. 4Child Annual Report 2009.* Oxford: National Perinatal Epidemiology Unit, 2009.)

Neonatology at a Glance, Third Edition. Edited by Tom Lissauer, Avroy A. Fanaroff, Lawrence Miall and Jonathan Fanaroff.
© 2016 John Wiley & Sons, Ltd. Published 2016 by John Wiley & Sons, Ltd.

Table 38.1 Definitions of disability for use at 18–24 months of corrected age in follow-up of very preterm infants. (Source: *Classification of Health Status at 2 Years as a Perinatal Outcome*. London: BAPM, 2008.)

	Severe neurodevelopmental disability	Moderate neurodevelopmental disability
Domain	**Any one of below:**	**Any one of below:**
Motor	Cerebral palsy with GMFCS level 3, 4 or 5	Cerebral palsy with GMFCS level 2
Cognitive function	Score <3 standard deviations below norm (DQ <55)	Score <2 standard deviations below norm (DQ 55–70)
Hearing	No useful hearing even with aids (profound >90 dBHL)	Hearing loss corrected with aids (usually moderate 40–70 dBHL) or Some hearing but loss not corrected by aids (usually severe 70–90 dBHL)
Speech and language	No meaningful words/signs or unable to comprehend cued sign	Some but fewer than 5 words or signs and able to comprehend cued sign
Vision	Blind or can only perceive light	Moderately reduced vision or blind in one eye
Other disabilities		
Respiratory	Requires continued respiratory support or oxygen	Limited exercise tolerance
Gastrointestinal	Requires PN, NG or PEG feeding	On special diet or has stoma
Renal	Requires dialysis or awaiting transplant	Renal impairment requiring treatment or special diet

GMFCS (Gross Motor Function Classification System): level 2 – walks with limitations; level 3 – walks using hand-held mobility device; level 4 – self-mobility with limitations, may use powered wheelchair; level 5 – manual wheelchair.
DQ, developmental quotient; PN, parenteral nutrition; NG, nasogastric; PEG, percutaneous endoscopic gastrostomy.

- abstract reasoning, e.g. mathematics
- processing several tasks simultaneously.

Deficits in working memory and processing of information seem to underpin many of the difficulties found at middle school age.

Behavioral outcomes

Children born very preterm have more behavioral difficulties than their term peers. Some have autism spectrum disorder. Although uncommon, a typical phenotype has been characterized with ADHD-I, where inattention rather than hyperactivity predominates, as well as anxiety and reduced social skills. The prevalence of behavioral difficulties is related to gestational age, as with learning outcomes; indeed, there is much comorbidity (Fig. 38.4).

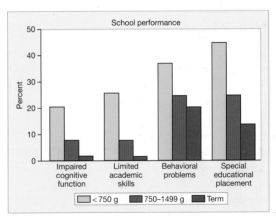

Fig. 38.4 Increased incidence of impaired cognitive function, academic skills, behavioral problems and special education placement in infants with birthweight below 750 g and 750–1499 g compared with term infants. (Adapted from Hack M. *et al.* School-age outcomes in children with birthweights under 750 g. *N Engl J Med* 1994; **331**: 753–759.)

School performance

Many very preterm children are either not ready to start school at the standard chronological age, or are kept back a year. At school age, problems with low IQ, poor executive function and behavior are evident in the need for special educational support. Around two-thirds of UK children born at <26 weeks of gestation have special needs at 11 years, including learning, behavior and physical support needs, and 13% require separate educational provision (Fig. 8.2).

Strategies to support the specific educational difficulties of very preterm infants are being developed.

There are also concerns about adult mental health outcomes following childhood behavioral disorders; this will be clarified by longitudinal studies which are now evaluating survivors into their fourth decade.

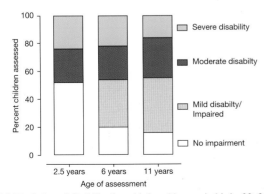

Fig. 38.3 Evolution of disability from birth to 11 years in births 22–25 weeks of gestation in the UK. About 55% have moderate or severe impairment at 11 years, after allowing for loss of children with severe disability from follow-up. (Source: Johnson S. *et al. Pediatrics* 2009; **124**: e249–e257.)

Overview

The clinical features of respiratory distress are shown in Fig. 39.1.

Monitoring
- Oxygen saturation (maintain >95% in term infants).
- Respiratory rate, heart rate, BP, temperature.
- Arterial blood gases if needing oxygen >30%.

Investigations
- Chest X-ray – confirms respiratory disease, look for pneumothorax, diaphragmatic hernia, lung malformations.
- Complete blood count, blood cultures, C-reactive protein, consider lumbar puncture.

Management
- Airway and breathing – oxygen/nasal high-flow therapy/CPAP/mechanical ventilation as required.
- Circulatory support if necessary.
- Intravenous fluids or frequent nasogastric feeds.
- Intravenous antibiotics – broad-spectrum coverage.

Respiratory distress:
Tachypnea (RR >60/min)
+
Nasal flaring
+
Grunting (prolonged expiration against closed glottis)
+
Chest retraction
– suprasternal
– intercostal
– subcostal
+
Cyanosis (if severe)

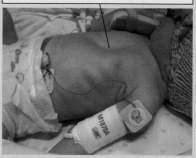

Fig. 39.1 Clinical features of respiratory distress (**see video: Signs of respiratory distress**).

Causes (Fig. 39.2)

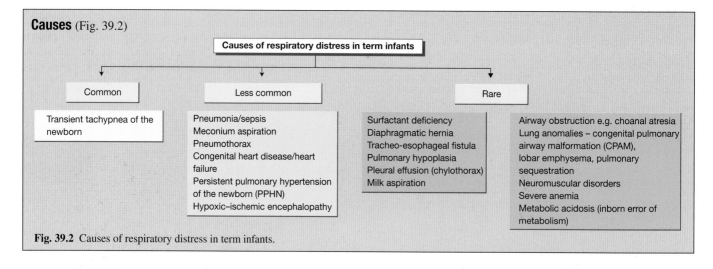

Causes of respiratory distress in term infants

Common

Transient tachypnea of the newborn

Less common

Pneumonia/sepsis
Meconium aspiration
Pneumothorax
Congenital heart disease/heart failure
Persistent pulmonary hypertension of the newborn (PPHN)
Hypoxic–ischemic encephalopathy

Surfactant deficiency
Diaphragmatic hernia
Tracheo-esophageal fistula
Pulmonary hypoplasia
Pleural effusion (chylothorax)
Milk aspiration

Rare

Airway obstruction e.g. choanal atresia
Lung anomalies – congenital pulmonary airway malformation (CPAM), lobar emphysema, pulmonary sequestration
Neuromuscular disorders
Severe anemia
Metabolic acidosis (inborn error of metabolism)

Fig. 39.2 Causes of respiratory distress in term infants.

Common causes

Transient tachypnea of the newborn (TTNB)

This is by far the most common cause of respiratory distress in term infants. Caused by delay in the absorption of lung liquid (Figs. 39.3 and 39.4), especially following elective cesarean section. Absence of pressure on the thorax squeezing lung liquid from the chest is thought to be a factor. However, clearance of fetal lung fluid is largely dependent on reabsorption of alveolar fluid via sodium channels in the lung epithelium, which is influenced by the level of circulating catecholamines. The lower concentration of circulating catecholamines, particularly following elective delivery, results in reduced absorption of lung liquid. Usually settles within first day or two of life, but may have low oxygen requirement and tachypnea for several days.

Neonatology at a Glance, Third Edition. Edited by Tom Lissauer, Avroy A. Fanaroff, Lawrence Miall and Jonathan Fanaroff.
© 2016 John Wiley & Sons, Ltd. Published 2016 by John Wiley & Sons, Ltd.

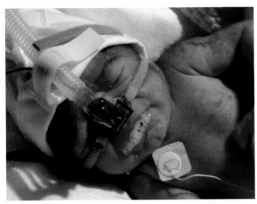

Fig. 39.3 Lung liquid in the mouth of a newborn term infant with transient tachypnea of the newborn receiving nasal CPAP.

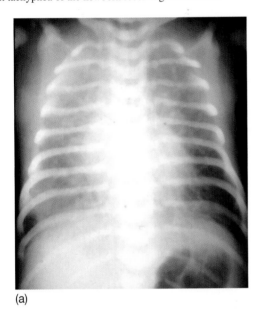

(a)

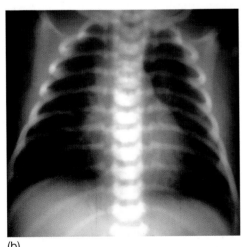

(b)

Fig. 39.4 Chest X-ray in transient tachypnea of the newborn showing fluid in the horizontal fissure and some streaky infiltrates with hyperinflation and perihilar haziness (a). Some hours later, the perihilar haziness has cleared, but there is still fluid in the horizontal fissure and hyperinflation (b).

Less common causes

Pneumonia

• Risk factors – prolonged rupture of the membranes (PROM), maternal fever, chorioamnionitis.
• All infants with respiratory distress should be started on broad-spectrum antibiotics until the results of the blood culture, C-reactive protein (CRP), complete blood count (CBC), lumbar puncture (if performed) are known.
• Group B streptococcus is the most common cause.

Meconium aspiration

The proportion of infants who pass meconium at birth increases with gestational age, affecting 20–25% at 42 weeks. Asphyxiated infants may start gasping and aspirate meconium before delivery. At birth infants may inhale thick meconium (see Chapter 13) which results in mechanical obstruction, chemical pneumonitis and inactivation of surfactant (Fig. 39.5). There is a high incidence of air leak (pneumothorax). Surfactant therapy may be beneficial. Mechanical ventilation is often required. Accompanying persistent pulmonary hypertension (PPHN) may require nitric oxide and sometimes ECMO (extracorporeal membrane oxygenation), i.e. cardiopulmonary bypass. Sildenafil may be considered.

Pneumothorax (see Chapter 29)

May occur spontaneously or more commonly as a complication of mechanical ventilation or CPAP. Diagnosed clinically, with unilateral decreased breath sounds or by transillumination of the chest (Fig. 39.6) or on chest X-ray.

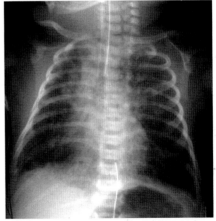

Fig. 39.5 Chest X-ray in meconium aspiration. There is hyperinflation of the lungs, flattened diaphragm and widespread patchy areas of collapse evident in coarse irregular densities with areas of overinflation. There is a tracheal tube and umbilical artery catheter. (Courtesy of Dr Sheila Berlin.)

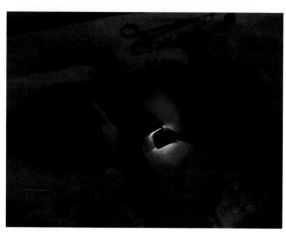

Fig. 39.6 Transillumination of the chest showing the presence of pneumothorax.

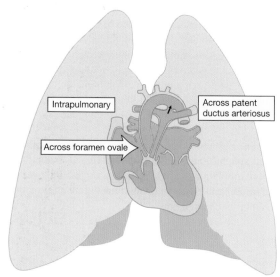

Fig. 39.7 Pulmonary hypertension leads to right-to-left shunting.

Heart failure (see Chapter 49)

Check for evidence of heart failure – including active precordium, enlarged heart, gallop rhythm, heart murmurs and enlarged liver. and that femoral pulses are palpable (reduced in coarctation of the aorta, hypoplastic left heart syndrome).

Persistent pulmonary hypertension of the newborn (PPHN)

Pulmonary hypertension leads to right-to-left shunting of blood (Fig. 39.7):

- across the patent foramen ovale
- across the patent ductus arteriosus
- intrapulmonary.

Causes

Usually secondary to:

- birth asphyxia
- meconium aspiration
- sepsis
- diaphragmatic hernia.

Occasionally it is the primary disorder.

Presentation

- Cyanosis or difficulty in oxygenation.
- Reduction between pre and post ductal saturations.

Specific investigations

- Chest X-ray – shows underlying cause or may be normal or show pulmonary oligemia (diminished vascularity).
- Echocardiography is needed to exclude congenital heart disease. It can also allow estimation of the magnitude of pulmonary hypertension (see Chapter 82).

Management

- Oxygen.
- Optimize mechanical ventilation.
- Circulatory support as required.
- Consider surfactant therapy.
- Pulmonary vasodilator – inhaled nitric oxide (NO). Oral or i.v. sildenafil may be considered.
- Consider high-frequency oscillatory ventilation (HFOV).
- Extracorporeal membrane oxygenation (ECMO) as rescue therapy for severe respiratory failure.

Rare causes

Surfactant deficiency

Rare in term infants. May occur in infants of maternal diabetes or with surfactant protein B deficiency, a rare genetic disorder.

Diaphragmatic hernia

Main problems

- Pulmonary hypoplasia, as herniated bowel reduces lung development in the fetus.
- Lung compression by the bowel, which increases in size as air enters it.
- Pulmonary hypertension (PPHN) – pulmonary arterioles reduced in number and size, and smooth muscle is hypertrophied.
- Other anomalies – present in 15–25%.

Incidence

1 in 4000 births.

Most common site

Left-sided hernia of bowel through the posterolateral foramen of the diaphragm (Bochdalek).

Presentation
- **Prenatal** – on ultrasound screening, polyhydramnios. Most identified antenatally. For antenatal management with fetal endoscopic tracheal occlusion see Chapter 4.
- **Resuscitation** – failure to respond; deteriorates with bag and mask ventilation.
- **Respiratory distress** – but onset may be delayed if underlying lung well developed.

Physical signs
- Respiratory distress.
- Asymmetry of chest.
- Reduced air entry on affected side.
- Apex beat displaced.
- Scaphoid abdomen – from reduced content of bowel.

Diagnosis
X-ray-chest and abdomen (Fig. 39.8).

Management
- Intubate and ventilate from birth. Gentle ventilation, allowing permissive hypercapnia, i.e. $PaCO_2 > 60\,mmHg$ ($8kPa$) but maintaining pH >7.25. Avoid mask ventilation.
- Pass large nasogastric tube and apply suction.
- Stabilize and support circulation.
- Early PN (parenteral nutrition).
- Surgical repair – delay until stable and PPHN is resolving.
- Nitric oxide for PPHN; sildenafil may be considered.
- Extracorporeal membrane oxygenation (ECMO) – pre- and post-surgery in selected cases.

Mortality
20–30%.

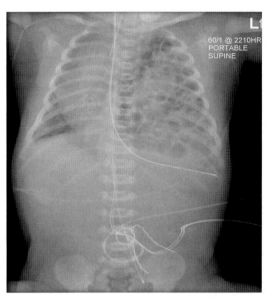

Fig. 39.8 Chest X-ray showing diaphragmatic hernia. There is bowel in the left chest and the heart and trachea are displaced to the right. There is a gavage (nasogastric) tube, umbilical artery and venous catheters and a radio-opaque umbilical tie.

Milk aspiration

Risk of aspiration if infant has cleft palate, neurologic disorder affecting sucking and swallowing or has respiratory distress. Infants with bronchopulmonary dysplasia often have gastroesophageal reflux, which predisposes to aspiration.

40 Upper airway disorders

Cleft lip and palate

Incidence – 1 in 1000 live births.
Inheritance – polygenic, but increased risk if family history.
Varies in severity from a mild unilateral cleft lip to severe bilateral cleft palate (Figs. 40.1 and 40.2).

It is increasingly diagnosed on antenatal ultrasound scanning. This allows counseling of the parents and family before birth. Showing parents photographs is often helpful to minimize the shock at birth as the defect is unsightly; photos after surgery provide reassurance that the defect can be corrected (Fig. 40.3).

A specialist multidisciplinary team from a tertiary center is required to provide:
• a key worker, usually a specialist nurse, for advice and to act as advocate for the child and family. Will visit the parents shortly after birth and also gives advice about feeding.
• craniofacial surgeon, orthodontist, speech and language therapist and audiologist.
• surgical repair of the lip, usually at 3 months of age for best long-term results, but some centers perform it immediately after birth. The palate is usually repaired at 6–12 months of age. Further surgery may be required when the child is older.

Long-term complications include middle ear infection and otitis media with effusion, difficulties with speech and orthodontic problems.

There are active self-help groups for parents who provide information and practical help. In the US there is Wide Smiles; in the UK it is CLAPA, the Cleft Lip and Palate Association.

Questions

Can babies with a cleft lip and palate breast-feed?
Yes, it is often possible, with expert assistance and encouragement.
What help with feeding can be provided for parents if their infant has a cleft lip and palate?
Special nipples (teats) are available and a dental plate may need to be made to occlude the cleft palate.

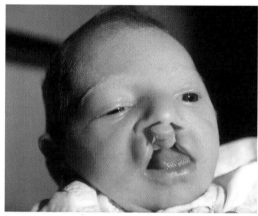

Fig. 40.2 Bilateral cleft lip and palate. The deformity looks very unsightly. Antenatal ultrasound diagnosis allows preparation before birth.

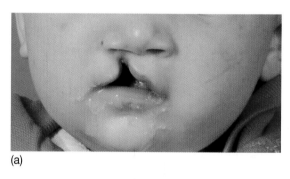
(a)

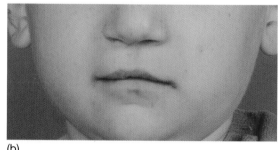
(b)

Fig. 40.3 Showing parents photographs (a) before and (b) after cleft lip surgery is reassuring. (Courtesy of Mr Alistair Smyth.)

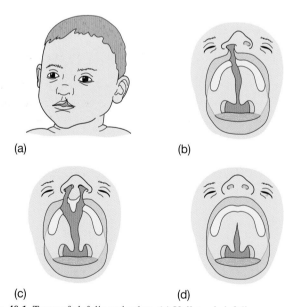

(a)

(b)

(c)

(d)

Fig. 40.1 Types of cleft lip and palate. (a) Unilateral cleft lip. (b) Unilateral cleft lip and palate. (c) Bilateral cleft lip and palate. (d) Cleft palate.

Neonatology at a Glance, Third Edition. Edited by Tom Lissauer, Avroy A. Fanaroff, Lawrence Miall and Jonathan Fanaroff.
© 2016 John Wiley & Sons, Ltd. Published 2016 by John Wiley & Sons, Ltd.

Choanal atresia

The condition

A rare bony obstruction between the nasal cavity and the naso-pharynx (Fig. 40.4).

Main problem

Bilateral lesions cause respiratory distress and cyanosis immediately after birth due to airways obstruction as newborn infants are obligatory nose breathers. The airway obstruction is relieved on crying or opening the mouth.

Treatment

- Initial – insert oral airway or tracheal tube.
- Definitive – surgical correction.

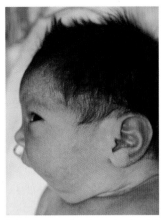

Fig. 40.5 Pierre Robin sequence showing micrognathia. (Courtesy of Dr David Clark.)

Pierre Robin sequence

This comprises (Fig. 40.5):
- micrognathia (small jaw)
- posteriorly displaced tongue
- posterior palatal defect
- increased incidence of other anomalies, especially of the heart.

Most serious complication is respiratory obstruction; may lead to hypoxia and cor pulmonale (pulmonary hypertension).

Management

- Avoid obstruction by the tongue:
  – nurse prone
  – may need CPAP (continuous positive airway pressure) via nasopharyngeal tube.
- Micrognathia and airway obstruction improve over the first 2 years.
- Surgery to the posterior palate is usually performed at about 1 year.
- Feeding can be problematic and initially gavage (nasogastric) feeding may be required.

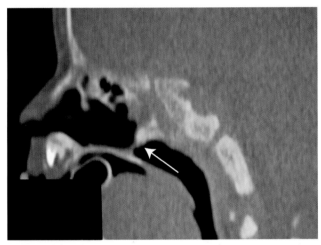

Fig. 40.4 Choanal atresia on MRI scan. There is a bony bar across the posterior nasal space (arrow).

41 Jaundice

Visible jaundice occurs in more than 80% of term and preterm infants during the first week. Bilirubin metabolism is shown in Fig. 41.1. Elevated bilirubin levels are due to:
- High hemoglobin (Hb) concentration at birth, so considerable heme degradation.
- A newborn's red blood cell lifespan in shorter than an adult's.
- Liver enzyme conjugation is reduced.
- Enterohepatic circulation is enhanced. This 'physiologic' jaundice peaks at 2–5 days and then usually clears by 14 days, but may persist for several weeks in breast-fed infants.

Significance of severe hyperbilirubinemia

Kernicterus describes bilirubin encephalopathy. In acute bilirubin encephalopathy there may be hyptonia, lethargy, poor feeding, irritability, high-pitched cry, fever, apnea, hypertonia with arching of

Question

What level of bilirubin is safe?

There is no single level of bilirubin that causes kernicterus, but in term infants it is extremely uncommon with bilirubin levels below 26 mg/dL (450 μmol/L). It may occur at lower levels if infants are preterm, or sepsis, hypoxia, seizures, acidosis or hypoalbuminemia are present.

the neck and trunk-opisthotonus (Fig. 41.2), seizures, coma and death. In chronic bilirubin encephalopathy there is permanent neurologic injury resulting from the deposition of unconjugated bilirubin in the basal ganglia and brainstem nuclei (Fig. 41.3). Long-term consequences include dental dysplasia with yellow staining of the teeth, high-frequency sensorineural hearing loss (auditory neuropathy), paralysis of upward gaze of the eyes, choreoathetoid cerebral palsy and learning difficulties. Kernicterus is rare in developed countries.

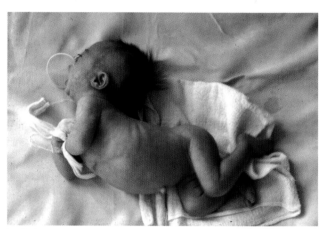

Fig. 41.2 Opisthotonus from kernicterus. This is now rarely seen in developed countries.

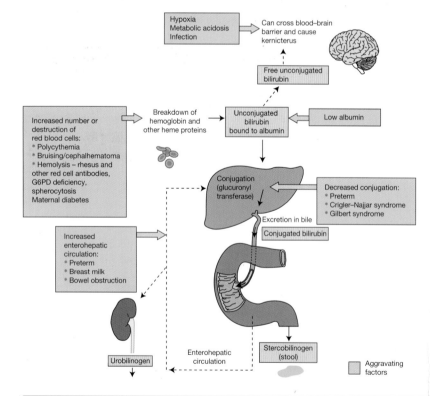

Fig. 41.1 Metabolism of bilirubin. Bilirubin is the product of the metabolism of hemoglobin and other heme proteins. The initial breakdown product is unconjugated bilirubin (indirect bilirubin), which is carried in the blood bound to albumin. When the albumin binding is saturated, free, unconjugated, lipid-soluble bilirubin can cross the blood–brain barrier. Unconjugated bilirubin bound to albumin is conjugated in the liver (direct bilirubin), which is excreted via the biliary tract into the gut. Some bilirubin is reabsorbed from the gut (enterohepatic circulation). Risk factors for jaundice are shown in green.

Neonatology at a Glance, Third Edition. Edited by Tom Lissauer, Avroy A. Fanaroff, Lawrence Miall and Jonathan Fanaroff.
© 2016 John Wiley & Sons, Ltd. Published 2016 by John Wiley & Sons, Ltd.

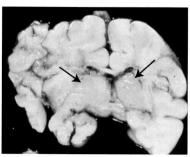

Fig. 41.3 Cross-section of the brain at autopsy showing yellow staining, predominantly in basal ganglia from deposition of unconjugated bilirubin.

Table 41.1 Causes of jaundice by age of onset.

<24 hours old	24 hours to 2 weeks old	Prolonged jaundice
Hemolytic:	Breast-feeding jaundice	Unconjugated:
• Rhesus disease	Hemolytic	• Breast milk
• ABO	Infection	jaundice
incompatibility	Bruising/	• Hypothyroidism
• Minor antigen	cephalhematoma	• Gastrointestinal
incompatibility	Gastrointestinal	obstruction
• G6PD deficiency	obstruction	• Sepsis
• Hereditary	Polycythemia	• Liver enzyme
spherocytosis	Metabolic disorders	defects
Congenital infection	Liver enzyme defects	Conjugated:
		• Neonatal hepatitis
		syndrome
		• Biliary atresia

Causes of early-onset jaundice (<24 hours) (Table 41.1)

Hemolysis

Jaundice within 24 hours of birth is most likely to be hemolytic. Bilirubin levels may rise rapidly.

Rhesus disease (see Chapter 5)

This is the most severe form of hemolytic disease with onset *in utero*. At birth, infants may have anemia, hydrops (edema), jaundice and hepatosplenomegaly. It is now uncommon because of anti-D prophylaxis (0–2/100 000 live births in developed countries but more common in resource-limited countries).

ABO incompatibility

• Mother's blood type O, infant's blood type A or B. Maternal anti-A or anti-B IgG crosses the placenta, causing hemolysis.
• Direct antibody test (DAT or Coombs test) is positive, but positive test is poor predictor of significant jaundice.
• Generally less severe than rhesus, but can still cause significant hemolysis and jaundice. Onset is after birth.
• Hemolysis may progress during the first few weeks of life, and requires monitoring for anemia.

Minor antigen Incompatibility (Kell, Duffy, Kidd, etc.)

• Infant's direct antibody test (DAT or Coombs test) is positive.
• Usually moderate hemolysis and jaundice.

G6PD (glucose-6-phosphate dehydrogenase) deficiency

This X-linked disorder is the most common enzyme defect in the world, affecting 200–400 million people. It affects males, but females can have a mild form, especially if they also have Gilbert syndrome (liver enzyme defect). It can cause severe jaundice and kernicterus in people originating from central Africa, the Mediterranean or Middle or Far East. It is diagnosed by measuring G6PD activity in red blood cells. However, during hemolytic crises this may be misleadingly elevated owing to the increased reticulo-cytes, which have a higher enzyme concentration. A repeat assay is required to avoid missing the diagnosis. Affected infants should avoid certain medications, i.e. some antimalarials and antibiotics, contact with mothballs (naphthalene) and eating fava (broad) beans when older.

Hereditary spherocytosis

Red blood cells are spherical with limited deformability, causing splenic sequestration and hemolysis. Autosomal dominant inheritance – family history positive in 75%. Uncommon.

Congenital infection

Increases hemolysis and may impair conjugation, causing elevated conjugated bilirubin. Other stigmata of congenital infection will be present.

Causes of jaundice 24 hours to 2 weeks

Breast-feeding jaundice

Common. Exacerbated if there is difficulty in establishing breast-feeding. Cause uncertain; may be related to low volume of breast milk and increased enterohepatic circulation of bilirubin. Breast-feeding should be continued but support may be needed. Continues beyond 2 weeks of age in up to 15% of breast fed infants.

Infection

Always consider infection, including urinary tract infection. Jaundice occurs because of hemolysis, impaired conjugation, reduced fluid intake and increased enterohepatic circulation.

Other causes

These include:
• hemolysis – may develop after first 24 hours of life
• bruising, cephalhematoma
• polycythemia
• liver enzyme defects, e.g. Crigler–Najjar syndrome, Gilbert syndrome
• gastrointestinal obstruction, e.g. pyloric stenosis
• metabolic disorders, e.g. galactosemia.

Clinical examination and assessment

Jaundice is clinically detectable from skin color on blanching the skin with digital pressure or yellow color of the sclerae when bilirubin exceeds 5 mg/dL (85 μmol/L).

It starts on the head, spreads to the abdomen and then to the limbs. It is harder to detect in preterm and dark-skinned infants. The severity of jaundice cannot be reliably assessed by clinical examination. However, an infant who is not jaundiced clinically is unlikely to have significant hyperbilirubinemia.

If jaundiced, also check for:
- pallor
- evidence of infection
- bruising, cephalhematoma
- hepatosplenomegaly (hemolysis)
- weight loss, dehydration
- family history of neonatal jaundice.

Investigations

Term infants who become jaundiced should have a transcutaneous bilirubin (TcB) measured. However, a serum measurement should be obtained if:
- the infant is <24 hours old
- transcutaneous bilirubinometer measurement >13 mg/dL (230 μmol/L) (>14.5 mg/dL, 250 μmol/L in the UK)
- transcutaneous bilirubinometer (TcB) not available
- infant ≤34 weeks' gestational age
- on phototherapy treatment.

Further tests, other than total bilirubin, that may be required (but in most infants no pathologic cause is found)

- direct (conjugated) bilirubin
- complete blood count, reticulocyte count and smear for red cell morphology
- blood packed cell volume or hematocrit
- blood group (mother and baby)
- direct antibody test (DAT or Coombs test)
- G6PD testing
- microbiological cultures of blood, urine and/or cerebrospinal fluid for infection.

Management

The need for treatment is determined by plotting the total bilirubin level on a gestation-specific graph of bilirubin against age. This will determine whether:
- no treatment is needed
- bilirubin should be repeated in 6–12 hours
- to start phototherapy
- to perform exchange transfusion.

Treatment will change according to the absolute level of bilirubin reached and the rate of rise on serial measurements (start if bilirubin rising at >0.5 mg/dL/h, 8.5 μmol/L/h). The evidence for treatment thresholds is very limited but national guidelines assist uniformity of practice (see American Academy of Pediatrics in US – Table 41.2; NICE guidelines in the UK). Different cut-off criteria are used for preterm infants, for whom the treatment threshold is lower (NICE guidelines include graphs for different gestational ages – see Appendix).

If an exchange transfusion is being considered, a low serum albumin may be an additional risk factor for kernicterus.

Other treatment to be considered:
- Ensure baby is well hydrated.
- Sepsis – requires investigation and treatment.

Phototherapy

Conventional phototherapy units use a blue–green light (wavelength 425–475 nm) above the baby, which converts unconjugated bilirubin to harmless isomers. If the bilirubin is rising rapidly or does not fall after 6 hours of treatment, then add in multiple units, ideally with one source underneath the infant. Phototherapy is most effective when there is an effective light source (LED lights), high irradiance (usually ≥30 μW/cm²/nm), the light is as close to the infant as possible (if LED lights are used, can be as close as 10 cm from the infant) with maximum skin exposure.

Disadvantages of phototherapy:
- Separates baby and parents.
- Eyes need to be covered.
- Bronze-baby syndrome if phototherapy given with elevated conjugated bilirubin.
- Unstable temperature while in open crib (cot) with majority of skin exposed.
- Increased insensible water loss (less with modern LED light sources).
- Slightly loose, more frequent stools.

Exchange transfusion

Baby's blood is removed in aliquots (usually twice blood volume, 'double volume exchange' = 2 × 90 mL/kg) and replaced with transfused blood (see Chapter 78). Removes bilirubin and hemolytic antibodies and corrects anemia. Complications include thrombosis, embolus, volume overload or depletion, metabolic abnormalities, infection, coagulation abnormalities and death (<1%).

Intravenous immunoglobulin (IVIG)

Can be used in rhesus disease or ABO incompatibility when total bilirubin levels are rising despite continuous multiple phototherapy to try to prevent the need for exchange transfusion.

Discharge and follow-up

In view of the re-emergence of kernicterus in otherwise healthy infants, particularly at 35–37 weeks' gestation, the American Academy of Pediatrics (2004) recommends predischarge measurement of bilirubin and/or assessment of clinical risk

Table 41.2 Indications for phototherapy and exchange transfusion in infants ≥35 weeks' gestation. (Adapted from American Academy of Pediatrics Subcommittee on Hyperbilirubinemia. Management of hyperbilirubinemia in the newborn infant 35 or more weeks of gestation. *Pediatrics* 2004; **114**: 297–316.)

Age (hours)	Phototherapy			Exchange transfusion		
	Higher risk	Medium risk	Lower risk	Higher risk	Medium risk	Lower risk
24	>8 mg/dL (137 μmol/L)	>10 mg/dL (171 μmol/L)	>12 mg/dL (205 μmol/L)	>15 mg/dL (257 μmol/L)	>17 mg/dL (291 μmol/L)	>19 mg/dL (325 μmol/L)
48	>11 mg/dL (188 μmol/L)	>13 mg/dL (222 μmol/L)	>15 mg/dL (257 μmol/L)	>17 mg/dL (291 μmol/L)	>19 mg/dL (325 μmol/L)	>22 mg/dL (376 μmol/L)
72	>13 mg/dL (222 μmol/L)	>15 mg/dL (257 μmol/L)	>18 mg/dL (308 μmol/L)	>18 mg/dL (308 μmol/L)	>21 mg/dL (359 μmol/L)	>24 mg/dL (410 μmol/L)
96	>14 mg/dL (239 μmol/L)	>17 mg/dL (291 μmol/L)	>20 mg/dL (342 μmol/L)	>19 mg/dL (325 μmol/L)	>22 mg/dL (376 μmol/L)	>25 mg/dL (428 μmol/L)

Lower risk: ≥38 weeks and well. Medium risk: ≥38 weeks and risk factor listed below or 35–37 weeks and well. Higher risk: 35–37 weeks and risk factor listed below.

Risk factors: isoimmune hemolytic disease, G6PD deficiency, asphyxia, significant lethargy, temperature instability, sepsis, acidosis or albumin <3.0 g/dL (30 g/L) if measured.

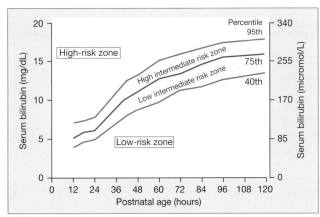

Fig. 41.4 Nomogram for determination of risk of development of severe hyperbilirubinemia for infants ≥35 weeks' gestation and ≥2.5 kg birthweight. (From Bhutani V.K. *et al.* Predictive ability of a predischarge hour-specific serum bilirubin for subsequent significant bilirubinemia in healthy term and near-term newborns. *Pediatrics* 1999; **103**: 6–14.)

factors for the development of jaundice for all infants. The risk of developing significant hyperbilirubinemia in healthy term and near-term newborns can be determined by plotting the bilirubin level on an hour-specific chart (Fig. 41.4). It also recommends a follow-up assessment for jaundice depending on their length of stay in the nursery:
- discharge at <24 hours, follow-up by 72 hours of life
- discharge at 24–48 hours, follow-up by 96 hours of life
- discharge at 48–72 hours, follow-up by 120 hours of life.

Earlier assessment may be needed if risk factors are present.

In the UK, the recommendation is further assessment by 48 hours of age if risk factors are present (gestational age <38 weeks, a previous sibling had neonatal jaundice requiring phototherapy, breast-fed, visible jaundice in the first 24 hours of life), otherwise by 72 hours of age.

Parents should also be given written and verbal information about jaundice.

Prolonged jaundice (>14 days)

Jaundice present at more than 2 weeks of age for term or 3 weeks for preterm infants can be considered prolonged jaundice and requires further assessment. First, it needs to be determined if the jaundice is unconjugated or conjugated.

Unconjugated jaundice
Causes are:
- breast milk jaundice – due to increased enteric reabsoption; can last for several months
- hypothyroidism – usually identified on newborn blood spot screening
- gastrointestinal obstruction, e.g. pyloric stenosis
- sepsis
- liver enzyme disorders.

Conjugated jaundice (direct bilirubin >1.5 mg/dL, 25 μmol/L)

The infant will pass pale, clay-colored stools (no stercobilinogen) and dark urine (from bilirubin).
Caused by:
- biliary atresia – uncommon, but important to identify as delay in surgery adversely affects outcome
- neonatal hepatitis syndrome.

Detailed investigation of infants with conjugated jaundice is required.

This is a common and serious problem in the neonatal period, affecting 1–5/1000 live births (Fig. 42.1). The highest incidence is in very low birthweight (VLBW) infants (see Chapter 34). Congenital infections are considered in Chapter 11.

Key point

Infection needs to be considered in all sick newborn infants. If suspected, a blood culture and other investigations should be performed and antibiotics and supportive therapy started immediately as it may progress and disseminate very rapidly.

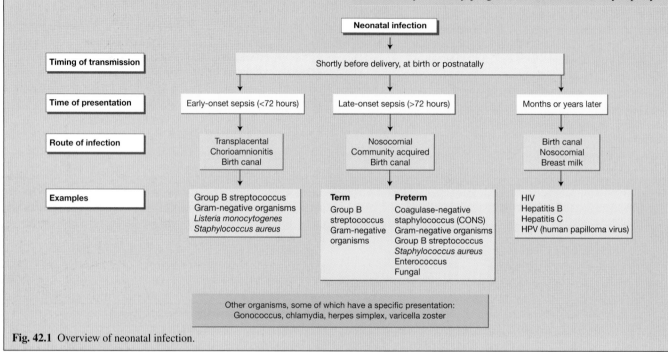

Fig. 42.1 Overview of neonatal infection.

Bacterial sepsis

Newborn infants are particularly susceptible to bacterial sepsis (clinical features of systemic infection with positive bacterial blood culture).

Early-onset sepsis (EOS): <72 hours of birth

Results from vertical exposure to high bacterial load during birth and few protective antibodies.

Late-onset sepsis (LOS): >72 hours after birth

Within the hospital, mostly from organisms acquired by nosocomial transmission from person to person. May also be caused by community-acquired organisms.

Risk factors

Early-onset infection

- Preterm.
- Prolonged rupture of membranes (>18 hours).
- Maternal fever in labor (>38 °C).
- Chorioamnionitis.
- Maternal colonization with Group B streptococcus (GBS).
- Previous infant with invasive GBS disease.

Late-onset nosocomial infection

- Preterm.
- Indwelling venous or arterial catheters or tracheal tube.
- Prolonged antibiotics, parenteral nutrition, gastric acid suppression therapy.
- Damage to skin from tape, skin probes, etc.

Clinical presentation

- Usually non-specific deterioration.
- Apnea and bradycardia.
- Respiratory distress/increased ventilatory requirements.
- Slow feeding/vomiting/abdominal distension.
- Fever/hypothermia/temperature instability.
- Tachycardia/collapse/shock.

Neonatology at a Glance, Third Edition. Edited by Tom Lissauer, Avroy A. Fanaroff, Lawrence Miall and Jonathan Fanaroff.
© 2016 John Wiley & Sons, Ltd. Published 2016 by John Wiley & Sons, Ltd.

- Purpura or bruising from disseminated intravascular coagulation (DIC).
- Irritability/lethargy/seizures.
- Jaundice.
- Rash.
- Reduced limb movement in bone or joint.
- In meningitis (late signs):
  - tense or bulging fontanel
  - head retraction (opisthotonus).
- On monitoring:
  - hypo/hyperglycemia
  - neutropenia, neutrophilia, left shift, i.e. increase in immature neutrophils, thrombocytopenia
  - acute phase reactants – raised C-reactive protein (CRP) or procalcitonin.
  - thrombocytopenia, coagulopathy

Investigations

Sepsis work-up:
- complete blood count (CBC), differential, platelets
- C-reactive protein/procalcitonin
- blood culture
- urine – microscopy and culture for LOS
- cerebrospinal fluid (CSF), if indicated
- chest X-ray, if indicated
- sites of infection – consider needle aspirate or biopsy for Gram stain and direct microscopy
- tracheal aspirate if ventilated.
  Consider:
- placental tissue culture and histopathology
- rapid antigen screen
- blood gases
- coagulation screen.

Question

When should a lumbar puncture (LP) be performed?
  If blood culture is positive.
  If there are clinical features of meningitis.
  Consider whenever performing sepsis work-up, but delay if infant clinically unstable.

Interpretation of laboratory investigations

Blood cultures:

- Gold standard but may be negative if insufficient volume of blood or maternal treatment with intrapartum antibiotics.
- If central line sepsis suspected, also take blood sample from it.

Blood count – infection is suggested by:

- neutropenia or neutrophilia
- increased ratio of immature (bands): total neutrophils
- thrombocytopenia.

C-reactive protein/procalcitonin

- Raised in infection (12 hours after onset); also following meconium aspiration, asphyxia, post-surgery.
- Takes time to rise – may be normal initially.

CSF – in meningitis:

- More than 30/mm^3 white blood cells (30×10^9/L); but more than 20/mm^3 white blood cells (20×10^9/L) and more than 5/mm^3 (5×10^9/L) neutrophils is suspicious of meningitis.
- Protein – term infants >200 mg/dL (>2 g/L).
- Glucose – less than 30% of blood glucose.
- May be able to observe group B streptococci on Gram stain even without any white cells present.

Treatment

- Supportive care – **A**irway, **B**reathing, **C**irculation. Check blood glucose.
- Treat with antibiotics immediately on suspicion of sepsis, immediately after taking cultures but whilst awaiting results.
- Antibiotic choice depends on local incidence and practice.

Early-onset sepsis
Cover Gram-positive and Gram-negative organisms.
  For example:
- penicillin/ampicillin + aminoglycoside (e.g. gentamicin/tobramycin).

Late-onset sepsis
Need to also cover coagulase-negative staphylococcus and enterococcus.
  For example:
- nafcillin/flucloxacillin + gentamicin
- or cephalosporin, e.g. ceftazidime/gentamicin + vancomycin.
  If central venous catheter in place, remove it if unresponsive to antibiotics, persistent positive culture, Gram-negative organisms cultured or seriously ill.

Questions

How long should antibiotics be continued?
  If blood cultures are negative and CRP/procalcitonin remains normal and no clinical signs of sepsis – stop antibiotics at 36–48 hours.
  If blood cultures negative but CRP/procalcitonin significantly raised – treat as infected.
  If blood cultures are positive – treat until clinical improvement and CRP has returned to normal (7–10 days, longer if Gram-negative or *Staphylococcus aureus* infection).
  Meningitis – 14–21 days.
  Septic arthritis/osteomyelitis – 6 weeks.

What supportive strategies are being evaluated?
  Early studies suggest that specific IgG- and IgM-enriched immunoglobulin may be of benefit.

43 Specific bacterial infections

Group B streptococcal (GBS) infection

This is the leading cause of bacterial sepsis in term infants.
- Early-onset infection usually presents with respiratory distress and septicemia; more than 90% present in first 24 hours.
- Late-onset infection – higher proportion with meningitis; also causes focal infection in bones or joints.

It is a serious disease, with 4% mortality. Before active prevention, the incidence in the US was approximately 1.5/1000 live births for early-onset disease, 0.35/1000 for late-onset disease, causing a total of 7600 cases of invasive disease per year, with 300 deaths. Now, the early-onset infection rate has declined to 0.35/1000 live births.

Up to 30% of pregnant women have rectal or vaginal carriage of group B streptococcus.

The 2010 CDC (Centers for Disease Control and Prevention) guideline recommends active prevention by culturing all mothers at 35–37 weeks and offering intrapartum prophylactic antibiotics to those who are positive for group B streptococcus (Fig. 43.1). However, the efficacy of this practice has not been demonstrated in a systematic review of well-designed clinical trials. Most infected infants are now preterm or born to unscreened mothers.

Question

What is the GBS policy in the UK?

In the UK the incidence of early-onset GBS is about 0.5/1000 live births and routine culturing of mothers is not recommended (UK National Screening Committee, 2012). Their recommendation is that intrapartum antibiotics:
- should be offered if previous baby with GBS infection
- should be considered if preterm labor, prolonged rupture of membranes (PROM) >18 hours, or fever in labor >38 °C.

Listeria monocytogenes

- Rare. From maternal ingestion of unpasteurized milk, soft cheeses and undercooked poultry.
- Mother develops flu-like symptoms. Fetal infection acquired transplacentally or from birth canal.
- Causes abortion, preterm delivery. Green staining of liquor before term has been claimed to be characteristic.
- Early-onset infection – usually with pneumonia, septicemia and widespread rash. Mortality 30%.
- Late-onset infection – mostly with meningitis.

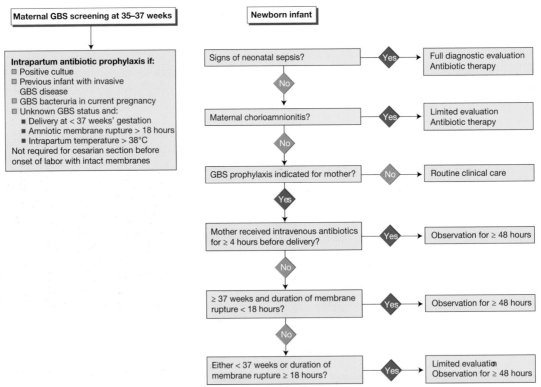

Fig. 43.1 Group B streptococcal (GBS) prophylaxis guidelines in the US. Full diagnostic evaluation: blood culture, complete blood count (CBC) including white blood cell differential and platelet count, chest radiograph (if respiratory distress) and lumbar puncture (if stable and sepsis suspected). Limited evaluation: blood culture (at birth) and CBC with differential and platelets (at birth and/or at 6–12 hours of life). (Based on revised CDC guidelines, 2010.)

Neonatology at a Glance, Third Edition. Edited by Tom Lissauer, Avroy A. Fanaroff, Lawrence Miall and Jonathan Fanaroff.
© 2016 John Wiley & Sons, Ltd. Published 2016 by John Wiley & Sons, Ltd.

Some specific sites of bacterial infection (Fig. 43.2)

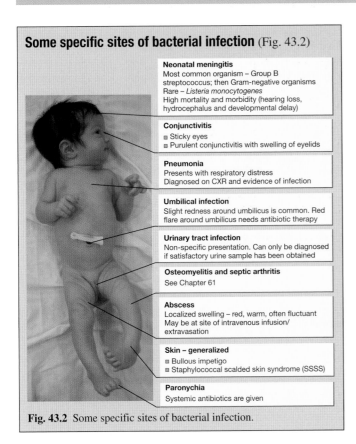

Neonatal meningitis
Most common organism – Group B streptococcus; then Gram-negative organisms
Rare – *Listeria monocytogenes*
High mortality and morbidity (hearing loss, hydrocephalus and developmental delay)

Conjunctivitis
▫ Sticky eyes
▫ Purulent conjunctivitis with swelling of eyelids

Pneumonia
Presents with respiratory distress
Diagnosed on CXR and evidence of infection

Umbilical infection
Slight redness around umbilicus is common. Red flare around umbilicus needs antibiotic therapy

Urinary tract infection
Non-specific presentation. Can only be diagnosed if satisfactory urine sample has been obtained

Osteomyelitis and septic arthritis
See Chapter 61

Abscess
Localized swelling – red, warm, often fluctuant
May be at site of intravenous infusion/extravasation

Skin – generalized
▫ Bullous impetigo
▫ Staphylococcal scalded skin syndrome (SSSS)

Paronychia
Systemic antibiotics are given

Fig. 43.2 Some specific sites of bacterial infection.

Gram-negative infection

- Less common than group B streptococcal infection.
- Presents as early- or late-onset infection.
- Significant morbidity and mortality.

Conjunctivitis

Sticky but white eyes

Common, 3rd–5th day of life. Clean with sterile water. If eye becomes red, may be staphylococcal or streptococcal infection so treat with a topical antibiotic ointment, e.g. neomycin. If persistent sticky eye but conjunctiva is white and uninflamed then usually due to obstruction of the nasolacrimal duct.

Purulent conjunctivitis with swelling of eyelids (Fig. 43.3)

If onset within 48 hours of birth, likely to be gonococcal (ophthalmia neonatorum). The discharge should be Gram-stained and cultured, and systemic treatment started immediately. Where penicillin resistance is common, as in the US and UK, a third-generation cephalosporin is given. The eye is cleaned frequently.

In the US all infants are given eye prophylaxis with erythromycin eye ointment. In the UK no prophylaxis is given, but the condition is rare.

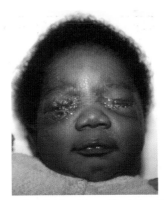

Fig. 43.3 Purulent conjunctivitis with swelling of eyelids at 6 days from *Chlamydia trachomatis*.

Chlamydia trachomatis can cause a similar condition, usually at the end of the first week; may coexist with gonococcal infection. The diagnosis is made with a monoclonal antibody test or culture of the discharge. Treatment is with oral erythromycin. No topical treatment required. These conditions must be treated promptly to avoid damage to the eye. The mother and her partner also need treatment.

Herpes simplex must also be considered with this presentation.

Skin

Bullous impetigo

Superficial blisters, readily burst, leaving denuded skin (Fig. 43.4) with crust formation.

Staphylococcus aureus or streptococcal. Give systemic antibiotics to prevent spread. Remove crusts with warm water. Identify and treat source. Usually from nasal colonization. The condition needs to be differentiated from transient pustular melanosis, which is benign (see Chapter 21).

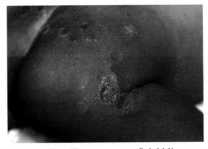

Fig. 43.4 Bullous impetigo. There are superficial blisters; some have been denuded.

Staphylococcal scalded skin syndrome (SSSS)

- Rare but serious infection. Toxin mediated.
- Fever.
- Bullae with shedding of skin leaving raw areas.
- Requires systemic antibiotics.
- Congenital candida may resemble SSSS.

44 Viral infections

Herpes simplex virus (HSV)

Infection in the newborn is rare; the incidence in the US is only 5–33/100000 live births; in the UK about 2/100000 live births. Most (85%) are HSV type II in US, but in UK a relatively higher proportion are HSV type I, associated with increased genital HSV type I infection. Seroconversion rate in pregnancy is 4%.

At any time in pregnancy, 1% of HSV-2 seropositive women are excreting virus in genital tract.

Most infections (85%) are acquired by passage through an infected birth canal, 10% are acquired postnatally from infected caregiver, and 5% are true intrauterine infections.

Risk of vertical transmission

• High (50–60%) with primary maternal infection, which is usually asymptomatic but is rarely symptomatic, with fever, systemic illness and painful genital lesions. Risk of transmission is increased if membranes have ruptured for more than 6 hours or following birth canal interventions, e.g. scalp electrode. However, in 70% of infected neonates maternal infection is undiagnosed.
• Low (2%) with recurrent maternal infection, which is often asymptomatic or genital lesions are localized.

Potential interventions to reduce transmission of symptomatic primary infection are:
• delivery by cesarean section
• maternal aciclovir (acyclovir) therapy for primary infection.
• Reduced use of invasive obstetric procedures (mechanically assisted deliveries, fetal scalp electrodes) during delivery.

Neonatal infection

There are three modes of presentation:
• **Disseminated infection** – presents at 10–12 days with pneumonia, hepatic failure, DIC (disseminated intravascular coagulation). Two-thirds develop encephalitis.
• **Encephalitis** – presents in second week. Lethargy is a prominent clinical feature, as well as focal or generalized seizures and coma
• **Localized lesions** – skin, eye or mouth – presents with vesicles at 10–11 days. One-third progress to encephalitis.

Rarely there may be congenital infection – presents at birth with triad of eye, skin and neurologic signs.

Diagnosis

Difficult, as maternal infection often undiagnosed and vesicles are present in only 60–80% of disseminated disease or encephalitis.

Rapid diagnosis with PCR (polymerase chain reaction) of infant's blood, CSF (cerebrospinal fluid), nasopharyngeal aspirates or local lesions.

Management

Infected infant:
• Intensive care support if required.

• High-dose intravenous aciclovir (acyclovir) therapy for 3 weeks. Suppressive oral treatment is subsequently given for 6–12 months to prevent relapse.
• In spite of treatment, morbidity, mortality and risk of relapse remain high.

Maternal HSV lesions at delivery:
– History of genital herpes before pregnancy:
• Low transmission risk. Surface viral cultures and blood DNA PCR at 24 hours (delay to avoid contamination from maternal secretions). Observe. Only treat if positive results or clinical features.
– No history of genital herpes before pregnancy:
• May be high transmission risk. Investigations as above, but include CSF PCR. Start intravenous aciclovir (acyclovir).

Hepatitis B (HBV)

• Highest incidence in the Far East and sub-Saharan Africa (Fig. 44.1). Increased risk with intravenous drug use.
• Screening of all mothers for HBsAg (hepatitis B surface antigen) is universal in the US and UK.
• HBV is transmitted from mother to infant during labor or at birth from ingestion of maternal blood and from breast milk. Also horizontal spread within families during childhood can occur.
• Infants are at high risk if their mother is hepatitis B e-antigen positive (HBeAg positive) or has high HBV viral load; the risk is markedly reduced if e-antibodies are present.
• Infants who become infected are usually asymptomatic during childhood, but 30–50% develop chronic HBV liver disease, which in 10% progresses to cirrhosis. There is also a long-term risk of hepatocellular carcinoma.

Prevention

All infants born to HBsAg-positive mothers should be given HBV vaccination as soon as possible after birth with boosters during infancy. In the US this is part of the standard immunization program; in the UK it is restricted to these high-risk infants.

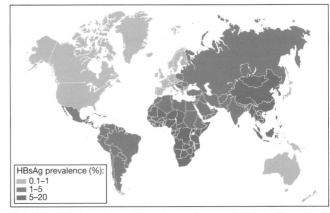

HBsAg prevalence (%):
◻ 0.1–1
◼ 1–5
◼ 5–20

Fig. 44.1 Global overview of prevalence of maternal HbsAg (hepatitis B surface antigen).

Neonatology at a Glance, Third Edition. Edited by Tom Lissauer, Avroy A. Fanaroff, Lawrence Miall and Jonathan Fanaroff.
© 2016 John Wiley & Sons, Ltd. Published 2016 by John Wiley & Sons, Ltd.

In the US, HBIG (hepatitis B immunoglobulin) for short-term protection from passive antibody is given within 12 hours of birth to infants of HBsAg-positive mothers or, for infants <2 kg, when maternal HepB status is unknown; in the UK it is confined to infants of mothers who are HBeAg-positive.

Immunization protects more than 90% of infants. There is no contraindication to breast-feeding when the infant is immunized.

Hepatitis C

Vertical transmission is uncommon and almost exclusively in women with high Hep C viral load in late pregnancy (<5%) unless there is co-infection with HIV (when it is 10–20%). Although viral DNA is present in breast milk, transmission via breast milk has not been proven, so breast-feeding is not contraindicated. Carriers are at risk of chronic liver disease and hepatocellular carcinoma in later life.

HIV

The global prevalence of HIV infection in children is shown in Fig. 44.2 and the annual incidence in children is shown in Fig. 44.3.

Main route of vertical transmission is at birth, but also transplacental and via breast-feeding.

Vertical transmission rate where mothers breast-feed and without any intervention is 25–40%.

Factors which increase transmission

- Advanced maternal disease.
- High maternal plasma viral load.
- Primary infection during pregnancy or breast-feeding.
- Concomitant sexually transmitted infections.
- Rupture of the membranes longer than 4 hours.
- Chorioamnionitis.
- Vaginal delivery with a detectable viral load.
- Blood exposure/instrumental delivery.

Interventions that reduce transmission

- Combination antiretroviral therapy is given to the mother to fully suppress plasma viral load antenatally and during delivery.
- Treat other maternal sexually transmitted infections to reduce birth canal transmission.
- Elective cesarean section with avoidance of labor and contact with the birth canal if the mother still has detectable viral load. Mothers with fully suppressed plasma viral load may have a vaginal delivery.
- Post-exposure prophylaxis (PEP) antiretroviral therapy to the infant for 4 weeks. Where the mother has a fully suppressed viral load monotherapy may be used, but if the mother has detectable viral load the infant should receive triple antiretroviral therapy for 4 weeks.
- In a resource-rich setting, mothers are advised to formula feed the infant to reduce all risk of postnatal infection.
- These interventions can reduce transmission rate below 0.5%.
- Refer to national guidelines for details of treatment of infants.
- In a resource-poor setting, mothers may breast-feed exclusively if they are on combination antiretroviral therapy with fully suppressed plasma viral load. If not, the baby should continue on daily post-exposure antiretroviral therapy during the entire period of breast-feeding. See Chapter 73 for further details.

Diagnosis

A first test for evidence of *in utero* infection is undertaken at birth. Confirmation that the infant is uninfected then relies on at least two further negative tests for the viral genome (DNA/RNA PCR) after cessation of PEP, or in the breast-feeding infant after cessation of breast-feeding. The HIV antibody test cannot be used until 18 months as maternal antibody is still present.

Management

Infants at high risk of infection (i.e. those born to mothers with significant viral load) should receive cotrimoxazole as prophylaxis against *Pneumocystis jiroveci (carinii)* pneumonia (PCP) from 4 weeks of age until negative HIV results are available.

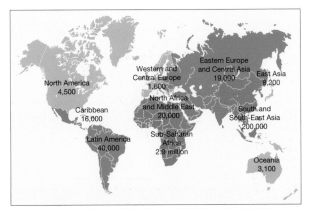

Total: 3.3 million children living with HIV infection in 2012

Fig. 44.2 Number of children <15 years old living with HIV infection in 2012. (UNAIDS, WHO, 2013.)

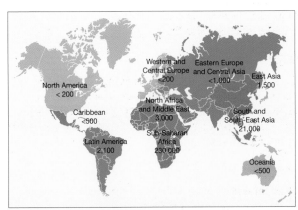

Total: 260 000 newly infected children in 2012

Fig. 44.3 Estimated number of newly HIV-infected children <15 years old during 2012. Most are in sub-Saharan Africa. (UNAIDS, WHO, 2013.)

45 Hypoglycemia and hyperglycemia

Hypoglycemia

Prolonged symptomatic hypoglycemia can cause neurologic damage. However, during the first few days of life many breastfed infants have low blood glucose levels but are asymptomatic; they are able to utilize ketones and other energy substrates. Therefore, the definition of hypoglycemia in the neonatal period has been the source of considerable controversy.

A serum glucose level of less than 45 mg/dL (<2.6 mmol/L) during the first days of life is currently accepted as a useful cut-off to establish the diagnosis of hypoglycemia and to initiate active evaluation and treatment (Fig. 45.1). Normal newborn infants require 4–5 mg/kg/min (0.22–0.28 mmol/kg/min) of glucose in order to maintain glucose homeostasis.

Risk factors

Maternal
- Maternal diabetes mellitus (Fig. 45.2) and obesity.
- Large or rapid infusions of glucose immediately before delivery.
- Maternal β-adrenergic agonist or antagonist therapy.

Neonatal
- IUGR (intrauterine growth restriction (Fig. 45.3).
- Small for gestational age (birthweight <10th centile)
- Large for gestational age (birthweight >90th centile).
- Preterm.
- Ill infant – sepsis, etc.
- Iatrogenic – reduced feeds with inadequate intravenous glucose.
- Polycythemia.
- Hypoxic–ischemic encephalopathy (HIE).
- Hypothermia.
- Rhesus disease.

Causes

Risk factors for transient hypoglycemia are listed above. Persistent hypoglycemia is uncommon; its causes are shown in Fig. 45.4.

Clinical features

Most are asymptomatic. Clinical features include:
- jitteriness/irritability/high-pitched cry
- depressed consciousness/lethargy/hypotonia
- apnea
- seizures.

Some abnormal physical signs may assist in identifying the cause (Table 45.1).

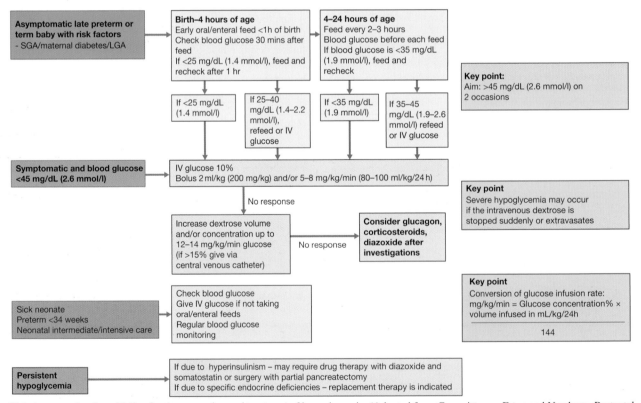

Fig. 45.1 An example of a guideline for the prevention and treatment of hypoglycemia. (Adapted from Committee on Fetus and Newborn. Postnatal blood glucose homeostasis in late-preterm and term infants. *Pediatrics* 2011; **127**: 575–579.)

Neonatology at a Glance, Third Edition. Edited by Tom Lissauer, Avroy A. Fanaroff, Lawrence Miall and Jonathan Fanaroff.
© 2016 John Wiley & Sons, Ltd. Published 2016 by John Wiley & Sons, Ltd.

Monitoring

Infants with risk factors should be fed regularly and frequently (at least every 3h) and their blood glucose monitored until it is above 45 mg/dL (>2.6 mmol/L) on two occasions (Fig. 45.1). Blood glucose should not be monitored in appropriately grown term infants establishing breast-feeding. All infants requiring intermediate or intensive care should have their blood glucose monitored.

Blood glucose determination should be performed at the bedside with a glucometer and hypoglycemia confirmed by the laboratory as bedside monitors are not designed to measure low glucose levels accurately.

Investigation

These are performed for persistent or symptomatic hypoglycemia.

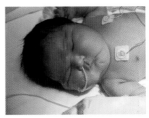

Fig. 45.2 Macrosomic infant of mother with diabetes mellitus. Maternal hyperglycemia causes β-cell hyperplasia of pancreas and hyperinsulinism in the fetus that lasts for up to 48 hours after birth.

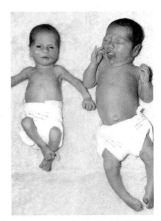

Fig. 45.3 Term twins, the one on the left with IUGR (intrauterine growth restriction). IUGR newborn infants are prone to hypoglycemia.

Blood tests
- Plasma glucose concentration – true (laboratory) measurement.
- Serum insulin concentration.
  If no features of hyperinsulinism (e.g. excessive glucose requirements to prevent hypoglycaemia), check:
- pituitary hormones
- for inborn error of metabolism and acylcarnitine (see Chapter 46).

Other investigations that may be indicated
- Ultrasound of brain and/or MRI – for structural anomaly.
- Ultrasound adrenals – for adrenal hemorrhage.
- Ophthalmologic examination – for septo-optic dysplasia.

Management

Prevention and treatment of hypoglycemia are shown in Fig. 45.1.

Hyperglycemia

No agreed definition, but >125–180 mg/dL (>7–10 mmol/L) on two occasions. Frequent in extremely preterm infants.
  Often associated with:
- higher than required rate of IV glucose infusion (>9 mg/kg/min) from dextrose infusion or parenteral nutrition
- sepsis (often associated with fungal infections)
- corticosteroid therapy (high doses) or cortisol response to stress
- insufficient insulin secretion – neonatal diabetes (rare).
  Management – check infusion rates, then treat cause or administer insulin therapy (but avoid hypoglycemia).

Table 45.1 Clinical features associated with specific causes of persistent hypoglycemia.

Clinical feature	Cause
Hepatomegaly with or without splenomegaly	Glycogen storage disease, infection
Hepatomegaly, large tongue, omphalocele, horizontal ear lobe crease	Beckwith–Wiedemann syndrome
Micropenis, hypoplastic optic disk	Panhypopituitarism
	Need to rule out midline brain defects, e.g. septo-optic dysplasia
Lethargy, coma, vomiting, unusual body odor	Hyperammonemia, lactic acidosis, urea cycle disorders or other inborn error of metabolism

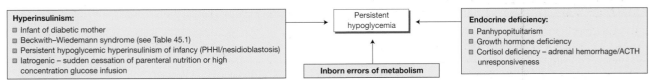

Fig. 45.4 Causes of persistent hypoglycemia.

Hyperinsulinism:
- Infant of diabetic mother
- Beckwith–Wiedemann syndrome (see Table 45.1)
- Persistent hypoglycemic hyperinsulinism of infancy (PHHI/nesidioblastosis)
- Iatrogenic – sudden cessation of parenteral nutrition or high concentration glucose infusion

Persistent hypoglycemia

Inborn errors of metabolism

Endocrine deficiency:
- Panhypopituitarism
- Growth hormone deficiency
- Cortisol deficiency – adrenal hemorrhage/ACTH unresponsiveness

46 Inborn errors of metabolism

Inborn errors of metabolism are individually rare (Table 46.1) but almost 100 may present in the neonatal period (Table 46.2). Delay in diagnosis can result in irreversible neurologic sequelae or death. In the US, tandem mass spectrometry on blood screening spots is used to identify a wide range of disorders; in the UK, metabolic screening is currently limited to phenylketonuria (PKU), medium-chain acyl-CoA dehydrogenase deficiency (MCAD), maple syrup urine disease (MSUD), isovaleric aciduria (IVA), glutaric aciduria type I (GA1) and homocystinuria (HCU).

Age of presentation

Inborn errors can present at any age to adulthood, including *in utero* as hydrops fetalis. Presentation is often non-specific with a wide differential diagnosis (see below). A characteristic presentation is with acute deterioration or sudden death in the first 3–7 days of life when a previously well term infant who is feeding accumulates toxic metabolites of intermediary metabolism that were previously removed by the placenta. However, feeding is not an obligatory trigger, except for galactosemia.

Table 46.1 Examples of inborn errors of metabolism that may present in the neonatal period with incidence.

Amino acid disorders	Urea cycle – ornithine transcarbamylase
	Maple syrup urine disease (MSUD)
Carbohydrate disorders	Galactosemia
	Glycogen storage disease
Organic acidemias	Propionic acidemia (PA)
	Methylmalonic acidemia (MMA)
Fatty acid oxidation defects	LCAD (long-chain acyl-CoA dehydrogenase deficiency)
	MCAD (medium-chain acyl-CoA dehydrogenase deficiency)
Energy defects	Lactic acidosis (LA)

Table 46.2 Incidence of some inborn errors of metabolism.

Disorder	Incidence
Phenylketonuria	1 in 10 000–20 000
Homocystinuria	1 in 200 000–335 000
Galactosemia	1 in 30 000–60 000
Maple syrup urine disease	1 in 185 000
If screened with tandem mass spectrometry:	
Amino acid disorders	1 in 4800
Fatty acid oxidation defects	1 in 14 000
Organic acid disorders	1 in 20 000

When to suspect an inborn error of metabolism

Clinical features

- Neurologic:
  - poor feeding, vomiting
  - apnea, tachypnea (secondary to central respiratory stimulation by hyperammonemia or acidosis)
  - irritability, progressive lethargy, hypotonia, seizures, encephalopathy, coma.
- Acid–base abnormality:
  - persistent, unexplained metabolic acidosis or lactic acidosis
  - respiratory alkalosis secondary to hyperammonemia
  - respiratory distress (from metabolic acidosis).
- Hypoglycemia – severe and persistent.
- Acute liver disease:
  - conjugated hyperbilirubinemia, coagulopathy, hepatomegaly or hepatosplenomegaly.
- Cardiac disease:
  - cardiac failure or arrest from arrhythmias or cardiomyopathy.
- Dysmorphic features.
- Failure to gain weight.
- Abnormal body or urine odor.

Suggestive clues

- Positive family history.
- Parental consanguinity.
- Sibling or family members with unexplained severe illness, recurrent miscarriages or neonatal death.
- Maternal fatty liver of pregnancy (in fetal fatty acid oxidation defects).
- Sudden onset of symptoms in previously well term infant.
- Progressive deterioration or death despite supportive treatment.

Differential diagnosis

- Sepsis – ill with non-specific features.
- Congenital heart disease – heart failure, low oxygen saturation.
- CNS disease – seizures, encephalopathy, infection (herpes simplex virus), intracranial hemorrhage, non-accidental injury.
- Gastrointestinal – vomiting from obstruction, liver disease.
- Endocrine – hyperinsulinism, hypopituitarism, adrenal insufficiency.
- Hypoxic–ischemic encephalopathy (HIE) – seizures and encephalopathy.

Management

- Early intervention (Table 46.5) is imperative to prevent neurologic sequelae or death. Families will need genetic counseling, which may include screening siblings.

Neonatology at a Glance, Third Edition. Edited by Tom Lissauer, Avroy A. Fanaroff, Lawrence Miall and Jonathan Fanaroff.
© 2016 John Wiley & Sons, Ltd. Published 2016 by John Wiley & Sons, Ltd.

Investigations (Tables 46.3 and 46.4, Fig. 46.1)

Table 46.3 First-line investigations when inborn error of metabolism is suspected.

Investigation	Abnormality	Possible disorder
Blood gas	Metabolic acidosis	Organic acidemia, disorders of carbohydrate metabolism, mitochondrial disorder
	Respiratory alkalosis (due to hyperammonemia)	Urea cycle disorder
Glucose	Hypoglycemia with ketosis	Organic acidemias; glycogen storage
	Hypoglycemia without ketosis	Fatty acid oxidation, hyperinsulinism
Ammonia	Hyperammonemia (Fig. 46.1)	See Fig 46.1
Lactate	High	Respiratory chain defects, pyruvate dehydrogenase deficiency, pyruvate carboxylase deficiency, hypoxia
Blood urea nitrogen (urea)	Low	Urea cycle
Electrolytes	Raised anion gap	Lactic acidosis, organic acidemia
Liver transaminases	High	Tyrosinemia, galactosemia
Complete blood count	Neutropenia Thrombocytopenia	Organic acidemias
Coagulation	Prolonged	Liver disease, galactosemia, tyrosinemia
Urine	Abnormal odor	Organic acidemia, PKU, MSUD
Urine reducing substances	Negative for glucose	Galactosemia
Urine ketones	Positive	Organic acidemias including MSUD
	Low/negative	Fatty acid oxidation disorders

(MSUD – maple syrup urine disease, PKU – phenylketonuria.)

Table 46.4 Second-line investigations, guided by clinical picture and discussion with specialist.

Urine organic acids
Urine amino acids
Plasma uric acid
Plasma amino acids
Plasma carnitine and acylcarnitine
Biotinidase
Galactosemia screening tests
CSF glucose and lactate (paired with venous samples done pre-lumbar puncture) and amino acids, neurotransmitters
Blood for mutation analysis or enzyme assay
Biopsies: e.g. enzyme assay on skin fibroblasts or blood cells, DNA mutation analysis, metabolite assays, mitochondrial studies and histochemistry on muscle or liver biopsy.

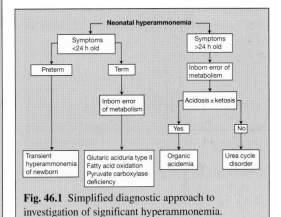

Fig. 46.1 Simplified diagnostic approach to investigation of significant hyperammonemia.

Table 46.5 Approach to management.

Basic support	Cardiorespiratory support, treat sepsis, anticonvulsants as required
Nutrition	Stop protein-containing feeds
	Stop galactose-containing feed if galactosemia possible.
	Avoid catabolism – give intravenous dextrose (minimum 10%) to ensure normoglycemia
	Consider insulin to control blood glucose and to promote anabolism, rather than reduce glucose intake
	Consider use of vitamin therapies, Table 46.6
Fluids	Consider bicarbonate to correct acidosis
Toxin removal	Ammonia scavenging medications (sodium benzoate, sodium phenylbutyrate or carglumic acid)
	Substrate support with arginine and/or carnitine
	Consider hemodialysis or hemodiafiltration

Table 46.6 Examples of vitamins used to treat IEM.

Carnitine
Pyridoxine and pyridoxal phosphate for seizure control
Vitamin B_{12}
Biotin (for biotinidase deficiency)
Hydroxycobalamin (for vitamin B_{12}-responsive methylmalonic acid)
Riboflavin (for glutaric aciduria type II)
Thiamin for pyruvate dehydrogenase deficiency
Also coenzyme Q for respiratory chain support, sodium benzoate, biopterin

Key point

If an inborn error of metabolism is suspected, consult a specialized center for advice on management.

Key point

Measure ammonia in any patient with unexplained lethargy or altered conscious level.

47 Gastrointestinal disorders

Vomiting

This is the forceful return of gastric contents through the mouth or nose. In contrast to regurgitation or possetting, the effortless return of small quantities of milk, which is very common during the first few months of life.

The significance of the vomiting will depend on:
- infant's age
- frequency, amount and characteristics of vomiting, e.g. if projectile
- presence of bile or blood (Fig. 47.1)
- abdominal distension (Fig. 47.2)
- stool characteristics – delayed passage of meconium or absent transitional stools
- presence of dehydration, weight loss
- evidence of a systemic illness – poor feeding, fever, lethargy.

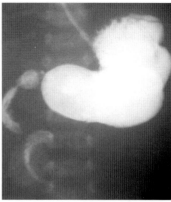

Fig. 47.1 This infant presented with blood-stained vomiting at 12 hours of age. Water-soluble contrast upper gastrointestinal study demonstrates coiled corkscrew appearance of second and third parts of duodenum due to midgut volvulus from malrotation. (Courtesy of Dr Annemarie Jeanes.)

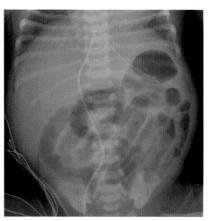

Fig. 47.2 Abdominal X-ray showing distended loops of bowel in an infant with persistent vomiting.

Causes

Physiologic:
- Gastroesophageal reflux
- Ingestion of maternal blood
- Overfeeding
- Incorrectly positioned nasogastric tube

Infection:
- Systemic – septicemia, urinary tract infection, meningitis
- Local – gastroenteritis

Mechanical/surgical:
- Intestinal obstruction – see Chapter 48
- Paralytic ileus – sepsis, electrolyte disturbance
- Necrotizing enterocolitis – see Chapter 36

CNS:
- Raised intracranial pressure – cerebral edema, intracranial or subdural bleed, hydrocephalus
- Kernicterus

Drugs:
- Side-effects – caffeine, theophylline, antibiotics
- Withdrawal (abstinence) – heroin, methadone

Cow's milk protein intolerance

Inborn errors of metabolism (rare)

Endocrine:
- Congenital adrenal hyperplasia (rare)

Diagnostic clues

Bile-stained vomiting (yellow–green)
Causes:
- Intestinal obstruction – distal to ampulla of Vater.
- Necrotizing enterocolitis.
- Incorrectly positioned nasogastric tube.
- Feeding intolerance in extreme preterm infants establishing feeds (common and presence of bile not significant unless there is abdominal distension or features of necrotizing enterocolitis).

Vomiting with abdominal distension
Causes:
- Intestinal obstruction (Fig. 47.3).
- Paralytic ileus – sepsis, electrolyte disturbance.
- Necrotizing enterocolitis.

Blood-stained vomiting
Flecks of fresh blood or dark-brown coffee grounds not uncommon in otherwise well infants and usually resolve spontaneously.

Key point

Bile-stained vomiting in term infants should always be regarded as intestinal obstruction until proven otherwise.

Neonatology at a Glance, Third Edition. Edited by Tom Lissauer, Avroy A. Fanaroff, Lawrence Miall and Jonathan Fanaroff.
© 2016 John Wiley & Sons, Ltd. Published 2016 by John Wiley & Sons, Ltd.

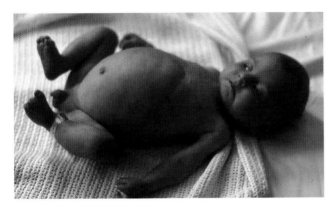

Fig. 47.3 Abdominal distension from Hirschsprung disease.

Causes:
• Swallowed maternal blood – from delivery or cracked nipple. Can be differentiated from fetal blood with the Apt test (see Table 47.1).
• Trauma – laryngoscopy at resuscitation, passing a nasogastric tube.
• Malrotation – uncommon but important to diagnose early (Fig. 47.2).
• Stress ulcer – hypoxic–ischemic encephalopathy.
• Abnormal coagulation–thrombocytopenia, vitamin K deficient bleeding, liver disease, DIC (disseminated intravascular coagulation), etc.
• Drug-induced – corticosteroids, indomethacin, ibuprofen.

Investigations

Most infants will require no or limited investigations. Those to be considered are listed in Table 47.1.

Management

Depends upon severity and cause. Intravenous fluids may be required to correct electrolyte disturbances, acid–base imbalance and dehydration.

Gastroesophageal reflux

Incidence is increased in:
• preterm infants, particularly with bronchopulmonary dysplasia or on caffeine
• following necrotizing enterocolitis and tracheoesophageal fistula repair
• infants with neurodevelopmental delay, e.g. following hypoxic–ischemic encephalopathy or hypotonia.

Associated features

• Failure to thrive.
• Irritability, arching of the back from esophagitis.
• Anemia (iron deficiency).
• Aspiration pneumonia.
• Apnea.
• Acute life-threatening events (ALTE).

Investigations

• Usually clinical diagnosis.
• Esophageal pH study, impedance study may show non-acid reflux, sometimes upper gastrointestinal contrast or endoscopy.

Management

Most do not need treatment. If required, use stepwise approach.
• Reduce interval between feeds, thicken feeds, alginate/antacid (Gaviscon), upright positioning.
• Prokinetic e.g. domperidone, but concerns about arrhythmias.
• H_2 receptor antagonist, e.g. ranitidine; proton pump inhibitors, e.g. omeprazole – reduce gastric acidity.
• Surgery – fundoplication with or without gastrostomy.
• Evidence of efficacy of medication in neonates is limited.

Table 47.1 Vomiting – investigations to consider and their purpose.

Imaging	Blood tests	Urine and stool tests
Plain abdominal X-ray: • intestinal obstruction – distended loops of bowel, bowel perforation • NEC (necrotizing enterocolitis) Ultrasound scans: • cranial for hemorrhage, ventricular dilatation • abdominal for pyloric stenosis, intra-abdominal fluid collections and cysts. Contrast X-rays: • malrotation, strictures • site of intestinal obstruction	Electrolytes and acid-base – for imbalance Sepsis work-up – to exclude infection Creatinine/blood urea nitrogen (urea) – for dehydration and renal function Glucose – for hypoglycemia Calcium, magnesium, phosphorus, liver function tests Coagulation screen – if blood in vomit or sepsis Consider: • 17-hydroxyprogesterone – for congenital adrenal hyperplasia • blood ammonia – for urea cycle abnormalities • drug screen – for drug overdose or withdrawal	Urine – microscopy and culture Stool – for blood Other: • Apt test of vomit/stool – to differentiate between maternal and fetal blood. Fetal hemoglobin is alkali-resistant (remains pink on addition of sodium hydroxide)

Esophageal atresia

- More than 85% associated with tracheoesophageal fistula (Fig. 47.4).
- 1 in 3500 live births.
- Often associated with other abnormalities, e.g. VACTERL syndrome (**v**ertebral **a**nomalies, **a**nal atresia, **c**ardiac, **t**racheo**e**sophageal, **r**enal, **l**imb).

Presentation

- Prenatal – polyhydramnios, absent stomach bubble, associated abnormalities.
- Birth onwards – frothing of oral secretions (Fig. 47.5) with choking and cyanosis.

Investigations

- Unable to pass wide-bore orogastric tube; confirmed on chest X-ray, shows tube curled in esophageal pouch. Air in the stomach indicates a distal fistula is present.

Management

- Pass large orogastric tube and aspirate pouch to avoid aspiration pneumonia.
- Intravenous fluids for resuscitation and maintenance. Early PN (parenteral nutrition).
- Surgical correction is required.

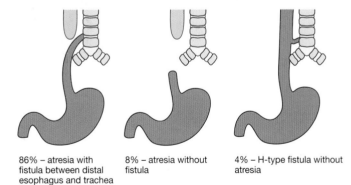

86% – atresia with fistula between distal esophagus and trachea

8% – atresia without fistula

4% – H-type fistula without atresia

Fig. 47.4 Different types of esophageal atresia and tracheoesophageal fistula.

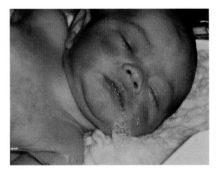

Fig. 47.5 Frothing of oral secretions after birth from esophageal atresia.

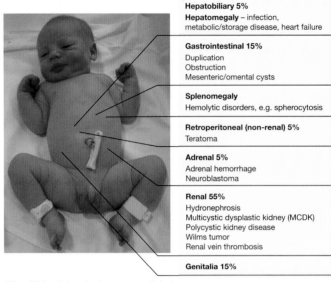

Hepatobiliary 5%
Hepatomegaly – infection, metabolic/storage disease, heart failure

Gastrointestinal 15%
Duplication
Obstruction
Mesenteric/omental cysts

Splenomegaly
Hemolytic disorders, e.g. spherocytosis

Retroperitoneal (non-renal) 5%
Teratoma

Adrenal 5%
Adrenal hemorrhage
Neuroblastoma

Renal 55%
Hydronephrosis
Multicystic dysplastic kidney (MCDK)
Polycystic kidney disease
Wilms tumor
Renal vein thrombosis

Genitalia 15%

Fig. 47.6 Abdominal masses and their causes.

Abdominal masses

Often detected *in utero* on ultrasound screening. The causes are shown in Fig. 47.6.

Abdominal wall defects

Omphalocele (Exomphalos)

Defect in umbilicus with herniation of abdominal contents. The bowel is covered by peritoneum and amnion (Fig. 47.7). Vary in size, from small defects where some bowel herniates into the umbilical cord to large defects where there is herniation of both bowel and liver. Occurs in 1 in 5000 fetuses. Most are diagnosed on prenatal ultrasound screening (see Fig. 3.2); 40% are associated with trisomy 13 or 18, Beckwith–Wiedemann (see Chapter 45) or other syndromes.

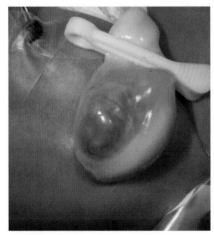

Fig. 47.7 Omphalocele.

Management (see video: Gastroschisis)

• Pass a large-caliber nasogastric tube at delivery to limit passage of air into the bowel, and nothing by mouth.
• Place infant's lower body into a sterile plastic wrap (bag) to limit heat and fluid loss and protect the bowel from damage and infection.
• Give intravenous fluids.
• Check for other anomalies, including echocardiography.
• Surgical repair is usually performed on the first day of life. If the defect is large, the viscera may be placed in a silastic silo, and gradually placed in the abdomen over several days.

Gastroschisis

Defect in anterior abdominal wall, usually to right of umbilicus, with herniation of the bowel (Fig. 47.8). In contrast to omphalocele, there is no protective covering of the bowel and the incidence of associated anomalies is low, other than intestinal atresia. The condition is usually diagnosed on prenatal ultrasound screening (Fig. 47.9).

Management

• The infant's lower body is placed into a sterile plastic wrap (bag or cling film).
• Pass a large-caliber nasogastric tube at delivery to limit passage of air into the bowel.
• Give intravenous fluids; colloid may be required to replace fluid losses from the exposed bowel. Closely monitor electrolytes. Give broad-spectrum antibiotics.
• Surgical repair can be performed directly or the abdominal contents can be gradually reduced after placing into a silo (Fig. 47.10).
• Prolonged parenteral nutrition is usually required to establish feeds. Prognosis is good.

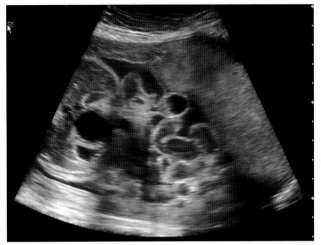

Fig. 47.9 Gastroschisis on prenatal ultrasound scan. (Courtesy of Dr David Lissauer.)

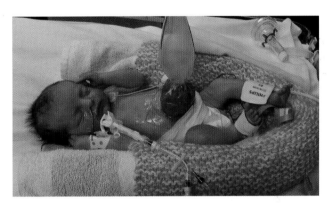

Fig. 47.10 Gastroschisis in silastic silo. There is also a central venous catheter for PN.

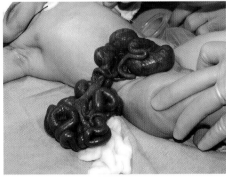

Fig. 47.8 Gastroschisis.

Imperforate anus

• Incidence 1 in 5000 births. Associated anomalies of genitourinary and gastrointestinal tract common, and seen in VACTERL association.
• In boys most often with fistula to urethra, in girls to vestibule adjacent to vagina-so may still pass meconium. Some lesions are complex.
• Surgery is with anoplasty or colostomy followed by repair.

48 Gastrointestinal obstruction

Most of the conditions causing gastrointestinal obstructions are serious but their prognosis has improved with advances in medical, anesthetic and surgical care. They are relatively uncommon but are important to recognize because:
• failure or delay in diagnosis may result in electrolyte imbalance, dehydration and shock
• malrotation with midgut volvulus is a surgical emergency in order to avoid bowel necrosis.

Causes – see Fig. 48.1

Diagnostic clues

Prenatal:
• **Polyhydramnios** – from obstruction to the passage of amniotic fluid through the gastrointestinal tract.
• **Abnormal ultrasound** – dilated bowel, hyperechoic bowel, ascites, calcified lesions. May be difficult to diagnose.
• **Fetus with trisomy 21 (Down syndrome)** – 30% have associated duodenal atresia.
• **Family history of cystic fibrosis** – associated with meconium ileus.
Delivery room:
• **Bubbly oral secretions** – esophageal atresia.
• **Peri-umbilical abdominal wall discoloration** – *in utero* bowel perforation.

Clinical presentation

• Vomiting – usually bile (yellow-green) stained. Bile is present if the obstruction is distal to ampulla of Vater. Presents within 24–48 hours of birth with high gastrointestinal lesions, may be delayed for several days for lower lesions. Hematemesis (blood-stained vomit) may occur with malrotation.
• Feeding intolerance.

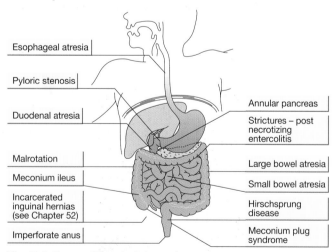

Esophageal atresia
Pyloric stenosis
Duodenal atresia
Malrotation
Meconium ileus
Incarcerated inguinal hernias (see Chapter 52)
Imperforate anus
Annular pancreas
Strictures – post necrotizing enterocolitis
Large bowel atresia
Small bowel atresia
Hirschsprung disease
Meconium plug syndrome

Fig. 48.1 Causes of intestinal obstruction.

• Abdomen – distension with visible loops of bowel or peristalsis, erythema/edema of abdominal wall, abdominal mass, peritonitis and shock.
• Failure to pass meconium within 48 hours of birth.
• Blood in stool (fresh or altered).

Diagnosis

Abdominal X-ray:
• Bowel obstruction – distended loops of bowel with air-fluid levels, with absence of gas distally (see Fig. 47.2).
• Bowel perforation – free air under diaphragm, intrahepatic or around falciform ligament.

Management

• Abdominal decompression with nasal or orogastric tube. In esophageal atresia, aspirate pouch to avoid aspiration pneumonia.
• Intravenous fluids for resuscitation and maintenance. Early parenteral nutrition (PN).
• Antibiotics preoperatively.
• Evaluate and correct bleeding diathesis.
• Surgical intervention for most lesions.
• Evaluate for other anomalies. Karyotype and microarray analysis may be necessary.

Some specific conditions

Esophageal atresia (Chapter 47)

Pyloric stenosis

Hypertrophy of circular smooth muscle of pylorus of stomach.
• **Presentation** – projectile vomiting in a hungry infant at 4–8 weeks of age. Occurs at same age in preterm infants.
• **Examination** – visible peristalsis. A firm, olive-like mass is palpable in right upper abdomen during feeds.
• **Investigation** – abdominal ultrasound – hypertrophy of pylorus.
• **Management** – correct electrolyte imbalance (hypochloremic hypokalemic alkalosis). Surgery-muscle incision (pyloromyotomy).

Duodenal atresia

• **Lesion** – obstruction may be due to atresia, webs, stenosis or fibrous cord.
• **Incidence** – 1 in 7500 births. Check for trisomy 21 and other anomalies.
• **Antenatal** – polyhydramnios, distended fluid-filled stomach on ultrasound.
• **Presentation** – vomiting – bilious or non-bilious, upper abdominal distension and feeding intolerance.
• **Diagnosis** – double bubble on X-ray (Fig. 48.2). May be accentuated by injecting 20 mL of air through gastric tube.

Neonatology at a Glance, Third Edition. Edited by Tom Lissauer, Avroy A. Fanaroff, Lawrence Miall and Jonathan Fanaroff.
© 2016 John Wiley & Sons, Ltd. Published 2016 by John Wiley & Sons, Ltd.

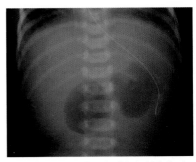

Fig. 48.2 Abdominal X-ray showing double bubble in duodenal atresia. (Courtesy of Dr Sheila Berlin.)

Malrotation

Failure of the developing bowel to undergo the normal counter-clockwise rotation during the 4th to 10th weeks of embryogenesis. Peritoneal bands (which normally attach the bowel to the central body axis posteriorly and are also known as Ladd bands) compress the duodenum, partially obstructing it. Because the mesentery is not fixed, malrotation predisposes to midgut volvulus (twisting of a loop of bowel around its mesenteric attachment). In addition to intestinal obstruction, compression of the superior mesenteric artery leads to ischemia of the small bowel.

Presentation

Sudden bilious vomiting is malrotation until proven otherwise. Usually in first few weeks of life but can occur at any age. With acute volvulus also abdominal distension and tenderness followed by shock. Hematemesis may occur.

Investigation

Doppler ultrasound of mesenteric vessels may be helpful at the bedside. Upper gastrointestinal exam (contrast swallow) is diagnostic. The normal position of the duodenal-jejunal junction (Treitz angle) is to the left of the spine. Any other position indicates malrotation. Volvulus classically appears as a spiral corkscrew of the duodenum (see Fig. 47.1).

Management

Volvulus is a surgical emergency. Ischemia can lead to small bowel infarction requiring bowel resection. Extensive resection of the small bowel carries a poor prognosis.

To relieve the obstruction, the peritoneal bands around the duodenum are divided. Appendectomy is also performed to avoid future confusion if the child has abdominal pain.

Meconium ileus

• Small bowel obstruction from inspissated, putty-like, sticky meconium.
• Affects 10–15% of patients with cystic fibrosis, whereas 95% of infants with meconium ileus have cystic fibrosis.

Presentation

Bilious vomiting, failure to pass meconium, abdominal distension, abdominal mass. Edema of abdominal wall suggests peritonitis. Complications include volvulus and perforation.

Investigation and management

• Abdominal X-ray – dilated loops of bowel, air fluid levels and ground glass soap-bubble appearance of meconium.
• Intra-abdominal calcification indicates intrauterine perforation and peritonitis.
• Gastrograffin (water-soluble contrast) enema may wash out the meconium, otherwise surgery is required.
• Test for cystic fibrosis.

Meconium plug syndrome

Presentation – low bowel obstruction, as in Hirschsprung disease.

Hirschsprung disease

• Congenital absence of ganglionic cells in the myenteric plexus secondary to defective migration of ganglion cell precursors from neural crest to hind gut. Abnormal bowel extends from rectum for variable distance of large bowel. Proximal bowel is normal.
• Incidence – 1 in 5000 births, male: female ratio 5:1.
• May be associated with trisomy 21 (Down syndrome).
• Accounts for 20–25% of cases of neonatal intestinal obstruction.

Presentation

• Delayed passage of stools – more than 50% do not stool for 48 hours.
• About 50% of affected children present with abdominal distension (see Fig. 47.3) and vomiting in neonatal period, others when older with constipation.
• May present with enterocolitis – explosive liquid stools, fever and shock.

Investigation

Abdominal X-ray shows distal bowel obstruction – multiple distended loops of bowel with lack of air in the rectum.

Diagnosis

• Rectal suction biopsy for histology.
• Barium enema – excludes other causes of intestinal obstruction and may show transition zone between normal and aganglionic bowel (Fig. 48.3).

Treatment

Rectal washouts, followed by surgical repair.

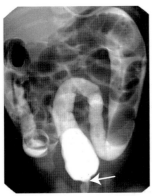

Fig. 48.3 Barium enema showing transition zone between normal and aganglionic bowel in Hirschsprung disease. (Courtesy of Dr Sheila Berlin.)

Congenital heart disease:

Is the most common group of structural malformations, accounting for 30% of all congenital abnormalities
• affects 6–9 per 1000 live births.

In children with congenital heart disease:
• 10–15% have complex heart disease with multiple lesions
• 10–15% have abnormalities of other systems.
A classification is shown in Table 49.1.

Risk factors

• Chromosomal disorders and syndromes, e.g. trisomy 21 (AVSD or VSD), chromosome 22q11 microdeletion (aortic arch abnormality), Turner (coarctation of aorta), Noonan (pulmonary stenosis), Williams (supravalvular aortic stenosis) and others.
• Maternal – diabetes mellitus (TGA), teratogenic drugs, e.g. anticonvulsants, lithium, fetal alcohol syndrome.
• Congenital infection, e.g. rubella.
• Siblings of affected child – only slight increase in risk.

Presentation

• Antenatal detection on ultrasound screening.
• Detection of a heart murmur on newborn examination.
• Heart failure – respiratory distress or shock.
• Cyanosis.
• Postnatal detection with oxygen saturation screening.

Antenatal diagnosis

About 70% of major lesions are diagnosed antenatally, especially those detectable on the four-chamber view used for antenatal ultrasound screening (Fig. 49.1), e.g. hypoplastic left heart. Lesions such as transposition of the great arteries and coarctation of the aorta are more difficult to identify. If an abnormality is suspected, referral to a perinatal cardiac specialist is indicated. Antenatal detection allows parents to be counseled and delivery to be planned in a cardiac center if indicated.

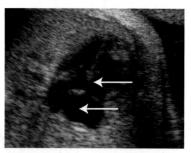

Fig. 49.1 Fetal ultrasound showing atrioventricular septal defect (AVSD).

Table 49.1 Classification of congenital heart disease, with examples and frequency of more common lesions (%).

Acyanotic	Cyanotic
Shunts ('holes'), left-to-right shunting • VSD (ventricular septal defect) 32% • PDA (patent ductus arteriosus) 12% • ASD (atrial septal defect) 6% • AVSD (atrioventricular septal defect)	**Right-to-left shunting (reduced pulmonary blood flow):** • Tetralogy of Fallot (6%) • Pulmonary atresia • Tricuspid atresia
Obstruction ('narrowing') • Pulmonary stenosis 8% • Coarctation of the aorta (6%) • Aortic stenosis (5%) • Hypoplastic left heart	**Transposition of the great arteries (TGA) (5%)** **Common mixing:** • Truncus arteriosus • Double outlet right ventricle
Pump failure • Supraventricular tachycardia (SVT) • Cardiomyopathy	**Total anomalous pulmonary venous connection (TAPVC)**

Key point

Acyanotic lesions usually present with shock or with heart failure and breathlessness.

Key point

Cyanotic lesions usually present with cyanosis at birth or when the duct closes.

Key point

About one-quarter of infants with congenital heart disease present in the neonatal period and usually have severe lesions.

Heart Murmur

Heart murmurs are heard in 1–2% of infants during routine examination of the newborn. May be due to:
• **A transient flow murmur** related to circulatory changes following birth. The murmur is soft, systolic, at the left sternal edge or pulmonary area in a well infant whose examination, including four-limb blood pressure measurements and oxygen saturation, is otherwise normal.
• **Branch pulmonary artery stenosis**. The murmur is best heard in the pulmonary area and radiates to the axilla and back, with otherwise normal examination. Resolves in a few weeks.
• **Congenital heart disease**. Murmurs due to turbulence through narrowed valves (e.g. aortic or pulmonary stenosis) or shunts (e.g. VSD). Although uncommon, the most worrying of these are duct-dependent lesions, which may result in circulatory failure or cyanosis when the ductus arteriosus closes soon after birth.

The definitive diagnosis is by echocardiography. A chest X-ray and ECG are of limited value. Pulse oximetry will establish if the arterial oxygen saturation is normal (>95%). If there are features of an innocent flow murmur, the infant should be reassessed within days to

Neonatology at a Glance, Third Edition. Edited by Tom Lissauer, Avroy A. Fanaroff, Lawrence Miall and Jonathan Fanaroff.
© 2016 John Wiley & Sons, Ltd. Published 2016 by John Wiley & Sons, Ltd.

check that the murmur has disappeared. The parents need to be informed that they should seek medical assistance should the infant develop symptoms suggestive of heart failure (Fig. 49.2). If the murmur persists or has pathologic features or the infant has other abnormal clinical signs, referral to a pediatric cardiologist is indicated.

> ### Key point
>
> The absence of a murmur does not exclude congenital heart disease.

Heart failure

The main cardiac causes are considered below. Non-cardiac causes include severe anemia or polycythemia or rarely arteriovenous malformation, e.g. vein of Galen in the brain.

Left-to-right shunting (high-output failure)

Usually presents with clinical features of heart failure (Fig. 49.2) several weeks after birth when the pulmonary vascular resistance falls and pulmonary blood flow increases.

Patent ductus arteriosus in preterm infants
See Chapter 33.

Atrioventricular septal defect (AV canal defect)
- Common (40%) in trisomy 21 (Down syndrome).
- Surgery at 2–4 months.
  Isolated atrial septal defects rarely cause heart failure.

Large ventricular septal defect
- Typically presents at about 1–3 months, when pulmonary vascular resistance is low and left-to-right shunt is maximal.
- Small muscular ventricular septal defects close spontaneously, but large perimembranous defects may require surgery if medical therapy fails.

Left ventricular outflow obstruction

Presents with low-output heart failure/shock when duct closes (Fig. 49.2). Key is to maintain ductal patency with prostaglandin infusion until surgery can be performed.

Severe coarctation of the aorta/interruption of the aortic arch
Key clinical sign is weak or absent femoral pulses. Blood pressure in the arms is markedly higher than in the legs (>20 mmHg). Post ductal saturation is low. Blood lactate may be elevated.
Prostaglandin infusion, then cardiac catheter aortoplasty or surgical repair is required.
Less severe lesions may present as hypertension in adults.

Hypoplastic left heart (Fig. 49.3)
Presents with signs of low cardiac output when ductus arteriosus closes. Pulses are weak at presentation, and there is severe metabolic acidosis. Fatal without treatment – options include a series of palliative operations (Norwood procedure) or heart transplantation.

Pump failure

Supraventricular tachycardia
- Heart rate 220–300 beats/min (Fig. 49.4).
- Heart is usually structurally normal, but accessory pathway (Wolff–Parkinson–White syndrome) is present in 40%.
- Place ice pack on face, give rapid bolus of intravenous adenosine. If these measures unsuccessful, perform DC cardioversion.

Cyanosis

Central cyanosis
- is clinically detectable if there is over 5 g/dL of reduced hemoglobin, so apparent cyanosis may be seen in polycythemia.
- is best detected in tongue/mucous membranes
- in the absence of respiratory distress is usually due to cyanotic congenital heart disease (Table 49.1).

Hypoplastic left heart

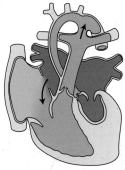

Fig. 49.3 Hypoplastic left heart syndrome.

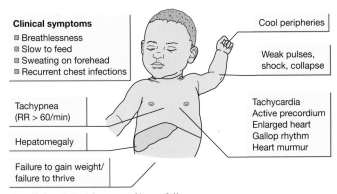

Clinical symptoms
- Breathlessness
- Slow to feed
- Sweating on forehead
- Recurrent chest infections

Tachypnea (RR > 60/min)

Hepatomegaly

Failure to gain weight/ failure to thrive

Cool peripheries

Weak pulses, shock, collapse

Tachycardia
Active precordium
Enlarged heart
Gallop rhythm
Heart murmur

Fig. 49.2 Clinical features of heart failure.

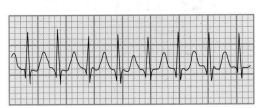

Fig. 49.4 ECG showing supraventricular tachycardia.

If there is respiratory distress, the cause may be:
- congenital heart disease
- pulmonary disease
- PPHN (persistent pulmonary hypertension of the newborn).

Peripheral cyanosis (acrocyanosis)

Hands and feet are blue. Common in infants in the first couple of days of life and in children of any age when cold. The tongue and mucous membranes are pink. Oxygen saturation is normal. It is of no clinical significance in the absence of hypovolemia or shock.

'Traumatic' cyanosis

Apparent cyanosis of the head from venous congestion, often accompanied by petechiae. Causes include umbilical cord around neck or face presentation. Tongue is pink. Oxygen saturation is normal. Resolves spontaneously.

Selected causes of cyanotic congenital heart disease (Table 49.1)

Transposition of the great arteries

In transposition of the great arteries there are two parallel circulations – the aorta arises from the right ventricle and the pulmonary artery from the left ventricle (Fig. 49.5). For survival, mixing of blood between the two circulations must occur, e.g. via the foramen ovale or ductus arteriosus. The less mixing between the circulations, the more severe the cyanosis and the earlier the presentation.

Presentation

Profound cyanosis occurs in the first day or two of life when the duct closes, but may be delayed if there is appreciable mixing of blood from an associated anomaly, e.g. ventricular or atrial septal defect.

Management

This is to promote mixing of the two circulations:
- maintain ductal patency with a prostaglandin infusion
- perform a balloon atrial septostomy to enlarge the foramen ovale (Fig. 49.6).

A definitive 'switch' operation is usually performed within the first 2 weeks, in which the pulmonary artery and aorta are switched

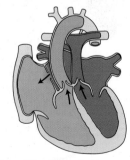

Complete transposition of the great arteries

Fig. 49.5 Transposition of the great arteries.

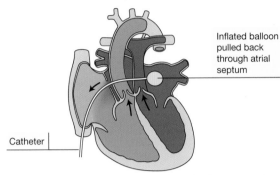

Balloon septostomy

Inflated balloon pulled back through atrial septum

Catheter

Fig. 49.6 Balloon atrial septostomy to enlarge the foramen ovale.

over. The coronary arteries also have to be transferred to the new aorta, which is technically challenging. Outcome is good.

Total anomalous pulmonary venous connection (TAPVC)

Instead of connecting to the left atrium, the pulmonary veins connect into the right atrium, sometimes via a shunt below the diaphragm. If the connection is narrow (obstructed) presentation is with cyanosis, respiratory distress and poor cardiac output. May be difficult to distinguish from respiratory distress syndrome. Treatment is surgical, sometimes as an emergency.

Oxygen saturation screening for critical congenital heart disease

An increasing number of centers perform oxygen saturation screening in the first 24 hours of life to identify duct-dependent congenital heart disease. Either a postductal oxygen saturation of <95% or a pre- (right arm) and postductal (either foot) oxygen saturation drop of >3% is used as cut-off to prompt medical review and echocardiography. False-positive results may occur, but many with low oxygen saturation have respiratory problems or sepsis. Early diagnosis of duct-dependent lesions is important as it can prevent collapse when the duct closes 24–48 hours after birth.

Key point

Oxygen saturation screening enables infants with duct-dependent lesions to be detected while still asymptomatic.

Investigations

The immediate problem in symptomatic neonates is usually to distinguish between a respiratory disorder, congenital heart disease (CHD) and persistent pulmonary hypertension of the newborn (PPHN).

Chest X-ray

Helpful to exclude pulmonary disease, but rarely diagnostic of congenital heart disease as heart size and shape and pulmonary vasculature are difficult to determine in the neonatal period. An enlarged heart border may be due to normal thymus. However, a chest radiograph may show:
• Cardiomegaly (>60% diameter of thorax), e.g. outflow obstruction from coarctation of the aorta or volume overload (patent ductus arteriosus).
• Abnormal shape (e.g. boot shape with tetralogy of Fallot, 'egg on side' with TGA), but often only recognized retrospectively!
• Prominent pulmonary vascular markings (plethoric) from excess blood flow to the lungs, e.g. left-to-right shunt from patent ductus arteriosus.
• Reduced vascular markings (oligemic) from reduced pulmonary blood flow to the lungs, e.g. tetralogy of Fallot.

ECG

• Seldom diagnostic; interpretation requires considerable skill.
• Can be useful if there is a superior axis (e.g. AVSD, tricuspid atresia).
• Helpful for arrhythmias and as baseline.

Hyperoxia test

May be helpful to distinguish respiratory from cardiac causes, especially if echocardiography not readily available. The infant is placed in 100% oxygen for 10 minutes (Fig. 49.7).

Interpretation of right radial (preductal) artery oxygen tension is:
• If $PaO_2 > 110\,mmHg$ (15 kPa) – unlikely to be cyanotic heart disease – usually lung disease or PPHN (persistent pulmonary hypertension of the newborn).
• If $PaO_2 < 110\,mmHg$ (15 kPa) – likely to be cyanotic heart disease, but can be severe lung disease or PPHN.

Echocardiography with Doppler (see Chapter 79)

Allow definitive anatomic diagnosis and identification of shunts in most instances. Need experienced operator. Doppler will identify the direction of any shunting and patency of the ductus arteriosus.

Cardiac catheterization

Sometimes required for hemodynamic measurements and to confirm collateral blood vessels and increasingly used for interventional procedures, e.g. pulmonary valvuloplasty or placing an occlusion device within the ductus (in term infants).

Management of congenital heart disease

• Maintain **A**irway, **B**reathing, **C**irculation. Provide ventilatory support if necessary.
• Correct metabolic acidosis, hypoglycemia and hypocalcemia.
• If duct-dependent defect suspected or confirmed:
  – give prostaglandin intravenously to keep the ductus arteriosus patent (expect apnea after high-dose prostaglandin)
  – do not give additional oxygen unless SaO_2 falls below 75% (oxygen will make the duct more likely to close).
• If in heart failure:
  – high-output failure (after first week of life) – fluid restriction (acute only), diuretics, ACE inhibitors, e.g. captopril
  – low-output failure/shock – inotropes, volume support; arrhythmias require specific treatment.
• Refer to pediatric cardiac center for expert advice, diagnostic imaging and management.

Question

Why may giving prostaglandin be life-saving?
By keeping the ductus arteriosus patent when the circulation is duct-dependent. For example:
• with obstruction to outflow of the left ventricle, when the systemic circulation is maintained by blood flowing right to left across the patent ductus, e.g. severe coarctation of the aorta (Fig. 49.8)
• with reduced pulmonary blood flow, when the pulmonary circulation is maintained by blood flowing from left to right through the duct, e.g. pulmonary atresia (Fig. 49.9).

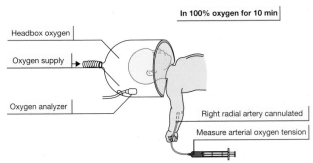

Fig. 49.7 Hyperoxia (nitrogen washout) test to identify cyanotic congenital heart disease.

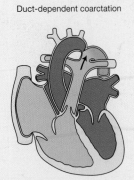

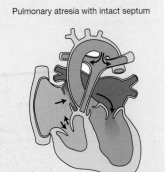

Fig. 49.8 Severe coarctation of the aorta, an example of duct-dependent systemic circulation.

Fig. 49.9 Pulmonary atresia, an example of duct-dependent pulmonary circulation.

50 Renal and urinary tract anomalies diagnosed prenatally

Most significant structural abnormalities of the kidneys and urinary tract are now identified prenatally on ultrasound screening. They account for 20–30% of all prenatally detected abnormalities. Early recognition and treatment may prevent or ameliorate complications such as urinary tract infection, failure to thrive and renal failure. When indicated, it may allow prenatal referral to a tertiary center. The disadvantage is that many minor or transient genitourinary anomalies are identified, resulting in unnecessary concern for the parents and additional investigations for the child.

Embryology

The kidneys and genitourinary tract are embryologically interdependent. If one system is abnormal, look for abnormalities of the other.

Structural abnormalities of the kidneys

Outflow obstruction

In the fetus with outflow obstruction (Fig. 50.1) there may be:
• hydronephrosis – unilateral or bilateral, with renal parenchyma that may be normal or malformed or dysplastic
• dilatation of the ureters and/or bladder
• reduced or absent amniotic fluid volume.

Unilateral hydronephrosis
• Hydronephrosis is dilatation of the proximal collecting system (Fig. 50.2).
• It is the commonest abnormality diagnosed antenatally, and accounts for 50% of all prenatally detected urologic anomalies. It occurs in 1 in 500–700 infants. Most common cause is physiologic hydronephrosis, but others are obstruction at the pelviureteric or vesicoureteric junction or urinary reflux.
• Management is shown in Fig. 50.3.
• Most but not all resolve spontaneously. Prognosis is dependent on degree of kidney damage resulting from obstruction.

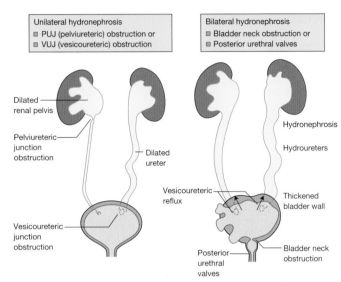

Fig. 50.1 Features of unilateral and bilateral outflow obstruction.

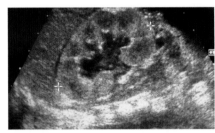

Fig. 50.2 Ultrasound showing unilateral hydronephrosis. As a measure of its severity, the anteroposterior renal pelvis diameter is measured. (Courtesy of Dr Annemarie Jeanes.)

• If the anteroposterior diameter does not exceed 15 mm either antenatally or postnatally, intervention is rarely needed.

Bilateral hydronephrosis
Less common than unilateral hydronephrosis but more likely to be serious.

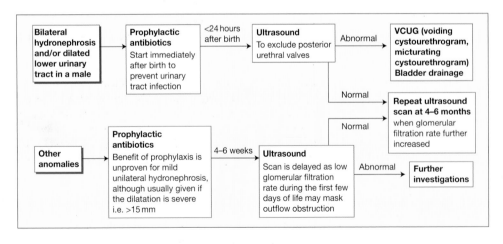

Fig. 50.3 Example of a guideline of the initial management of renal and urinary tract abnormalities detected on antenatal ultrasound.

Neonatology at a Glance, Third Edition. Edited by Tom Lissauer, Avroy A. Fanaroff, Lawrence Miall and Jonathan Fanaroff.
© 2016 John Wiley & Sons, Ltd. Published 2016 by John Wiley & Sons, Ltd.

Posterior urethral valves

- Mucosal folds or a membrane obstruct urine flow causing bilateral hydronephrosis, hydroureter and thickened bladder. One-third develop end-stage renal failure.
- Incidence is 1 in 5000–8000 live male births.
- Most are diagnosed on prenatal ultrasound, when antenatal intervention may be considered. Options include percutaneous vesicoamniotic shunt placement, bladder aspiration, and drainage of a severely distended kidney. However, outcome after intervention has been disappointing. As amniotic fluid is mainly derived from fetal urine, there may be severe oligohydramnios resulting in Potter syndrome/sequence (Fig. 50.4); the dominant features are from compression of the fetus and pulmonary hypoplasia resulting in stillbirth or early neonatal death.
- Presentation in the infant not diagnosed antenatally includes a palpable, distended bladder, poor urinary flow, renal and respiratory failure.
- Management postnatally is shown in Fig. 50.3. It is with prophylactic antibiotics, renal and urinary tract ultrasound within 24 hours of birth and VCUG (voiding cystourethrogram, micturating cystourethrogram, see Fig. 51.2).
- Treatment – drainage of the urinary tract, initially by urinary catheter, later by ablation of the valves. Careful fluid and electrolyte management.

Key point

Bilateral hydronephrosis with bladder distension in a boy should be assumed to be posterior urethral valves until proven otherwise.

Polycystic kidney disease

Autosomal dominant polycystic kidney disease (ADPKD)
(Fig. 50.5a)
- Common: 1 in 500–1000 live births.
- Wide spectrum of severity; usually asymptomatic in childhood, causes renal failure in late adulthood.
- Extrarenal features: cysts in liver and pancreas, cerebral aneurysms and mitral valve prolapse.

Autosomal recessive polycystic kidney disease (ARPKD)
(Fig. 50.5b)
- Rare: 1 in 10 000–40 000 live births.
- Cysts form in the collecting duct.

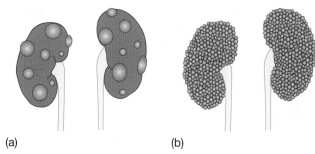

Fig. 50.5 (a) Autosomal dominant polycystic kidney disease (ADPKD). There are separate cysts of varying size between normal renal parenchyma. (b) Autosomal recessive polycystic kidney disease (ARPKD). There is diffuse bilateral enlargement of the kidneys.

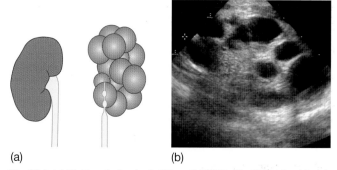

Fig. 50.6 (a) Multicystic dysplastic kidney (MCKD). The kidney is replaced by cysts of variable size, with atresia of the ureter. (b) Renal ultrasound shows discrete cysts of variable size in multicystic dysplastic kidney (MCKD).

- Neonates may present with pulmonary hypoplasia secondary to oligohydramnios (Potter syndrome/sequence, Fig. 50.4). May also present with abdominal masses, hypertension and renal failure.
- Associated with congenital hepatic fibrosis.
- May cause renal failure requiring renal transplant.

Multicystic dysplactic kidney (MCDK)

- Uncommon: 1 in 4000 live births.
- Renal parenchyma replaced by cysts of various sizes (Fig. 50.6a and b).
- Kidney is functionless, accompanied by atresia of the ureter.
- If bilateral, it leads to Potter syndrome/sequence.
- Kidney may be large and palpable, but more often is small. Contralateral kidney is usually normal, should have undergone compensatory hypertrophy, but at increased risk of vesicoureteric reflux.
- Half will have involuted by 2 years. Nephrectomy is only indicated if cysts increase in size or hypertension develops, both of which are rare.

Renal agenesis

- Unilateral agenesis (present in 1 in 1000 live births) is only significant if the contralateral kidney is abnormal.
- Bilateral agenesis (Potter syndrome) is fatal from pulmonary hypoplasia due to severe oligohydramnios (Fig. 50.4).

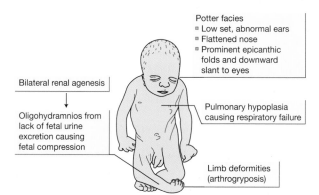

Potter facies
- Low set, abnormal ears
- Flattened nose
- Prominent epicanthic folds and downward slant to eyes

Bilateral renal agenesis

Oligohydramnios from lack of fetal urine excretion causing fetal compression

Pulmonary hypoplasia causing respiratory failure

Limb deformities (arthrogryposis)

Fig. 50.4 Potter syndrome (Potter sequence).

Renal function in the newborn

Almost all infants void by 24 hours of life. If it is suspected that urine has not been passed within the first day, it is usually that voiding has not been recorded, especially immediately after birth. Consider obstruction or intrinsic renal problem, but they are usually detected on antenatal ultrasound screening.

Some key points regarding renal function are listed in Fig. 51.1.

The fetal kidney plays no role in excretion or homeostasis – which is performed by the placenta	In the fetus, the function of the kidney is to produce amniotic fluid. The fetal circulation is in chemical equilibrium with that of the mother. Fetal or cord blood measurements of renal function, e.g. blood urea nitrogen (urea) or creatinine, reflect renal function of the mother, not the fetus
Glomerular filtration rate (GFR) is low in newborns, even if adjusted for body size	Glomerular filtration rate (GFR) in ▫ A preterm infant at 28 weeks – 10 mL/min/1.73 m² body surface area (BSA) ▫ A healthy, term infant – 30 mL/min/1.73 m² ▫ Adult – 120 mL/min/1.73 m² (range 80–120), reached by the second year of life. Some argue that it is more appropriate to quote GFR in infancy by weight, the mean value being 1 mL/min/kg (range 0.5–1.5 mL/min/kg)
The newborn kidney is optimized for retention of dietary solutes for growth, not for excretion	The healthy newborn infant grows very rapidly, i.e. is strongly anabolic. Breast milk is *just* sufficient to provide the nutrients needed for this growth. There is little excess dietary solute requiring excretion, so infants can thrive despite biochemical evidence of renal insufficiency that would be inadequate for an adult. There are two practical consequences of this: ▫ The newborn kidney is optimized for *retention*, not excretion, of essential substances such as sodium and other minerals ▫ If growth ceases, e.g. infection, the low renal reserve of the infant is exposed and biochemical derangements are common Both these are even more true of the preterm than of the term infant
The term kidney conserves sodium, the preterm kidney loses sodium	Term infants produce urine almost free of sodium, and can thrive on human milk that contains <10 mmol/L of sodium. This is not true of the preterm infant <32 weeks' gestational age fed mature human milk or an artificial formula of similar composition. Under these circumstances they are prone to become sodium-depleted and hyponatremic, typically at about 10 days postnatal age (late hyponatremia of prematurity). This can be prevented by increasing the dietary sodium intake to 4–6 mmol/kg/day for the vulnerable period of 4–14 postnatal days. Mature human milk would only provide 1.25 mmol/kg/day. Neonates with renal tract malformations such as dysplasia or obstructive uropathy are also prone to becoming hyponatraemic and acidotic and require sodium and bicarbonate supplements, respectively.
Reduced urine osmolality in the newborn is physiologic	Term infants are less able to concentrate urine than adults. This is even more pronounced in preterm infants

Fig. 51.1 Some key points about renal function in newborn infants.

Electrolyte problems

Sodium

Normal range 135–145 mmol/L.

Hyponatremia – Na <130 mmol/L

Results from excess water relative to sodium or insufficient sodium relative to water.

Key is to assess fluid status overall. If detailed assessment required, measure paired urinary and serum sodium, osmolality and creatinine to establish fractional excretion of sodium. (Fractional excretion of sodium, $FENa = UNa/PNa \times PCr/UCr \times 100$, where UNa is urinary sodium, PNa plasma sodium, PCr is plasma creatinine, UCr urinary creatinine).

Term infants, hyponatremia usually from giving excessive volume of IV dextrose containing no or insufficient sodium. Especially in first 48 hours of life and when there is intravascular

Neonatology at a Glance, Third Edition. Edited by Tom Lissauer, Avroy A. Fanaroff, Lawrence Miall and Jonathan Fanaroff.
© 2016 John Wiley & Sons, Ltd. Published 2016 by John Wiley & Sons, Ltd.

volume depletion with water reabsorption. Also excess IV fluids to mother during labor; oliguric renal failure (renal impairment with little urine output and fluid overload).

Preterm – marked Na loss in urine, poor at conserving sodium as tubular reabsorptive capacity not fully developed. This results in hyponatremia of prematurity (see Fig. 51.1).

Other causes include:
• insufficient Na supplementation (low FENa)
• gastrointestinal losses – diarrhea, vomiting (low FENa)
• renal losses – diuretics (high FENa), renal dysplasia, congenital adrenal hyperplasia, renal tubulopathies
• SIADH, syndrome of inappropriate antidiuretic hormone (high FENa, low POsm and high UOsm) – probably rare in newborn infants.

Hypernatremia – Na >150 mmol/L

Result of excessive water loss over sodium or excess sodium intake over water.

If detailed assessment required, assess fluid status and measure FENa.

Hypernatraemic dehydration may be from:
• insufficient input of fluids e.g. insufficient breast milk
• excessive water losses, e.g. evaporative through skin in extremely preterm, phototherapy, radiant heater or gastrointestinal losses
• excess sodium intake, e.g. sodium containing flushes of lines, sodium bicarbonate, sodium phosphate, etc (high UOsm and high FENa)

Rare causes – diabetes insipidus (central, e.g. septo-optic dysplasia or nephrogenic, no ADH or ADH effect) (low UOsm, low FENa), deliberate salt poisoning.

Question

What is the significance of hypernatremia in breast fed babies?

Most breast fed babies have a normal serum sodium. However, if there is insufficient intake of breast milk, the infant may develop hypernatremic dehydration. On examination the infants may not appear to have severe dehydration as the anterior fontanel may not be sunken and skin turgor may be normal as the extracellular fluid volume is relatively well maintained. However, the baby may be lethargic and quiet and feed poorly because of cerebral intracellular dehydration. Movement of water from brain cells may cause a decrease in brain volume and rupture of intracerebral veins and bridging blood vessels resulting in hemorrhage and seizures. The definitive sign is significant weight loss, often in excess of 12% birth weight.

Once recognized, it is important that the serum sodium is corrected slowly over 24-48 hours. Serum sodium may be extremely high (>160 mmol/L). Too rapid correction can result in seizures from too rapid expansion of cells in the brain. Lactation advice and support should be given to try to re-establish successful breastfeeding.

Hypernatremia has also been seen after accidental over-concentration of formula milk feeds or due to deliberate salt poisoning, although both are very rare.

Potassium (normal range 3.5–5.5 mmol/L)

Hyperkalemia – K >6.0 mmol/L

Serious condition as can result in arrhythmias and death. But most common reason is hemolyzed blood sample.

Other causes – renal impairment (transient is relatively common in extremely preterm infants), excess K supplementation, congenital adrenal hyperplasia.

Neonates tolerate hyperkalemia better than older children, so only treat if K >6.5 mmol/L. ECG monitoring is required.

Treatment involves giving calcium gluconate to stabilize myocardium, salbutamol IV or nebulized, correcting acidosis, stopping all K, changing to low K feed, infusion of glucose and insulin, calcium resonium orally or rectally but can cause gastrointestinal obstruction.

Question

What are the ECG changes in hyperkalemia?

ECG changes progress with increasing potassium concentration:
• Initial changes – prolonged PR interval, peaked T waves
• Progression – absent P waves, ST depression, peaked T waves
• Further progression – QRS widening, ST depression, peaked T waves; danger of ventricular fibrillation and other arrhythmias and asystole

Key point

Unexpected hyperkalemia – repeat measurement as often due to hemolyzed blood sample.

Hypokalaemia – K <3.0 mmol/L

Causes include insufficient supplementations, diuretics, diarrhea, vomiting, renal tubular losses (e.g. Bartter syndrome), drugs, e.g. amphotericin.

Calcium and phosphate

Hypocalcemia

Relatively common problem and can lead to seizures.

Causes: birth trauma/asphyxia, infants of diabetic mothers, exchange transfusion with blood reconstituted in citrate, maternal hyperparathyroidism, Di George syndrome, associated with hypomagnesemia, maternal vitamin D deficiency.

Hypophosphatemia

Usually results from insufficient supplementation in feeds or parenteral nutrition.

Urinary tract infection (UTI)

- Commoner in boys than in girls – the reverse of older children.
- Should be suspected in any infant who is non-specifically unwell.

Presentation

- Fever or sometimes low temperature or temperature instability
- Poor feeding
- Vomiting
- Prolonged jaundice
- Diarrhea
- Failure to thrive

Investigations

Urine – collecting urine samples:
- clean catch specimen
- urethral catheterization
- suprapubic aspiration (see Chapter 76).

Blood culture and sepsis work-up (with or without lumbar puncture) should be performed as urinary tract infection is often accompanied by septicemia in neonates.

Diagnosis

Is made by culture of a single strain of any organism on a catheter sample or suprapubic aspirate. However, may get false-positive suprapubic aspirate result from skin commensal or bowel perforation.

White cells may or may not be present on microscopy or urinalysis.

E. coli is the commonest organism (>75%); remainder caused by *Klebsiella, Proteus, Enterobacter*.

Management

Intravenous antibiotics – start immediately whilst awaiting the result of the urine culture. Subsequent choice of antibiotics will depend on the sensitivities of the cultured organism. Should be continued at full dosage until the infant has been well for 2–3 days

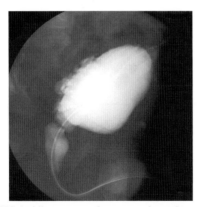

Fig. 51.2 VCUG (voiding cystourethrogram, micturating cystourethrogram) showing trabeculation of the bladder wall, hypertrophy of the bladder and dilated posterior urethra from posterior urethral valves.

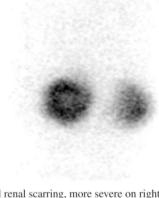

LT   RT

Fig. 51.3 Bilateral renal scarring, more severe on right, on DMSA radionuclide scan on investigation following a urinary tract infection.

and a negative follow-up urine culture obtained. Following treatment of culture positive UTI, oral prophylactic antibiotics, e.g. trimethoprim or cefalexin, should be given until the results of imaging of the kidneys and urinary tract are known.

Imaging – if culture is positive, ultrasound of the kidneys and urinary tract is performed to detect renal tract abnormalities. A VCUG (voiding cystourethrogram, micturating cystourethrogram) is performed to identify bladder outflow obstruction, e.g. from posterior urethral valves or vesicoureteral reflux (Fig. 51.2). A radionuclide scan (DMSA, dimercaptosuccinic acid) is performed 3 months later to identify renal scarring (Fig. 51.3).

Acute kidney injury, AKI (acute renal failure)

In acute kidney injury (acute renal failure) there is sudden impairment in renal function leading to inability of the kidney to excrete nitrogenous waste and electrolytes. It is defined as a rise in the plasma creatinine concentration to twice the upper limit of normal, i.e. 1.5 mg/dL (130 mmol/L) accompanied by a reduction in urine flow rate to <1 mL/kg/hour. However, renal failure can occur without oliguria. It results from a significant fall in glomerular filtration rate with failure of tubular reabsorption of salt and water.

Causes

Different in neonates from children and adults as usually prerenal (Table 51.1). Mild renal impairment is not uncommon in the first few days of life, particularly in preterm infants, and is usually transient.

Clinical features

- Creatinine concentration raised – at birth it reflects maternal creatinine, falls over the next 4-6 weeks; a rising creatinine after day 1 suggests acute kidney injury
- Urinary features – oliguria, hematuria, proteinuria
- Clinical features – edema, dehydration, vomiting, lethargy, seizures, hypertension

Table 51.1 Causes of acute kidney injury (acute renal failure) in neonates.

Prerenal	Renal	Postrenal
Hypovolemia Dehydration, sepsis, necrotizing enterocolitis Blood loss: antepartum, neonatal Heart failure Hypoxia including birth asphyxia	Acute tubular necrosis secondary to an uncorrected prerenal cause Congenital renal abnormality, e.g. polycystic kidney disease, renal agenesis, renal hypodysplasia Vascular insult – renal vein thrombosis, renal artery thrombosis (associated with use of umbilical arterial lines) Nephrotoxins, e.g. aminoglycosides Infection – pyelonephritis	Congenital obstructive uropathy – posterior urethral valves, etc. Neurogenic bladder

- Other biochemical features – hyperkalemia, acidosis, hyperphosphatemia and hypocalcemia

Investigations

Ultrasound of kidneys and urinary tract – identifies if there are abnormal kidneys, outflow obstruction, abnormal blood flow in renal arteries and veins.

Management

Prevention
- Monitor the creatinine, blood urea nitrogen (urea) and electrolytes of newborn infants who have been exposed to risk factors for acute kidney injury, such as birth asphyxia or sepsis
- Early treatment of hypovolemia
- Relief of obstruction
- Avoid nephrotoxic agents if possible

Electrolyte and fluid management
- Restrict sodium, potassium and phosphate. Use calcium carbonate as phosphate binder. Correct metabolic acidosis.

- High-dose furosemide 2–5 mg/kg to convert oliguric into non-oliguric renal failure.
- Nutritional support.
- Renal replacement therapy – rarely needed, only if fluid and metabolic abnormalities cannot be corrected. Peritoneal dialysis is preferable but may not be possible (e.g. abdominal wall defects or necrotizing enterocolitis). Hemodialysis is difficult due to vascular access and risks associated with anticoagulation. Continuous veno-venous hemofiltration is more gentle and better tolerated, especially in the sick neonate unable to tolerate intermittent hemodialysis.

Prognosis
Infants who develop acute kidney injury in the neonatal period have increased mortality, highest in extremely preterm.

Infants who have chronic kidney disease and need to start renal replacement therapy in the neonatal period have a 2-year survival rate of 81%, with infection being the most common cause of death. The 5-year survival rate is 76%. However, there is significant comorbidity in the survivors, with growth problems, anemia and hypertension.

52 Genital disorders

Features of the normal male genitalia are listed in Table 52.1. Most abnormalities arise from abnormal embryology (Fig. 52.1).

Inguinal hernia

This results from the processus vaginalis remaining patent. Much more common in males than females and usually on the right side.

Common in preterm infants, particularly those with bronchopulmonary dysplasia as they have weak muscles and increased intra-abdominal pressure.

Presents as a swelling in the groin or scrotum on crying (Fig. 52.2). It should be repaired promptly to avoid the risk of strangulation in both term and preterm infants, unless the anesthetic risk necessitates delaying the operation.

If the hernia becomes irreducible, the lump is firm and tender, the infant vomits or becomes unwell, then an attempt should be made to reduce it after sustained gentle compression together with opioid analgesia. If possible, surgery is delayed for 24–48 hours to allow the edema to resolve. If reduction is unsuccessful, emergency surgery is required to avoid bowel strangulation and damage to the testis.

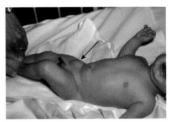

Fig. 52.2 Inguinal hernia in a newborn infant (arrow). (Courtesy of Dr Mike Coren.)

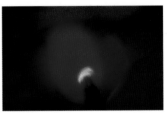

Fig. 52.3 Hydrocele on transillumination. (Courtesy of Dr Mike Coren.)

Hydrocele

This is fluid around the testis from a processus vaginalis that is wide enough to allow peritoneal fluid to flow down it but too narrow to form an inguinal hernia. Tense, transilluminates (Fig. 52.3). Often bilateral. Most resolve spontaneously.

Table 52.1 Features of normal male genitalia at term.

Length and diameter – normal size
Meatus – at tip
Testes – palpable in scrotum
Scrotum – rugae

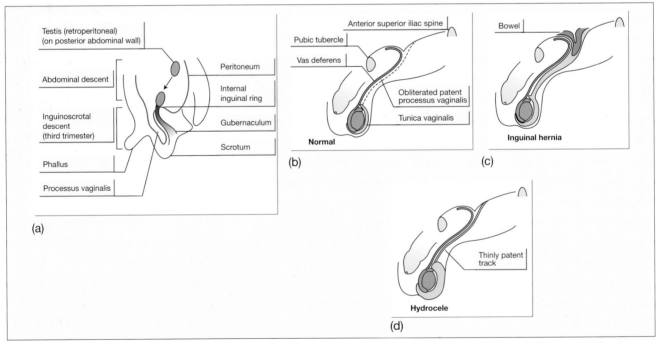

Fig. 52.1 (a) Embryology of testicular descent. The testis migrates from the posterior abdominal wall to the scrotum. It is preceded by a tongue of peritoneum, the processus vaginalis. This is obliterated in the normal infant (b). It remains widely patent in an inguinal hernia (c). With a hydrocele, it is patent but narrow (d).

Neonatology at a Glance, Third Edition. Edited by Tom Lissauer, Avroy A. Fanaroff, Lawrence Miall and Jonathan Fanaroff.
© 2016 John Wiley & Sons, Ltd. Published 2016 by John Wiley & Sons, Ltd.

Undescended testis

Failure of the testis to descend into the scrotum. Present in 5% of term male infants. Incidence is higher in preterm infants as testicular descent through the inguinal canal only occurs in the third trimester of pregnancy. Testicular descent may continue after birth; by 3 months of age only 1.5% are affected, but few descend thereafter.

Examination

With warm hands the contents of the inguinal canal are gently massaged towards the scrotum. If undescended, no testis is palpable in the scrotum, and the overlying scrotum is often poorly formed. The undescended testis may be palpable in the groin, but may sometimes be in the abdomen or outside the normal line of descent. A descended testis sometimes subsequently retracts upwards into the inguinal region (retractile testis).

Investigations

For bilateral undescended testes, pelvic ultrasound and karyotype may be needed to establish the infant's gender, i.e. male and not a virilized female. The presence of testicular tissue can be confirmed by detecting testosterone production after hormonal stimulation. Sometimes laparoscopy is required to locate the testis.

Management

Surgery to place the testis in the scrotum (orchidopexy) is performed soon after 6 months of age, definitely by 2 years because:
• fertility is optimized – the testis needs to be in the scrotum to be below body temperature
• malignancy – increased risk, which for a unilateral undescended testis is reduced to nearly the same as a normal testis
• it is cosmetic and avoids psychologic upset.

Torsion of the testis

There is interruption of the blood supply to the testis and epididymis. The testis and surrounding area may be inflamed and the scrotum is dark red or black. Must be differentiated from a strangulated hernia and scrotal hematoma. Doppler ultrasound of testicular blood supply is helpful to determine testicular viability. Torsion must be relieved promptly for testis to remain viable. Occasionally present at birth, when testis is seldom viable.

Hypospadias

Common, affecting 1 in 300 boys. In the fetus, the urethra is created by flat tissue folding over from the perineum towards the tip. If this is not completed, the meatal opening may not reach the normal site at the tip of the penis (Fig. 52.4).

In hypospadias there is:
• a ventral urethral meatus – usually on the glans of the penis, but can be on the shaft or perineum (Fig. 52.5)

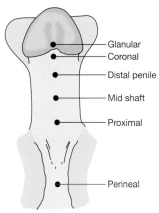
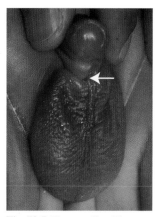

Fig. 52.4 Classification of hypospadias.

Fig. 52.5 Hypospadias. The arrow shows the urethral meatus.

• a hooded foreskin – from failure to fuse
• chordee – tethering resulting in ventral curvature of the penis, most obvious on erection. This is associated with the more severe forms.

Surgical correction is performed by 18 months of age so that the urethral meatus is at the tip of the penis, erection is straight and the penis looks normal. In most cases of hypospadias affecting only the glans, surgery is not required, except sometimes for cosmetic reasons.

Key point

Infants with hypospadias must not be circumcised as the foreskin may be needed at surgery.

Circumcision

At birth, the foreskin adheres to the surface of the glans penis. These adhesions subsequently separate, allowing the foreskin to become retractile. The foreskin cannot be retracted in 50% of boys at 1 year of age and in 10% at 4 years, but in only 1% by 16 years.

The advantages and disadvantages of circumcision are controversial and emotive.

Advantages are:
• hygiene – easier to keep clean
• prevents possibility of pathologic phimosis (scarring) or recurrent balanitis (infection) requiring circumcision when older
• slightly reduced incidence of urinary tract infection
• reduced risk of heterosexual HIV transmission as adults.

However, it is not a trivial operation, as healing can take up to 10 days. Complications of neonatal circumcision include:
• pain during and after the operation – adequate analgesia should be provided
• bleeding, infection, damage to glans penis, but this is uncommon.

In the US, circumcision is widely performed. In the UK, the main indication is religious, among Jews and Muslims. In countries in Sub-Saharan Africa with high HIV prevalence, the WHO recommends consideration as a component of HIV prevention.

53 Disorders of sex development

In newborn infants, disorders of sex development (DSD) present with ambiguous genitalia. There may be:
• virilized female – clitoromegaly, labial fusion
• undervirilized male – micropenis, bilateral undescended testes, poorly developed or bifid scrotum
• true hermaphrodite, now called ovotesticular DSD – complex external phenotype with both testicular and ovarian tissue present.

They are rare but require prompt evaluation and skilled management to avoid emotional turmoil for parents. Family support and counseling are of utmost importance.

Sex development

The fetal gonad is initially bipotential (Fig. 53.1).

The testis-determining gene on the Y chromosome (*SRY*) causes differentiation of gonads into testes. Production of testosterone and its metabolite dihydrotestosterone results in the development of male genitalia.

Undervirilization in the male may result from:
• inadequate androgen action from:
  – abnormal testes
  – inability to convert testosterone to dihydrotestosterone (5α-reductase deficiency)
  – abnormalities of the androgen receptor (androgen insensitivity syndrome)
• gonadotropin insufficiency from:
  – congenital pituitary dysfunction
  – several syndromes, e.g. Prader–Willi syndrome.

In the absence of the *SRY* gene the gonads become ovaries and the genitalia female.

Virilized female is from excessive androgens; the most common cause of this is congenital adrenal hyperplasia.

Ovotesticular DSD is from chromosomal rearrangement and is rare.

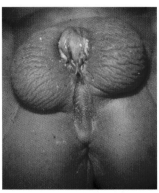

Fig. 53.2 Ambiguous genitalia at birth. Do not assign a gender before expert opinion. (Courtesy of Dr David Clark.)

Birth

When a baby is born, the parents immediately want to know if they have a girl or boy.

If the genitalia are ambiguous (Fig. 53.2), it is imperative not to guess but to inform the parents that further evaluation is needed. Birth registration must be delayed until this has been completed.

Investigations

Detailed assessment may include:
• karyotype
• sex and adrenal hormones:
  – blood glucose and electrolytes
  – 17α-hydroxyprogesterone
  – testosterone, dihydrotestosterone and androstenedione
  – hormone (GnRH or HCG) stimulation tests
• ultrasound of internal genitalia and gonads.

Laparoscopic examination and biopsy of internal structures are sometimes required.

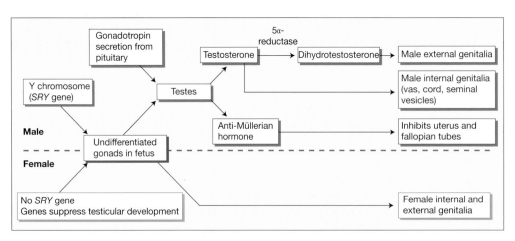

Fig. 53.1 Sex development in the fetus.

Neonatology at a Glance, Third Edition. Edited by Tom Lissauer, Avroy A. Fanaroff, Lawrence Miall and Jonathan Fanaroff.
© 2016 John Wiley & Sons, Ltd. Published 2016 by John Wiley & Sons, Ltd.

Management

Ensure good communication between all health-care professionals so that they do not ascribe a gender to the infant inadvertently.

Most are reared as females, as it is easier to create female external genitalia than a functioning penis, but it is increasingly recognized that this may not necessarily be in the long-term best interest of the child. There is increasing evidence of problems with gender identity as teenagers and adults of males reared as females, and evidence of good sexual functioning and satisfaction in males who had a poorly formed penis in the neonatal period. Early referral, expert multidisciplinary assessment and long-term management are required.

Congenital adrenal hyperplasia

- Autosomal recessive condition.
- About 1 in 5000 live births.
- Most common cause is a deficiency of an enzyme, 21-hydroxylase, required for cortisol biosynthesis (Fig. 53.3). There is a deficiency in the production of cortisol, aldosterone (salt loss) and an excess of adrenal steroids (virilization).

Presentation
May be with:
- virilization of female external genitalia (Fig. 53.4)
- enlarged penis and pigmented scrotum in male, but rarely recognized
- salt-losing adrenal crisis with hyponatremia and hyperkalemia at 1–3 weeks of age; there is vomiting, weight loss, circulatory collapse which may be fatal; may be accompanied by hypoglycemia
- tall stature, precocious puberty in males.

Diagnosis
Raised blood level of 17α-hydroxyprogesterone.

Management
Short term:
- Salt-losing crisis – requires intravenous saline, glucose, hydrocortisone.

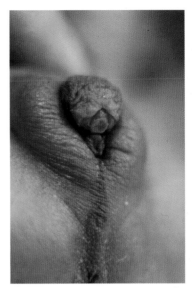

Fig. 53.4 Virilized female from congenital adrenal hyperplasia. There is clitoral hypertrophy and fusion of the labia. (Courtesy of Dr David Clark.)

- Corrective surgery of external genitalia in females is occasionally needed during infancy.

Long term:
- Glucocorticoids throughout life.
- Mineralocorticoids if salt loss; infants may need extra oral sodium chloride.
- Monitoring of growth and pubertal development.
- Additional hormone replacement (stress doses) if ill or prior to surgical procedures.
- Further corrective surgery in adolescence to external genitalia in females.
- Psychologic support.

Prenatal testing and screening
Prenatal testing and treatment of affected fetuses are available.

Screening (17α-hydroxyprogesterone concentration) is now performed in most routine biochemical screening programs of newborn infants in the US but not in the UK.

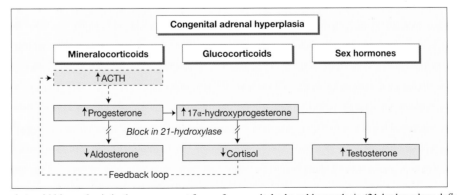

Fig. 53.3 Abnormal adrenal steroid biosynthesis in the commonest form of congenital adrenal hyperplasia (21-hydroxylase deficiency).

54 Anemia and polycythemia

Anemia

Physiology

In the fetus, the oxygen tension is low. The oxygen affinity of fetal red cells containing hemoglobin F (HbF) is increased compared to adult red cells (Fig. 54.1) and this favors uptake of more oxygen. The hemoglobin concentration (Hb) is also much higher than in adults.

After birth, the concentration of Hb is greatly affected by the time of cord clamping and the position of the infant relative to the placenta. Delaying cord clamping by more than 1 minute after birth may allow blood to flow from placenta to baby, significantly increasing Hb levels and iron stores and stability of blood pressure.

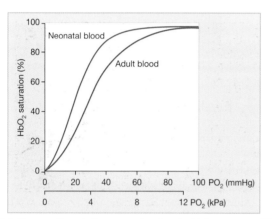

Fig. 54.1 Oxygen dissociation curve showing the higher oxygen affinity of neonatal than adult hemoglobin.

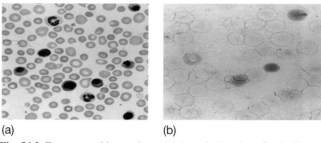

(a)   (b)

Fig. 54.3 Fetomaternal hemorrhage. (a) Anemia (number of red cells are reduced), nucleated red cells (erythroblasts) and reticulocytes on a blood smear (film) from a term neonate with severe anemia at birth (4.5 g/dL) due to fetomaternal hemorrhage. (b) Kleihauer test on maternal blood from of the same baby showing several intensely pink-stained cells containing HbF, which is resistant to acid lysis.

Clinical features (Table 54.1) and management

Blood transfusion

Kept to a minimum because of potential hazards unless there has been clinically significant blood loss, e.g placental abruption, placenta previa. Transfusion thresholds vary between neonatal units and are based on severity of illness of the infant and respiratory support required. Anemia of prematurity is considered in Chapter 34.

Oral folic acid

Given as prophylaxis if chronic hemolysis (e.g. hereditary spherocytosis). Some neonatal units prescribe it for VLBW infants for the first few months as their folate stores are low, the folate content of breast milk is low and there is increased demand from rapid growth.

Causes and investigation of anemia (Fig. 54.2)

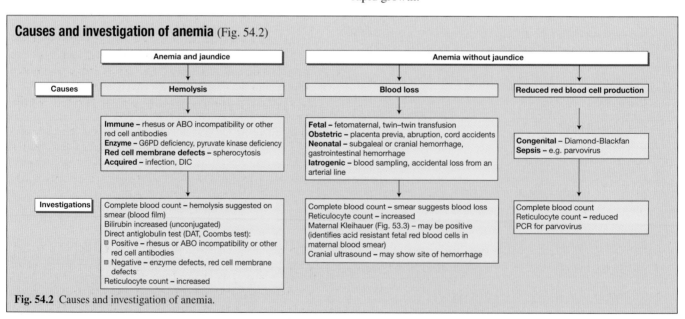

Anemia and jaundice		Anemia without jaundice	
Causes	Hemolysis	Blood loss	Reduced red blood cell production
	Immune – rhesus or ABO incompatibility or other red cell antibodies **Enzyme** – G6PD deficiency, pyruvate kinase deficiency **Red cell membrane defects** – spherocytosis **Acquired** – infection, DIC	**Fetal** – fetomaternal, twin–twin transfusion **Obstetric** – placenta previa, abruption, cord accidents **Neonatal** – subgaleal or cranial hemorrhage, gastrointestinal hemorrhage **Iatrogenic** – blood sampling, accidental loss from an arterial line	**Congenital** – Diamond-Blackfan **Sepsis** – e.g. parvovirus
Investigations	Complete blood count – hemolysis suggested on smear (blood film) Bilirubin increased (unconjugated) Direct antiglobulin test (DAT, Coombs test): ▪ Positive – rhesus or ABO incompatibility or other red cell antibodies ▪ Negative – enzyme defects, red cell membrane defects Reticulocyte count – increased	Complete blood count – smear suggests blood loss Reticulocyte count – increased Maternal Kleihauer (Fig. 53.3) – may be positive (identifies acid resistant fetal red blood cells in maternal blood smear) Cranial ultrasound – may show site of hemorrhage	Complete blood count Reticulocyte count – reduced PCR for parvovirus

Fig. 54.2 Causes and investigation of anemia.

Neonatology at a Glance, Third Edition. Edited by Tom Lissauer, Avroy A. Fanaroff, Lawrence Miall and Jonathan Fanaroff.
© 2016 John Wiley & Sons, Ltd. Published 2016 by John Wiley & Sons, Ltd.

Table 54.1 Clinical features of anemia.

History	Examination
History – blood loss	Pallor
Family history – anemia, jaundice, splenomegaly from hemolytic disease	Jaundice from hemolysis
	Apnea and bradycardia
	Tachycardia
Obstetric history – antepartum hemorrhage	Heart murmur – systolic flow murmur
Maternal blood type – rhesus or other red cell antibodies, potential for ABO incompatibility	Respiratory distress, heart failure
	Hepatomegaly and/or splenomegaly, hydrops
Ethnic origin – hemoglobinopathies and G6PD deficiency	Inadequate weight gain from poor feeding

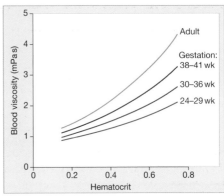

Fig. 54.4 Hematocrit is the main determinant of blood viscosity. Blood viscosity rises exponentially when hematocrit is >0.65.

Oral iron therapy

In preterm infants given after the age of 4–6 weeks to prevent anemia of prematurity. Not given if the infant has recently had a blood transfusion or is on iron-supplemented formula feeding.

Polycythemia

Usually defined as a venous hematocrit (Hct) above 0.65. The hematocrit depends on the site of sampling: capillary hematocrit > peripheral venous > central venous > arterial.

Potential danger of high hematocrit is hyperviscosity, which causes sludging of red blood cells and formation of microthrombi, leading to vascular occlusion (Fig. 54.4).

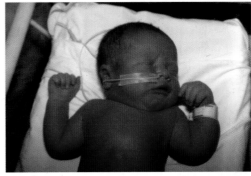

Fig. 54.5 Plethoric term infant. Nasogastric tube is because of poor feeding.

Causes

Increased erythropoietin production:
- Intrauterine hypoxia – IUGR (intrauterine growth restriction).
- Maternal diabetes.
- High altitude.

Trisomy 21 (Down syndrome)

Increased blood volume:
- Excessive placental transfusion from delayed cord clamping.
- Twin–twin transfusion.

Clinical features and complications (Table 54.2)

Table 54.2 Clinical features and complications of polycythemia.

Plethora (Fig. 54.5)	Respiratory distress
Hypoglycemia/hypocalcemia	Heart failure
Irritability, lethargy, seizures	Intestinal – necrotizing enterocolitis
Poor feeding	Renal – renal vein thrombosis, hematuria, oliguria
Hyperbilirubinemia	
Priapism	Thrombocytopenia
	Neurologic impairment.

Treatment

Treatment is to reduce the hematocrit by replacing a proportion of the infant's blood with 0.9% saline (plasma is no longer used to minimize blood product usage), by partial exchange transfusion (see Chapter 78).

As treatment has not been shown to be of long-term benefit, criteria are controversial:
- venous hematocrit > 0.65 and infant symptomatic or hematocrit > 0.70 even if asymptomatic – generally agreed that a partial dilutional exchange transfusion should be performed.
- If venous hematocrit 0.65–0.70 and asymptomatic – observe and treat only if becomes symptomatic.

Question

Should all babies be screened for polycythemia?

Screening all infants is not recommended because of lack of evidence of benefit of treatment (American Academy of Pediatrics).

55 Neutrophil and thrombotic disorders

Neutrophil disorders

There is a physiologic rise in neutrophils between 12 and 24 hours of life and thereafter the number falls (Fig. 55.1).

Neutrophilia

The most common causes are:
- acute bacterial infection
- maternal chorioamnionitis (usually without active infection in the baby).

Much less common causes are fungal infection and postnatal corticosteroid therapy. When neutrophilia is accompanied by a left shift, i.e. increase in immature neutrophils, such as band forms (Fig. 55.2), it is used as a marker for bacterial infection. The combination of an abnormal absolute neutrophil count and immature:total neutrophil ratio increases the likelihood of infection to about 65%. Neutrophilia from bacterial infections often develops 12–24 hours after the onset of infection. Serial measurements are more informative than isolated values. However, interpretation of the blood smear requires technical expertise. In the UK band counts have largely been replaced by measuring acute phase reactants (C-reactive protein or procalcitonin). In many units in the US both band counts and acute phase reactants are measured.

Neutropenia

This is a neutrophil count of less than 1500 cells/mm^3 (1.5×10^9/L). Neutropenia is usually caused by sepsis, necrotizing enterocolitis, cytomegalovirus (CMV) and other congenital infections, intrauterine growth restriction (IUGR), maternal preeclampsia and the chromosome trisomies (13, 18 and 21). Alloimmune neutropenia and inherited causes are uncommon. Most types of neonatal neutropenia are self-limiting and treatment is primarily of the underlying cause. Intravenous immunoglobulin is non-specific and has not been shown to be beneficial. The recombinant hematopoietic growth factor, G-CSF (granulocyte colony stimulating factor) will increase the neutrophil count, but has not been shown to improve outcome, except in the rare disorder severe congenital neutropenia. White cell transfusions are rarely effective.

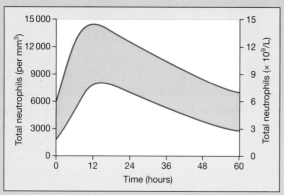

Fig. 55.1 Total neutrophil count, showing the rise with age and the normal range. (From Manroe B.L. *et al. J Pediatr* 1979; **95:** 89–98.)

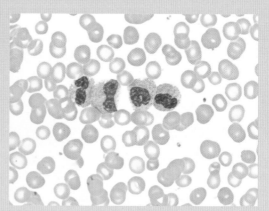

Fig. 55.2 Blood smear showing four neutrophil 'band' cells in a neonate with bacterial sepsis. The 'band' cells also show toxic granulation in the cytoplasm, another useful sign of acute bacterial infection.

Neonatology at a Glance, Third Edition. Edited by Tom Lissauer, Avroy A. Fanaroff, Lawrence Miall and Jonathan Fanaroff.
© 2016 John Wiley & Sons, Ltd. Published 2016 by John Wiley & Sons, Ltd.

Thrombotic disorders (thrombophilia)

These are a group of disorders characterized by an increased tendency for abnormal clot formation. Thrombosis occurs in approximately 5 per 100 000 births; 50% of episodes are arterial and 50% are venous.

Predisposing factors

These are:
- indwelling catheters (80–90% of episodes)
- acute bacterial and viral infection
- asphyxia (ischemia), shock
- cardiac abnormality
- polycythemia
- prematurity
- twin–twin transfusion
- genetic.

Maternal and familial conditions associated with thrombophilia

These include:
- multiple fetal losses
- anticardiolipin antibodies
- SLE (systemic lupus erythematosus)
- maternal diabetes
- placental abruption
- myocardial infarction
- deep venous thrombosis
- pulmonary embolism.

Inherited causes of thrombosis

Gene mutations have been identified for some of the most common thrombotic disorders:
- protein C deficiency (Fig. 55.3)
- protein S deficiency
- antithrombin deficiency
- factor V Leiden mutation (APC resistance)
- prothrombin gene mutation.

Diagnosis

Most thrombi are asymptomatic.

Clinical signs of thrombosis depend on location of the clot, which may embolize:
- Arterial – limb may become mottled in color, cool and discolored with reduced pulses. In time may become gangrenous with zone of demarcation (see Fig. 66.5). Thrombus in aorta may lead to heart failure or stroke.
- Venous – portal vein, renal vein thrombosis causing abdominal mass, hematuria, oliguria and hypertension. Thrombus in right atrium may lead to stroke.

Imaging
Depends on site:
- Ultrasound, echocardiography, MRI for diagnosis and follow-up.
- Angiography is the gold standard but may become difficult or impossible to perform or not justified, e.g. for stroke. MR angiography is now available.

Management

Options include:
- If catheter-related, may be due to arterial spasm or too large a catheter or hypovolemia. If does not respond promptly to partial withdrawal of the catheter or correction of hypovolemia, the catheter should be removed.
- Observe and follow up for increase in clot size and functional compromise.
- Anticoagulation with unfractionated or low molecular weight heparin (e.g. enoxaparin).
- Clot lysis with fibrinolytic agents (tissue plasminogen activator), but contraindicated if there has been a recent intraventricular hemorrhage.
- Surgical thrombectomy – rarely required or possible.
- Factor concentrate if thrombosis and inherited deficiency (e.g. protein C, antithrombin).

> ### Question
>
> **Which neonates should be screened for inherited thrombophilia?**
>
> Any neonate with clinically significant thrombosis, e.g. severe purpura, renal vein thrombosis, extensive thrombosis or a family history of severe neonatal purpura.

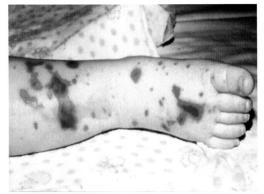

Fig. 55.3 Infant with microthrombi in the skin from protein C deficiency.

56 Coagulation disorders

In the newborn, abnormal bleeding may be due to:
- a platelet abnormality (number or function)
- abnormal coagulation system
- vascular endothelial damage/abnormality.

Thrombocytopenia

This is the most common platelet disorder. It is defined as a platelet count of less than $150\,000/mm^3$ ($150 \times 10^9/L$). It is usually identified on the complete blood count (CBC), but, if severe, may cause petechiae (Fig. 56.1) or bleeding.

A convenient classification is according to the time of onset (Table 56.1). The most common causes are maternal pre-eclampsia and diabetes mellitus, intrauterine growth restriction and neonatal infection.

Treatment is directed to the underlying cause.

For infants who are sick or septic, where production may be compromised, platelet transfusion is considered if:
- platelets $<30\,000/mm^3$ ($30 \times 10^9/L$) in term infants
- platelets $<50\,000/mm^3$ ($50 \times 10^9/L$) in preterm infants
- if actively bleeding or before surgery, platelets $<100\,000/mm^3$ ($100 \times 10^9/L$).

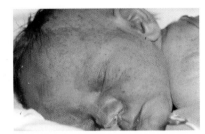

Fig. 56.1 Petechiae from thrombocytopenia in an infant.

Abnormal coagulation

Coagulation factors are a group of proteins that when activated will promote the formation of a fibrin-rich clot or hemostatic plug (Fig. 56.2). These proteins are formed early in gestation in the fetus and do not cross the placenta.

The most common acquired cause of coagulopathy is a combination of coagulation activation and poor liver reserve in a sick or septic infant.

Deficiency of certain coagulation factors will lead to bleeding disorders (Table 56.2).

Indications for performing clotting studies

These are:
- family history of bleeding disorder
- clinical signs of abnormal bleeding:
  - oozing from venepuncture/surgical sites
  - bleeding umbilical cord stump
  - extensive bruising or large cephalhematoma or subgaleal (subaponeurotic) bleed
  - gastrointestinal bleeding
- septic infant
- necrotizing enterocolitis

Table 56.1 Classification of fetal and neonatal thrombocytopenia (most common causes in bold type).

Time of presentation	Condition
Fetus	**Neonatal alloimmune thrombocytopenia (NAITP)**
	Maternal autoimmune thrombocytopenia (ITP, SLE)
	Congenital infection (CMV, rubella, herpes, syphilis)
	Severe rhesus disease
	Chromosome abnormalities (trisomy 21, 18, 13)
	Inherited (very rare)
Neonatal (<72 h)	**Placental insufficiency (PIH, IUGR, diabetes)**
	Neonatal infection
	Birth asphyxia
	Neonatal alloimmune thrombocytopenia (NAITP)
	Maternal autoimmune thrombocytopenia (ITP, SLE)
	Thrombosis (renal vein, aortic)
	Congenital infection (CMV, rubella, herpes, syphilis)
	Inherited (very rare)
Neonatal (>72 h)	**Late-onset bacterial infection, necrotizing enterocolitis**
	Disseminated intravascular coagulation (DIC)
	Giant hemangioma (Kasabach–Merritt syndrome)

ITP, idiopathic thrombocytopenic purpura; SLE, systemic lupus erythematosus; CMV, cytomegalovirus; PIH, pregnancy-induced hypertension; IUGR, intrauterine growth restriction.
Adapted from Murray N. *Semin Neonatol* 1999; **4**: 27–40.

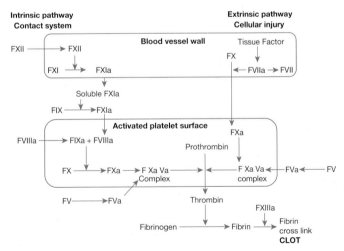

Fig. 56.2 The coagulation pathway.

Neonatology at a Glance, Third Edition. Edited by Tom Lissauer, Avroy A. Fanaroff, Lawrence Miall and Jonathan Fanaroff.
© 2016 John Wiley & Sons, Ltd. Published 2016 by John Wiley & Sons, Ltd.

Table 56.2 Bleeding disorders.

Deficiency	Disorder	Comments
Vitamin K	Vitamin K deficient bleeding (VKDB) (Hemorrhagic disease of newborn)	Deficiency of vitamin K-dependent coagulation factors (factors II, VII, IX and X) Associated with breast-feeding or severe liver disease in the infant or maternal use of anticonvulsants
Factor VIII	Classic hemophilia A	X-linked inheritance – positive family history in 80%. Mild and moderate forms usually asymptomatic during the newborn period, but 20% of cases present in the newborn, usually after circumcision or other surgery. Severe form may result in life-threatening hemorrhage
Factor IX	Christmas disease – hemophilia B	X-linked inheritance. Similar presentation to hemophilia A
Von Willebrand factor	Von Willebrand disease	Most common inherited bleeding disorder Autosomal dominant inheritance Only rare subtypes present in the newborn period

- rapidly falling platelet counts in a sick infant
- severe hypoxic–ischemic encephalopathy.

Investigations

Coagulation screen consists of:
- PT (prothrombin time)
- APTT (activated partial thromboplastin time)
- TT (thrombin time).
  May include:
- fibrinogen
- D-dimers – a measure of fibrin breakdown, may be useful for diagnosis of disseminated intravascular coagulation (DIC).

Interpretation of abnormal clotting studies (Table 56.3)

The normal values for preterm and term infants are derived locally, as different hospitals use different assays.

The coagulation values in preterm and term neonates differ significantly from older children and adults:
- Prothrombin time tends to be a few seconds longer at birth but will reach the normal adult range within a week.
- Activated partial thromboplastin time may not reach adult normal range for several months because of low levels of the 'liver' factors (e.g. IX, XI, XII).

- Thrombin time may be slightly prolonged in early life due to the presence of a fetal form of fibrinogen. This is of no clinical significance.

Management of abnormal clotting

If there is active bleeding a correct diagnosis must be established. Vitamin K should be given while results are awaited, and fresh-frozen plasma (FFP) if there is severe bleeding. Intramuscular injections must **not** be given to any neonate with a known or suspected major coagulation disorder (e.g. hemophilia), and care must also be taken after venepuncture and/or heelprick testing in such babies – pressure for >5 minutes is recommended.

If there is disseminated intravascular coagulation (DIC), treat the underlying cause. In the interim, platelets, FFP and cryoprecipitate (only if the fibrinogen level is low) may be indicated. Their need is determined by the coagulation tests, which should be repeated regularly as this is an evolving disorder.

FFP contains all coagulation factors and is suitable for emergencies, but does not contain sufficient of any single factor for severe single factor deficiencies. Replacement by a suitable concentrate is optimal, once a firm diagnosis has been established.

Severe congenital coagulation factor deficiencies – consult pediatric hematologist.

Table 56.3 Interpretation of abnormal clotting studies.

Test	Vitamin K deficiency	DIC	Liver impairment	Hemophilias
Platelets	Normal	Reduced	Normal	Normal
PT	Prolonged	Prolonged	Prolonged	Normal
PTT	Prolonged	Prolonged	Prolonged	Prolonged
TT	Normal	Prolonged	Prolonged	Normal
Fibrinogen	Normal	Reduced	Reduced	Normal

The prothrombin time (PT) may be reported by some laboratories in the form of an INR (international normalized ratio). Although this may be useful for adults, the INR is not a reliable measure of coagulation for neonates. PTT, partial thromboplastin time; TT, thrombin time.

Question

What is special about taking blood samples for coagulation studies?

Blood sample must be free-flowing. Squeezed and slow-flowing samples cause tissue activation and can give abnormal results, including a normal result in a baby with severe hemophilia.

If the sample is taken from a heparinized line, it may not be possible to interpret the thrombin time. Instead, fibrinogen levels and reptilase time must be used as they are unaffected by heparin.

If an inherited coagulation disorder is suspected, it is advisable to test the parents as well as the baby since neonatal coagulation tests are often difficult to interpret.

57 Dermatological disorders

Functions of the skin include:
- mechanical protection
- barrier against microorganisms and toxins
- thermoregulation and fluid balance
- sensory input and tactile communication with the environment.

There are marked differences in the structure and function of the skin of preterm infants, term infants and adults (Table 57.1).

Goals of neonatal skin care

- Avoid traumatic injury during routine care.
- Prevent skin dryness leading to cracking and fissures.
- Minimize exposure to topical agents that are potentially toxic when absorbed (Table 57.2).

Diaper (nappy) dermatitis

Much less of a problem since disposable diapers (nappies) used.
- Keep skin dry with super-absorbent diapers and frequent changes.
- Treat underlying cause-of excessive stooling, such as infectious diarrhea, malabsorption, opiate withdrawal.
- Apply zinc oxide and pectin paste barriers liberally to excoriated skin to prevent reinjury from fecal enzymes and allow skin to heal.
- Add 1% hydrocortisone if unresponsive.
- Identify candida dermatitis with distinctive pattern of redness on perineum, groin and thighs, and red pustular satellite lesions; apply antifungal ointment or cream. Consider oral antifungal treatment if mouth lesions present.

Table 57.2 Toxicity reported from topical antiseptic use in preterm infants.

Antiseptic	Toxicity
Hexachlorophene	Spongiform encephalopathy
Povidone-iodine	Hypothyroidism, goiter
Chlorhexidine in alcohol	Scalds (avoid alcohol containing solution in extreme preterm)

Question

What is the significance of a pustular rash in a newborn infant?

There is a wide differential diagnosis. By far the most common cause is erythema toxicum, which typically presents within the first week with new lesions rapidly appearing at different sites. Transient pustular melanosis may be present at birth and has a scaly halo around the pustule. Both are benign.

Herpes simplex infection and disseminated staphylococcal aureus infection - uncommon, but should be considered, especially if the infant is at all unwell.

Infection

- **Bacterial** – bullous impetigo, staphylococcal scalded skin syndrome (SSSS) (see Chapter 43).
- **Viral** – herpes simplex virus infection (see Chapter 44), CMV and rubella (see Chapter 11).
- **Fungal** – (see Chapter 34).

Table 57.1 Developmental differences between the skin of infants and adults.

Developmental differences	Significance
Stratum corneum *Term infants and adults:* 10–20 layers *<30 weeks of gestation:* 2–4 layers *24 weeks of gestation:* virtually no stratum corneum. Also, diminished cohesion between epidermis and dermis as fewer fibrils	*Preterm infants, susceptible to:* • evaporative and transepidermal water loss • transcutaneously transmitted infection and toxicity from topical agents • epidermal stripping with adhesives
Dermis *Term* – only 60% the depth of adults *Preterm* – even thinner dermis, less collagen and fewer fibrils	*Preterm* – excess fluid (edema) accumulates in the dermis, which is prone to injury
Sweating *Term* – limited ability during first few days *Preterm* – unable to sweat before 31 weeks' gestational age in response to heat, although sweat glands are present Emotional sweating of hands and feet – present at term, poorly developed in preterm infants	Thermal sweating in adults is important to avoid overheating, but newborn infants cannot do this Emotional sweating to measure response to pain – can be used in term infants, but not in preterm

Neonatology at a Glance, Third Edition. Edited by Tom Lissauer, Avroy A. Fanaroff, Lawrence Miall and Jonathan Fanaroff.
© 2016 John Wiley & Sons, Ltd. Published 2016 by John Wiley & Sons, Ltd.

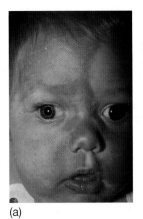
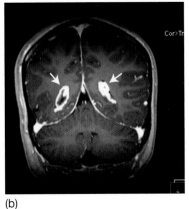

(a)   (b)

Fig. 57.1 (a) Port wine stain with trigeminal distribution (Sturge-Weber syndrome). (b) MRI scan following gadolinium administration showing choroidal enhancement from choroidal angiomas (arrows). Neuroimaging is only performed in infancy if specific ocular or neurological abnormalities are present. (MRI scan courtesy of Dr Sheila Berlin.)

Vascular skin lesions

Port wine stain (nevus flammeus)

Present at birth in 0.3% of newborns. Most often on the face. Permanent malformation of the capillaries in the dermis. Laser therapy may improve the appearance of disfiguring lesions.

Rare associations:
• trigeminal nerve distribution (Sturge–Weber syndrome) associated with intracranial vascular anomaly in 10% (Fig. 57.1a & b)
• severe limb and bone hypertrophy – (Klippel–Trenaunay syndrome).

Strawberry nevus (hemangioma)

Not usually present at birth. Appears in first month of life (Fig. 57.2). Preterm infants at increased risk. Increases in size until 8–18 months of age then gradually regresses. No treatment is indicated unless lesions are large with potential for disfigurement, ulcerating, threaten vital function e.g. vision, hearing, breathing or feeding. Oral propranolol, sometimes combined with laser therapy, has replaced corticosteroids as the treatment of choice for complicated lesions. Recently, topical beta-blocker therapy applied directly to the lesion has been shown to be beneficial.

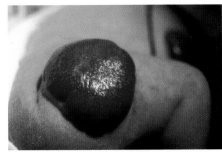

Fig. 57.2 Strawberry nevus. (Courtesy of Dr David Clark.)

Congenital melanocytic nevus (CMN) (pigmented nevus)

Small lesions (<1.5 cm) – observe; may remove when older for cosmetic reasons. Small but possible increased risk in malignant melanoma; this contrasts with the much higher risk in giant lesions (>20 cm) (Fig. 57.3), which are usually treated aggressively by surgical removal.

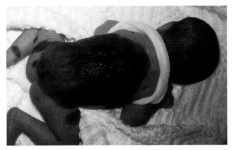

Fig. 57.3 Giant congenital melanocytic nevus (GCMN). Rare but serious condition because of 5–15% risk of malignant melanoma in first decade of life. The lesion may be hairy and satellite lesions are often present.

Genetic syndromes

There are a large number of rare conditions (Table 57.3).

Table 57.3 Some skin lesions associated with genetic syndromes.

Skin lesion	Diagnostic group
Unformed skin	Aplasia cutis (absent patch of skin ± bony defect); may be associated with trisomy 13
Thin skin	Dermal hypoplasia, collagen disorders
Blisters/erosions	Bullous disorders, e.g. epidermolysis bullosa (Fig. 57.4)
Thick/scaly skin	Ichthyoses, e.g. collodion infant, or more severe, harlequin ichthyosis
White skin/hair	Pigment deficient disorders, e.g. oculocutaneous albinism, piebaldism, tuberous sclerosis
Palpable brown patches	Syndromes with melanocytic nevi
Flat brown patches	Syndromes with café-au-lait macules, e.g. neurofibromatosis
Deficient hair, nails, sweat	Ectodermal dysplasias. Syndromes with abnormal hair

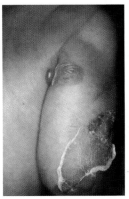

Fig. 57.4 Epidermolysis bullosa. Rare group of disorders. Bullae, or blisters, are caused by trauma or friction to the skin. There are scarring and non-scarring subgroups. (Courtesy of Prof. Julian Verbov.)

58 Seizures and perinatal strokes

Seizures (Table 58.1)

Table 58.1 Recognition, causes, investigation and management of seizures.

Recognition (see video: Seizures)	Seizures may present with clonic or tonic involuntary movements of one or more limbs. Often difficult to recognize with certainty, as manifestations are often subtle: • apnea or transient cyanosis, or episodes of oxygen desaturation • lip smacking • transient eye rolling, altered consciousness, floppiness.

Causes

Cerebral	Metabolic	Sepsis	Drugs	Others
Hypoxic–ischemic: • encephalopathy, birth trauma, • focal ischemia (arterial/venous) Subarachnoid or subdural hemorrhage Parenchymal hemorrhage in preterm infants Cerebral malformations of the brain, including vascular anomalies	Hypoglycemia Hypocalcemia Hypomagnesemia Hyponatremia Hypernatremia Hyperammonemia Inborn errors of metabolism	Septicemia Meningitis Encephalitis	Drug withdrawal: • maternal abuse • following neonatal narcotic therapy Side-effect of drugs	Kernicterus Pyridoxine dependent Benign genetic seizure disorders

Investigations

Always performed	EEG	To be considered
Blood glucose (immediate at bedside) Blood urea nitrogen (urea) and electrolytes Calcium and magnesium Complete blood count Blood cultures Lumbar puncture – protein, glucose, gram stain and culture Blood gases Cranial ultrasound to identify hemorrhage or parietal infarcts or cerebral malformation or abnormalities (may miss subarachnoid hemorrhage)	Multichannel EEG (Fig. 58.1) or aEEG (amplitude integrated EEG), preferably with video observation (See Fig. 14.4 for seizures on aEEG and Chapter 80 on aEEG.)	CT to identify hemorrhage, traumatic injury MRI to identify ischemia, malformations Metabolic screen – plasma for ammonia, amino acids, lactate; urine for amino acids and organic acids Screen for congenital infection Urine for drug toxicology Specific biochemical tests in suspected neurometabolic conditions

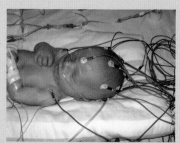

Fig. 58.1 EEG being performed.

Management	Airway, Breathing, Circulation. Check for hypoglycemia. Anticonvulsants: • Administer if seizure is prolonged (more than about 5 minutes) or clusters. Controversy about how aggressively to treat electrical seizures (seizures on EEG or aEEG but no clinical manifestations) • No drug shown to be superior to others. Those used include phenobarbital (most common first-line drug), phenytoin, levetiracetam, midazolam, clonazepam, lidocaine (lignocaine; with ECG monitoring). • Acute seizures often respond poorly. • Use as few anticonvulsants as possible. • Treat the underlying cause, if possible, e.g. sepsis. • If unresponsive to treatment, consider therapeutic trial of pyridoxine.
Prognosis	Depends on cause. Epilepsy in 15–20% and abnormal neurodevelopment in 25%. Poor prognosis – if poor response to initial anticonvulsant treatment, abnormal EEG background and presence of electro-clinical dissociation on EEG. If caused by acute brain insult, most seizures resolve and anticonvulsant therapy can usually be slowly withdrawn. If maintenance anticonvulsant therapy required – is usually with phenobarbital, clonazepam or sodium valproate.

Neonatology at a Glance, Third Edition. Edited by Tom Lissauer, Avroy A. Fanaroff, Lawrence Miall and Jonathan Fanaroff.
© 2016 John Wiley & Sons, Ltd. Published 2016 by John Wiley & Sons, Ltd.

Perinatal strokes

Defined as cerebral injury from vascular cause that originates between 20 weeks of gestation and 28 days of life. Occurs in as many as 0.2–1 per 1000 live births.

Types
- Perinatal arterial ischemic stroke (PAIS) – the most common site is left middle cerebral artery.
- Hemorrhage – may be parenchymal, subarachnoid or intraventricular.
- Cerebral sinovenous thrombosis (CSVT) – can cause venous infarction, often with hemorrhage.

Based on neuroimaging, strokes may be classified as fetal if diagnosed before birth, neonatal if diagnosed in the first 4 weeks of life or presumed perinatal ischemic stroke (PPIS) if diagnosed after 28 days of life.

Etiology
Complex and multifactorial. Often no maternal, fetal or neonatal risk factors can be identified.

Perinatal arterial ischemic stroke (PAIS) may be due to thrombo-embolism. The emboli may originate from thrombosis of placental vessels, from venous thrombi that cross the patent foramen ovale, from right-to-left shunts in congenital heart disease and from thrombi from umbilical vessel catheters. Sepsis or meningitis, trauma and prothrombotic disorders, e.g. protein C or protein S deficiency, may also contribute. Further details of prothrombotic disorders are considered in Chapter 56, Coagulation disorders. The contribution of maternal risk factors and intrapartum events is unclear.

Hemorrhagic stroke may result from intraparenchymal hemorrhage from vascular anomalies or hemorrhage into ischemic infarction; periventricular hemorrhagic infarction is associated with intraventricular hemorrhage in extremely preterm infants.

In cerebral sinovenous thrombosis (CSVT), perinatal complications such as hypoxia or prolonged rupture of membranes or maternal infection may be present. Head trauma during birth and prothrombotic disorders are other risk factors.

Clinical presentation
Most often with seizures within the first 3 days of life, usually focal but can be non-specific. Some present with encephalopathy. Many are asymptomatic in the neonatal period.

Specific investigations
- Cranial ultrasound is abnormal in most infants, but is not always diagnostic.
- MRI scan for accurate diagnosis and prognosis (Fig. 58.2).
- In focal cerebral infarction, investigations to rule out underlying thrombophilic disorders are indicated.

Management
Treatment of seizures with anticonvulsants and supportive therapy. The role of anticoagulation for neonates with cerebral venous thrombosis is controversial.

Prognosis
Nearly 50% of infants with perinatal stroke develop motor disability, often a hemiplegia on the contralateral side presenting in infancy or childhood, and cognitive dysfunction. Occipital lesions may be associated with visual impairment. Large lesions may lead to epilepsy.

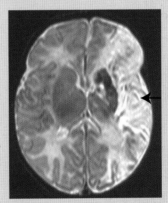

Fig. 58.2 MRI scan showing left cerebral infarct (see arrow). (Courtesy of Dr Frances Cowan.)

59 Neural tube defects and hydrocephalus

Neural tube defects

In the embryo, the flat neural plate folds to become the brain and spinal cord. Neural tube defects (NTDs) arise from a deficiency in this process:
• anencephaly – from failure of cranial development of most of the cranium and brain
• spina bifida – from failure of caudal development of the vertebral bodies
• midline defects – from failure of fusion, e.g. of the skull as an encephalocele.

Most are now diagnosed antenatally, by ultrasound or α-fetoprotein measurement in maternal serum.

Prevalence

NTDs result from a combination of environmental and genetic factors. The risk of having a second affected child is 3–5% and of a third 5–10%. The risk is increased 10–20-fold in mothers taking valproate. In the US, 7 per 10 000 pregnancies are affected, with a birth prevalence of 4 per 10 000 live births, and in the UK, 12 per 10 000 pregnancies, with a birth prevalence of 2 per 10 000 live births.

Maternal folic acid supplementation pre- and periconceptually and during early pregnancy has been shown to reduce prevalence. In the US, but not in the UK or most countries in Western Europe, cereal grain products are fortified with folic acid.

The prevalence of affected infants has decreased markedly over the last 30 years, with better maternal nutrition, folic acid supplements, food fortification in the US, prenatal screening with maternal ultrasound and raised maternal serum a-fetoprotein together with the option of termination of pregnancy.

Trial of open fetal surgery for myelomeningocele is described in Chapter 4.

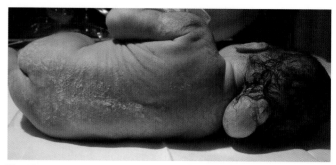

Fig. 59.1 Occipital encephalocele.

Anencephaly

The condition is lethal; most are stillborn. There has been considerable debate about the ethics of the use of their organs for donor transplantation. However, the situation rarely arises because few anencephalic infants are now born as most are diagnosed antenatally and parents opt for termination of pregnancy.

Encephalocele

Herniation of sac containing CSF and may contain brain, through a midline skull defect. Most are occipital (Fig. 59.1). Developmental impairment is likely if brain tissue is in the sac or there are other cerebral malformations.

Spina bifida

There is a spectrum, of increasing severity:
• spina bifida occulta (Fig. 59.2a)
• meningocele (Fig. 59.2b)
• myelomeningocele (Figs 59.2c and d).

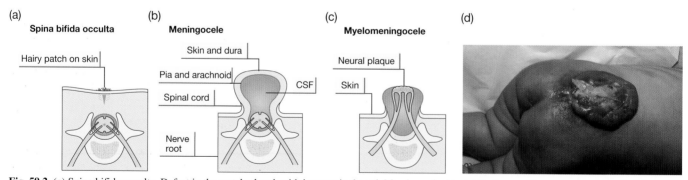

Fig. 59.2 (a) Spina bifida occulta. Defect in the vertebral arch with intact spinal cord. May be an incidental finding on X-rays – asymptomatic. More extensive lesions indicated by overlying patch of hair or nevus or other skin abnormality. (b) Meningocele. Bony defect with herniation of meninges but not the spinal cord. The lesion is covered with skin. (c) Myelomeningocele. Defect in the lumbar or thoracic spine with herniation of the meningeal sac and spinal cord tissue with leakage of CSF. (d) Photograph of myelomeningocele (myelo = cord; meninges = covering, cele = sac) showing exposed neural tissue and patulous, neuropathic anus.

Neonatology at a Glance, Third Edition. Edited by Tom Lissauer, Avroy A. Fanaroff, Lawrence Miall and Jonathan Fanaroff.
© 2016 John Wiley & Sons, Ltd. Published 2016 by John Wiley & Sons, Ltd.

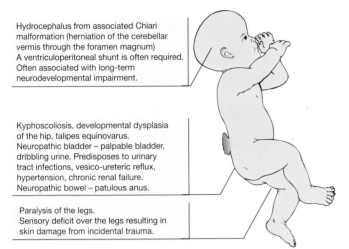

Hydrocephalus from associated Chiari malformation (herniation of the cerebellar vermis through the foramen magnum) A ventriculoperitoneal shunt is often required. Often associated with long-term neurodevelopmental impairment.

Kyphoscoliosis, developmental dysplasia of the hip, talipes equinovarus. Neuropathic bladder – palpable bladder, dribbling urine. Predisposes to urinary tract infections, vesico-ureteric reflux, hypertension, chronic renal failure. Neuropathic bowel – patulous anus.

Paralysis of the legs. Sensory deficit over the legs resulting in skin damage from incidental trauma.

Fig. 59.3 Complications associated with severe myelomeningocele. These depend on the extent and level of the lesion.

Spina bifida occulta

Spina bifida occulta is often suggested by a skin lesion over the lower spine and is confirmed with further diagnostic imagining such as spinal ultrasound and/or MRI. Usually, there is no neurologic deficit at birth but tethering of the spinal cord may occur during childhood. Neurosurgical opinion should be obtained. May be an incidental finding on X-rays.

Meningocele

Prognosis following surgery is usually good.

Myelomeningocele

Wide range of complications (Fig. 59.3). Most lesions are detected antenatally and a management plan made before the baby is born.

Management requires an extensive multidisciplinary team (pediatrics, orthopedics, neurosurgery, urology, child development) working with the family.

The back lesion is usually closed immediately after birth to minimize the risk of infection and surveillance performed for hydrocephalus.

Hydrocephalus

This is from an excessive volume of cerebrospinal fluid (CSF). It is usually from blockage of CSF flow or a defect in CSF reabsorption.

Causes

Congenital
- Aqueduct stenosis.
- Chiari malformation.
- Atresia of outflow foramina of fourth ventricle (Dandy–Walker syndrome).
- Congenital infection.

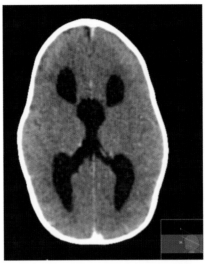

Fig. 59.4 CT scan axial view showing ventricular dilatation in a term infant with aqueductal stenoisis. (Courtesy of Dr Sheila Berlin.)

Acquired
- Post-intraventricular hemorrhage in preterm infants.
- Post-intracranial infection.
- Post-subdural/subarachnoid hemorrhage.

Clinical features

- Ventricular dilatation on imaging precedes symptoms or signs (Fig. 59.4).
- Increasing head circumference.
- Separation of sutures.
- Vomiting.
- Apnea, abnormal muscle tone, seizures, depressed consciousness.
- Dilatation of head veins.
- Sun-downing sign (setting-sun sign, eyes deviate downwards).
- Full then bulging fontanel.

Monitoring and treatment

In neonates, hydrocephalus is monitored by serial cranial ultrasound measurements of ventricular size and head circumference (See Chapter 79, Cranial ultrasound).

If severe and progressive or the infant becomes symptomatic, a ventriculoperitoneal shunt is inserted surgically. It carries a significant complication rate.

Hydrocephalus in preterm infants

Usually secondary to intraventricular hemorrhage causing fibrosis and impaired CSF reabsorption. Ventricular dilatation may need treatment if progressing rapidly or causing symptoms. Ventriculoperitoneal shunt insertion in small infants may be delayed because of the risk of skin breakdown or shunt blockage if the CSF protein is high. Instead, CSF may be removed by lumbar or ventricular puncture or from a neurosurgically inserted reservoir. No difference in long-term outcome between repeated lumbar/ventricular taps compared with removal of CSF only when symptomatic. Intraventricular fibrinolytics and acetazolamide, which reduce CSF production, have not been shown to be of benefit.

60 The hypotonic infant

The 'hypotonic infant' describes marked hypotonia or floppiness, i.e. less resistance to passive movement than normal, and is usually accompanied by muscle weakness (Fig. 60.1a, b and c). The cause of the hypotonia is either:
- **central** – central nervous system, or
- **peripheral** – lower motor neuron, neuromuscular junction or muscle disorders.

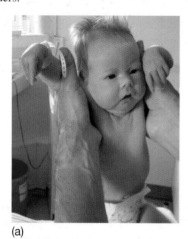

(a)

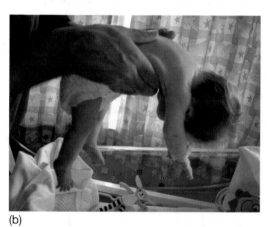

(b)

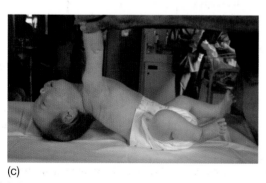

(c)

Fig. 60.1 (a) When held upright, the hypotonic infant slides through one's hands. (b) When held prone, the infant flops like a rag doll. (c) On traction of the arms, there is marked head lag.

Transient hypotonia may result from systemic infection, electrolyte disorders, hypermagnesemia, seizures or drugs administered to the infant or mother. Preterm infants have reduced tone and strength compared to term infants. These circumstances are not considered in this chapter.

Clues from the history

- Family history – consanguinity, unexplained deaths, multiple miscarriages.
- May be increasing severity with succeeding generations, e.g. muscular dystrophy.
- Clinical features in mother – ptosis in myasthenia gravis, absence of facial expression and weak grip in myotonic dystrophy and family history of cataracts.
- Pregnancy – polyhydramnios and reduced fetal movements.

Causes and clinical features (Table 60.1)

Table 60.1 Causes and clinical features of central and peripheral hypotonia.

	Central hypotonia	Peripheral hypotonia
Causes	Cerebral malformation Encephalopathy: • Hypoxic–ischemic encephalopathy • Meningitis/encephalitis • Hypoglycemia. Chromosomal/ syndromes: • Trisomy 21 (Down syndrome) • Prader–Willi syndrome Metabolic: • Hypothyroidism • Inborn errors of metabolism, e.g. hyperammonemia, amino acidopathy	Spinal cord injury Anterior horn cell: • Spinal muscular atrophy (Werdnig–Hoffmann syndrome) Neuromuscular junction: • Neonatal myasthenia gravis Muscles: • Congenital myopathies • Myotonic dystrophy
Clinical features	Antigravity movements present	Weak or absent antigravity movements from severe muscle weakness
	Normal or brisk tendon reflexes	Reduced or normal tendon reflexes
	Features of brain dysfunction may be present	Other features – see Fig. 60.2

Neonatology at a Glance, Third Edition. Edited by Tom Lissauer, Avroy A. Fanaroff, Lawrence Miall and Jonathan Fanaroff.
© 2016 John Wiley & Sons, Ltd. Published 2016 by John Wiley & Sons, Ltd.

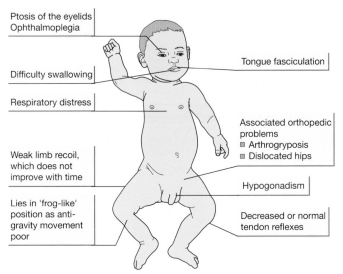

- Ptosis of the eyelids
- Ophthalmoplegia
- Difficulty swallowing
- Respiratory distress
- Weak limb recoil, which does not improve with time
- Lies in 'frog-like' position as anti-gravity movement poor
- Tongue fasciculation
- Associated orthopedic problems
  - ▪ Arthrogryposis
  - ▪ Dislocated hips
- Hypogonadism
- Decreased or normal tendon reflexes

Fig. 60.2 Clinical features that may be present with a peripheral neuromuscular disorder.

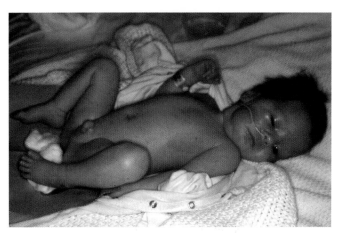

Fig. 60.3 Prader–Willi syndrome. Characteristic facies and hypogonadism. The nasogastric tube is required because of poor feeding. (Courtesy of Dr Mike Coren.)

Investigations

May include:
- karyotype/DNA analysis
- gene tests for specific disorders
- imaging of brain/spinal cord – MRI or ultrasound
- blood glucose, calcium, magnesium and lactate
- acid–base status, urine and plasma amino acids, urine organic acids, plasma ammonia, lactate, acylcarnitines, CSF lactate
- CPK (creatine phosphokinase) – raised in muscular dystrophy
- thyroid function tests
- congenital infection screening tests
- EMG (electromyogram)
- nerve conduction studies
- muscle biopsy.

Some specific conditions

Central

Hypoxic–ischemic encephalopathy
Hypotonia may be replaced by spasticity when older.

Prader–Willi syndrome
- 70% have partial chromosomal (15q) deletion (imprinting, where the deletion occurs on the active paternal chromosome 15 and the maternal copy is inactive). Also uniparental disomy (two maternal copies of the 15q region).
- Characteristic facies with narrow forehead, almond-shaped eyes and triangular mouth (Fig. 60.3).
- Hypotonia.
- Hypogonadism/cryptorchidism.
- Obesity after the neonatal period.
- Behavior problems, developmental delay.

Peripheral (rare)

Spinal muscular atrophy type 1 (Werdnig–Hoffmann syndrome)
- Autosomal recessive – anterior horn cell degeneration.
- Pregnancy – decreased or loss of fetal movements.
- At birth – arthrogryposis (contractures) may be present.
- Characteristic feature – fasciculation of tongue.
- Severe, progressive disorder, with death from respiratory failure during first year of life.
- DNA test available.

Neonatal myasthenia gravis
- Affects 10–20% of infants of mothers with myasthenia gravis.
- Transient condition, from maternal anti-acetylcholine IgG antibodies.
- Presentation – generalized weakness, facial diplegia, rarely ptosis, weak suck and cry, tendon reflexes normal.
- Use neostigmine, not tensilon, to confirm diagnosis.

Myotonic dystrophy
- Autosomal dominant – inherited from the mother (trinucleotide repeat expansion mutations). Earlier and more severe presentation in successive generations (anticipation).
- Pregnancy – polyhydramnios and decreased fetal movement.
- Neonate – weakness, edema and petechiae at birth with or without arthrogryposis.
- Facial diplegia, ptosis, tent-shaped mouth, talipes equinovarus.
- Brain abnormalities present in some forms of muscular dystrophies.
- Feeding difficulties due to poor gut motility.
- CPK may be elevated, EMG and biopsy are diagnostic.

Congenital myopathies
- Most are recessively inherited.
- Clinical features – weak, hypotonic, areflexic.
- Abnormal swallowing, normal extra-ocular movements.
- Muscle weakness usually slowly progressive.

61 Bone and joint disorders

Congenital abnormalities of the hip and feet

Developmental dysplasia of the hip, DDH

Hip is dislocatable, dislocated and/or has shallow acetabulum.

Incidence
- 6 per 1000 live births have abnormal clinical examination on screening.
- 0.5–2 per 1000 live births are treated.

Risk factors, clinical examination and initial management
These are described in Chapter 17.

Treatment
- Pavlik harness for 1–3 months (Fig. 61.1):
  - maintains flexion and abduction and limits adduction
  - redirects femoral head towards acetabulum.
- Orthoses or open reduction and derotation femoral osteotomy may be required.

Outcome
- 80–95% identified on screening do not need surgery.
- 5% of treated cases develop avascular necrosis (ischemic damage) of the femoral head.
- Impact of neonatal screening on need for surgery is uncertain.

Talipes equinovarus

Anatomy
Foot held in rigid equinovarus position (Fig. 61.2a and b). Needs to be distinguished from positional talipes (see Chapter 21).

Incidence
1 in 1000 live births. Bilateral in 50%.

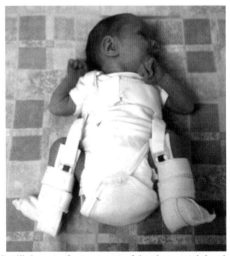

Fig. 61.1 Pavlik harness for treatment of developmental dysplasia of the hip.

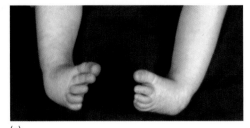

(a)

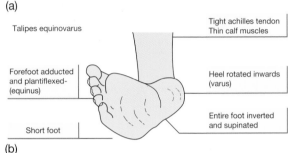

(b)

Fig. 61.2 (a and b) Talipes equinovarus. The foot is inverted and supinated and the forefoot is adducted. The affected foot is shorter and the calf muscles thinner than normal. The position of the foot is fixed and cannot be corrected by passive manipulation.

Risk factors
- Multifactorial inheritance.
- 3–4% risk if affected parent.
- 2% risk for subsequent siblings.
- May be secondary (20%):
  - oligohydramnios
  - neuromuscular disorder, e.g. spina bifida
  - malformation syndrome.
- May be associated with developmental dysplasia of the hip, but this has recently been questioned.

Management
- Refer to orthopedic surgeon as soon after birth as possible.
  Ponseti regimen now followed worldwide as highly successful and avoids surgical correction:
- Initially, foot is manipulated into the maximum position of correction and held in a plaster cast (Fig. 61.3). Changed regularly to correct deformity of the midfoot and forefoot.

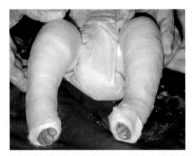

Fig. 61.3 Treatment of talipes equinovarus with serial plaster casts (courtesy of Mr Brian Scott).

Neonatology at a Glance, Third Edition. Edited by Tom Lissauer, Avroy A. Fanaroff, Lawrence Miall and Jonathan Fanaroff.
© 2016 John Wiley & Sons, Ltd. Published 2016 by John Wiley & Sons, Ltd.

- If foot still in equinus position, Achilles tenotomy performed.
- If correction is complete, "boots and bar" to hold feet abducted, externally rotated and dorsiflexed, worn all the time for about 3 months, then at night until 4 years old.
- Monitor for recurrence. Tibialis anterior tendon transfer may be required for supination of the forefoot.
- Foot should be supple and corrected; may be smaller and calf thinner than unaffected side.

Infection

Septic arthritis

- Rare in newborn.
- Usually via extension from underlying bone infection, rather than primary infection of the joint but can be from hematogenous spread.

Signs
- Decreased joint movement.
- Joint is swollen, warm, red (Fig. 61.4). Effusion may be present.

Diagnosis
Joint aspiration for cell count, >50 000 white blood cells/mm^3 (>50 white blood cells × 10^9/L), Gram stain, culture.

Imaging
- Ultrasound – fluid in joint space.
- Radionuclide bone scan, if indicated – hot spot.
- MRI scan of bone if necessary.
  Plain X-ray is of limited value – may show widened joint space.

Treatment
- Single or repeated joint aspiration.
- Surgical drainage of hip joint if no improvement.
- Antibiotics – prolonged course for 3–6 weeks.

Long-term complications
- Erosion of articular surface. Joint ankylosis.

Osteomyelitis

- Rare in newborn.
- Most are hematogenous in origin, in metaphysis.
- Usually presents within first 2 weeks of life.

Pathogens
Commonest are *Staphylococcus aureus* and streptococci.

Signs
- No movement (pseudoparalysis) of limb.
- Red, warm, swollen, painful limb.

Diagnosis
- Blood culture positive.
- Bone aspiration for cultures if indicated.

Imaging
- Ultrasound – periosteal elevation and soft tissue swelling.
- Radionuclide bone scan, if indicated – hot spot (needle aspiration does not produce positive bone scan).
- Plain X-ray – limited use at this stage, as only shows periosteal elevation and soft tissue swelling.
- MRI scan of bone if necessary.

Treatment
Antibiotics – prolonged course for approximately 6 weeks. Continued for 2–3 weeks after symptoms resolve and CRP normalizes.

Skeletal dysplasias

There are several hundred, with shortening of the limbs and spine resulting in short stature.

Achondroplasia

- Short bowed limbs, normal trunk, large head.
- Midface hypoplasia, frontal bossing.
- Trident hand (short and broad), protuberant abdomen.

Osteogenesis imperfecta

- Inherited disorder of type 1 collagen formation.
- Rare – 1 in 20 000 live births.

Clinical features
- Increased bone fragility, susceptibility to fracture from mild to lethal, depending on sub-type (Fig. 61.3), scoliosis and kyphosis.
- Blue sclerae, defective tooth formation in some patients.
- Hearing loss.

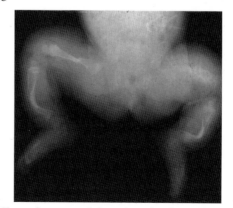

Fig. 61.5 X-ray of osteogenesis imperfecta showing multiple fractures.

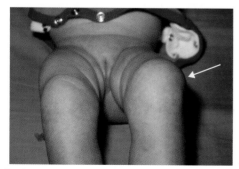

Fig. 61.4 Septic arthritis showing swollen left knee (arrow).

62 Hearing and vision

Hearing

Congenital hearing loss affects 1–2/1000 live births. If the infant receives neonatal intensive care, risk is increased 10-fold.

Hearing loss is:
- **conductive** – involves conduction of sound in the middle or outer ear, often occurs in childhood from secretory otitis media
- **sensorineural** – involves the hair cells of the cochlea in the inner ear, or the cochlear branch of cranial nerve VIII, as in congenital or neonatal hearing loss.

The speech and language of children with severe hearing impairment are delayed or do not develop. The earlier in life hearing can be restored or specialist assistance provided, the better the outcome. Screening infants with risk factors (Table 62.1) identifies only 40–60% of significant bilateral hearing loss. Universal screening in the first few days of life, and certainly by the age of 3 months is therefore conducted in both the US and UK (Table 62.2).

Table 62.1 Risk factors for hearing loss.

Family history
Syndromes with hearing loss
Malformations of the ears, including pits and tags
Perinatal
    Very low birthweight
    Congenital infection – e.g. CMV (cytomegalovirus), rubella
    Severe hyperbilirubinemia
    Ototoxic medications, e.g. furosemide, aminoglycosides
    Mechanical ventilation or extracorporeal membrane oxygenation
    Hypoxic–ischemic encephalopathy
    Bacterial meningitis

Table 62.2 Rationale for universal hearing screening.

Is hearing impairment common?
Yes – more common than hypothyroidism, phenylketonuria or
    hemoglobinopathy
Is the condition serious?
Yes. Results in marked speech and language delay
Is treatment available?
Yes. Sound amplification including hearing aids, cochlea implantation,
    finger-spelling, lip-reading, use of gestures and sign language to
    maximize early development of language skills
Are reliable screening tests available?
Yes. Acceptable sensitivity and specificity
Are other methods of detection available?
Other methods, e.g. parental concern, are unreliable
Does it improve outcome?
Yes. The earlier amplification and specialist intervention for infant and
    family, the better the outcome
Offers possibility of preventing progression in certain cases e.g. treatment if
    caused by congenital CMV
Can it be done at reasonable cost?
Yes, but requires skilled facilities for diagnostic confirmation and habilitation

Neonatal hearing screening

Performed using otoacoustic emissions (OAE) (Fig. 62.1). Repeated if necessary, followed by automated auditory brainstem response (AABR) (Fig. 62.2) if fails OAE. Some centers use AABR as initial test, or for high risk infants.

Otoacoustic emissions (OAE)

Stimuli generated from ear phones. The emissions are normal sound vibrations from the cochlea

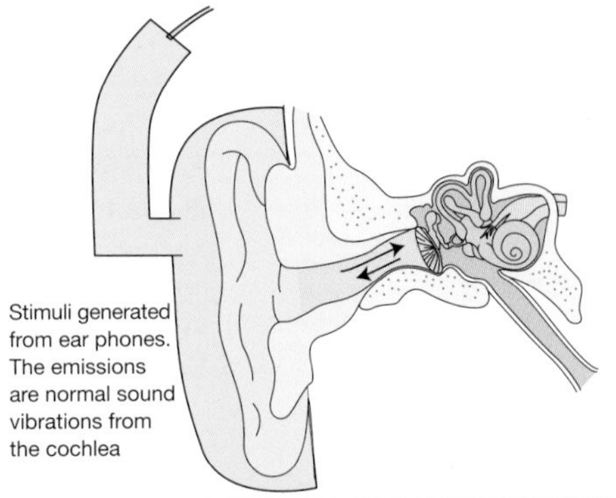

Advantages
- Simple and quick to perform, but affected by ambient noise

Disadvantages
- Misses auditory neuropathy
- False positive rate of up to 30% in first 24 hours after birth as vernix or amniotic fluid are still in ear canal
  Referral rate of 6–8%, with risk of loss to follow-up
  Can reduce referral rate to 1% by doing AABR if fail OAE testing but adds complexity to screening program

Fig. 62.1 Otoacoustic emissions (OAE).

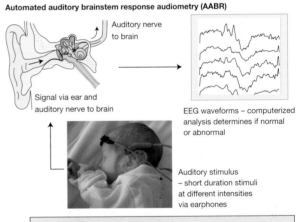

Automated auditory brainstem response audiometry (AABR)

Auditory nerve to brain

Signal via ear and auditory nerve to brain

EEG waveforms – computerized analysis determines if normal or abnormal

Auditory stimulus – short duration stimuli at different intensities via earphones

Advantages
- Screens hearing pathway from ear to brainstem; this test is required to identify auditory neuropathy
- Good for testing speech wavelengths
- Detects moderate hearing loss
- Few false negatives, false positive rate <3%

Disadvantages
- Affected by movement, so infants need to be asleep or very quiet, so time consuming
- Complex computerized equipment, but is mobile
- Requires electrodes applied to infant's head, which parents may dislike

Fig. 62.2 Automated auditory brainstem response (AABR).

Neonatology at a Glance, Third Edition. Edited by Tom Lissauer, Avroy A. Fanaroff, Lawrence Miall and Jonathan Fanaroff.
© 2016 John Wiley & Sons, Ltd. Published 2016 by John Wiley & Sons, Ltd.

Vision

The normal term infant will fix and follow horizontally a moving face, a brightly colored object (e.g. a red ball) or a picture of a target of black and white concentric circles by about 6 weeks. They prefer to look at high-contrast patterned objects rather than plain ones.

Visual acuity is initially reduced – only about 6/36. It improves over the first few months, to 6/18 at 4 months and 6/9 at 8 months, but adult visual acuity is not reached until about 3 years. At birth, many have mild hypermetropia (far-sightedness), which persists through early childhood; clarity of vision is achieved by accommodation. This contrasts with preterm infants, who often become myopic (nearsighted).

The eyes of newborn infants are often not aligned, and an intermittent squint (strabismus) is common during the first weeks of life. A constant squint or one persisting beyond 12 weeks post term should be referred to an ophthalmologist.

Lesions needing urgent ophthalmologic referral

During early childhood, failure of focused visual images to reach the retina, e.g. from a cataract or glaucoma, results in permanent loss of vision (amblyopia). Optimal vision is achieved if surgery and optical correction are performed soon after birth (by 6 weeks of age). Affected infants must therefore be referred urgently to an ophthalmologist for surgery.

Cataracts (Fig. 62.3)
Cataracts may be detected by parents or on checking the red reflex with an ophthalmoscope during the routine examination of the newborn, but may otherwise present with blindness at several months of age. Many are genetic, but congenital infection and other causes must be excluded. They are infrequent.

Congenital glaucoma (Fig. 62.4)
Intraocular pressure is raised. There is watering of the eyes, photophobia and irritability. The eye becomes enlarged and the cornea hazy. Most are bilateral.

Other congenital abnormalities

There are numerous, rare, congenital abnormalities of the eye, including:
- anophthalmos/microphthalmos (absent or extremely small eye)
- coloboma (Fig. 62.5) may affect iris, ciliary body, choroid and optic nerve. Vision may be normal in mild cases, but poor if optic nerve involved
- aniridia (absence of iris)
- albinism (lack of melanin pigment in iris and retina) – may be ocular or generalized, often resulting in macular hypoplasia, nystagmus and poor vision
- white pupil (leukocoria) or white reflex on ophthalmoscopy – causes include retinoblastoma, cataract, retinopathy of prematurity.

Affected infants should be referred to an ophthalmologist.

The causes of severe visual impairment and blindness in children are listed in Table 62.3. Most visually disabled children also have other disabilities.

Other eye conditions

- Retinopathy of prematurity – see Chapter 35.
- Conjunctivitis – see Chapter 43.
- Chorioretinitis in congenital infection – see Chapter 11.

Table 62.3 Sites and causes of severe visual impairment and blindness in children (<16 years).

Whole globe and anterior segment	7%
Glaucoma, cornea, lens (cataract)	10%
Congenital infection	2%
Retina	29%
Retinopathy of prematurity	3%
Oculocutaneous albinism	4%
Optic nerve, cerebral/visual pathways	76%

In some children there was more than one cause.
From Rahi J.S. *et al.* Severe visual impairment and blindness in children in the UK. *Lancet* 2003; **362**: 1359–1365.

Cataract

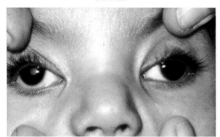

Fig. 62.3 Cataract in right eye of a newborn infant. (Courtesy of Prof. Alistair Fielder.)

Glaucoma

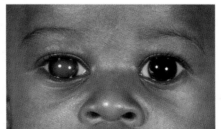

Fig. 62.4 Congenital glaucoma of right eye. (Courtesy of Prof. Alistair Fielder.)

Coloboma

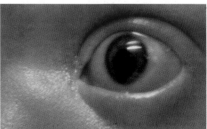

Fig. 62.5 Iris coloboma. Keyhole-shaped pupil due to defect of the iris inferiorly.

63 Pain

Pain is a subjective cortical experience. Newborn infants cannot describe a painful experience, but there is good evidence from physiologic and behavioral responses that they respond to pain and it causes distress (Table 63.1). Pain is one of the main parental concerns for infants in intensive care or undergoing procedures. Parents often also worry about long-term consequences. There is evidence that children who undergo repeated painful experiences as neonates show increased sensitivity to pain in childhood, e.g. to an immunization, and are more fearful of pain than their peers.

Development of pain pathways in the fetus and preterm infant

Pain pathways are well described in the fetus:
• 20 weeks – sensory receptors and cortical neurons have developed
• 24 weeks – cortical synapses are present
• 30 weeks – myelination of pain pathways and development of spinal cord synapses with sensory fibers.

This implies that even preterm infants have anatomic, neurophysiologic and hormonal components to perceive pain. Central descending inhibitory control is less well developed – so response to painful stimuli is actually greater than in older children and adults.

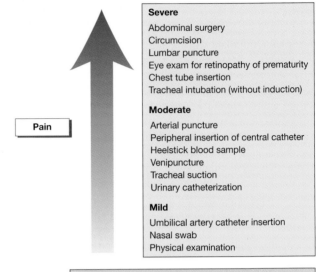

Fig. 63.1 Postulated hierarchy of pain from procedures. (Adapted from Porter F. *et al*. Procedural pain in newborn infants: the influence of intensity and development. *Pediatrics* 1999; **104**: 1–10.)

Factors that modify pain responses

Infants requiring intensive care are subjected to an average of 2–10 painful procedures per day. They are also repeatedly disturbed, e.g. for examination, nursing care.

The pain they experience will be affected by:
• procedure being performed (Fig. 63.1), the skill of the operator and their concern about minimizing discomfort
• gestational age and postnatal age
• behavioral state
• number of previous painful experiences
• time since last painful experience
• severity of their illness.

Table 63.1 Some early milestones in neonatal pain.

1987	Proven that surgical thoracotomy for PDA ligation caused greater physiologic and hormonal disturbance if performed without analgesia
2000	American Academy of Pediatrics Policy Statement on Prevention and Management of Pain and Stress in the Neonate. Updated 2006
2001	International Consensus Statement for the Prevention and Management of Pain in the Newborn

Assessment of pain

Pain can be assessed clinically according to:
• Physiologic responses:
  – heart rate, respiratory rate, oxygen requirement, blood pressure, palmar sweating.
• Behavioral responses:
  – facial expression, body movements, crying.
• Metabolic responses:
  – stress hormones, e.g. cortisol
  – blood glucose, lactate.

These may be used as proxy measures of pain. Obtaining reliable results is problematic and their interpretation is difficult.

Pain assessment scales

A variety of neonatal pain assessment scales have been developed (Table 63.2), mainly for clinical research or postoperative pain assessment (CRIES, NFCS, PIPP scores). The simpler scales can also be used for regular, systematic pain assessment for infants undergoing intensive care, or as guidance for staff on pain assessment (NPASS).

Neonatology at a Glance, Third Edition. Edited by Tom Lissauer, Avroy A. Fanaroff, Lawrence Miall and Jonathan Fanaroff.
© 2016 John Wiley & Sons, Ltd. Published 2016 by John Wiley & Sons, Ltd.

Table 63.2 Some validated pain assessment scales in newborn and preterm infants.

Neonatal Pain, Agitation and Sedation Scale (NPASS)	Premature Infant Pain Profile (PIPP)	Neonatal Facial Coding Scale (NFCS)	CRIES score
Behavioral cues: • Sleep in preceding hour • Facial expression of pain • Motor activity, tone • Consolability, cry Physiologic cues: • Heart rate • Systolic blood pressure • Respiratory frequency and pattern • Oxygen saturation	Gestational age Behavioral state Brow bulge Eye squeeze Nasolabial furrow Heart rate Oxygen saturation	Brow bulge Eye squeeze Nasolabial furrow Open lips Stretch mouth Lip purse Taut tongue Chin quiver Tongue protrusion	**C**rying **R**equires increased oxygen **I**ncreased vital signs **E**xpression **S**leeplessness

Minimizing pain

There are both non-pharmacologic and pharmacologic approaches. Always consider:
• Is the procedure really necessary?
• Timing the procedure for when the infant is awake, if possible.
• Grouping procedures together, *but* limit the number of procedures occurring within a short time of each other (as with physical training, we all need recovery time!).
• Using equipment or methods designed to minimize discomfort (e.g. appropriately sized heel lancets, non-invasive monitoring, venous or arterial catheters to avoid repeated skin punctures, avoiding intramuscular injections).

Non-pharmacologic

These include:
• Environmental modification:
 – quiet, low lighting, talking to baby, slow stroking, rocking, skin-to-skin contact.
• Non-nutritive sucking on a pacifier (dummy) or sucking on breast.

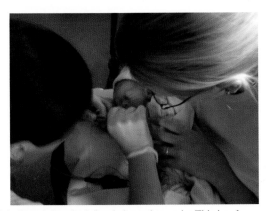

Fig. 63.2 Containing the infant helps reduce pain. This involves secure, supported, non-restrictive positioning, not tight swaddling to prevent moving. Here, during the insertion of a nasogastric tube, the mother is containing her baby and the infant is grasping the nurse's finger.

• Sucrose and breast milk both reduce pain responses.
• Positioning on side, swaddling, comfort holding with still hands (Fig. 63.2).

Pharmacologic approaches

Infants on mechanical ventilation
Use of analgesic/anesthetic agents differs between units. The most widely used are:
• morphine – side-effects include hypotension, respiratory depression and withdrawal syndrome if there is a too rapid dose reduction after prolonged use
• fentanyl – side-effects include respiratory depression, tolerance, occasionally tongue and chest wall rigidity.

Procedures
Optimal analgesia aims to prevent rather than treat pain. In the past, fear of side-effects limited the use of opioids and anesthetic agents, but it should now be possible to provide adequate pain relief, especially postoperatively. Options include:
• Opioids –continuous opioid infusion is preferable as intermittent boluses are associated with poor outcome.
• General anesthesia – all major or surgical procedures.
• Regional anesthesia – e.g. peripheral nerve blocks, spinal or epidural, local infiltration, e.g. for chest tube insertion.
• Non-opioids – e.g. acetaminophen (paracetamol); sometimes used for minor procedures or postoperatively.

Question

How can the pain of heelsticks be minimized?
 Pain is mainly from squeezing the foot, so keep this to the minimum.
 Autostylets are less painful than lancets. Venepuncture is less painful than heelsticks and adequate samples are obtained twice as often, but not suitable for repeated sampling.
 Topical analgesia – not effective for heelsticks and not licensed in the US in newborns.
 Analgesia – sucrose, breast milk or nurse at the breast.

64 Pharmacology

Pharmacology includes the study of:
- the effects of drugs on the body (pharmacodynamics)
- the effect of the body on drugs (pharmacokinetics – *a*bsorption, *d*istribution, *m*etabolism, *e*limination)
- the use of drugs.

The pharmacology, and in particular the pharmacokinetics of drugs in neonates differs significantly from that in children and adults. Primarily this is the result of their different physiology (Fig. 64.1).

Drug prescription and administration

The wide variation in absorption, metabolism, excretion and body composition is mainly related to the neonate's gestational age and postnatal age together with their variation in size, from less than 500 g in the extreme preterm to 5000 g in the large term infant. As a result, drug regimens are complex and vary according to age and are usually calculated as a dose per kilogram.

Drug monitoring

Monitoring plasma levels of drugs is useful if there is a known concentration range within which the drug works and has no toxicity. This applies to only a few drugs, but some of them are in routine use in neonatology (e.g. gentamicin, vancomycin). Monitoring may involve the measurement of peak and trough plasma concentrations, or trough levels only. Measurements are made once the drug has reached the steady state (Fig. 64.2).

Drugs in breast milk

Neonates may be exposed to maternal drugs through their consumption of breast milk. Breast milk has a lower pH than blood (pH 7.0 versus pH 7.4) and a high fat content and will therefore concentrate basic and fat-soluble drugs. Highly protein-bound drugs do not tend to transfer into milk as easily. The concentration

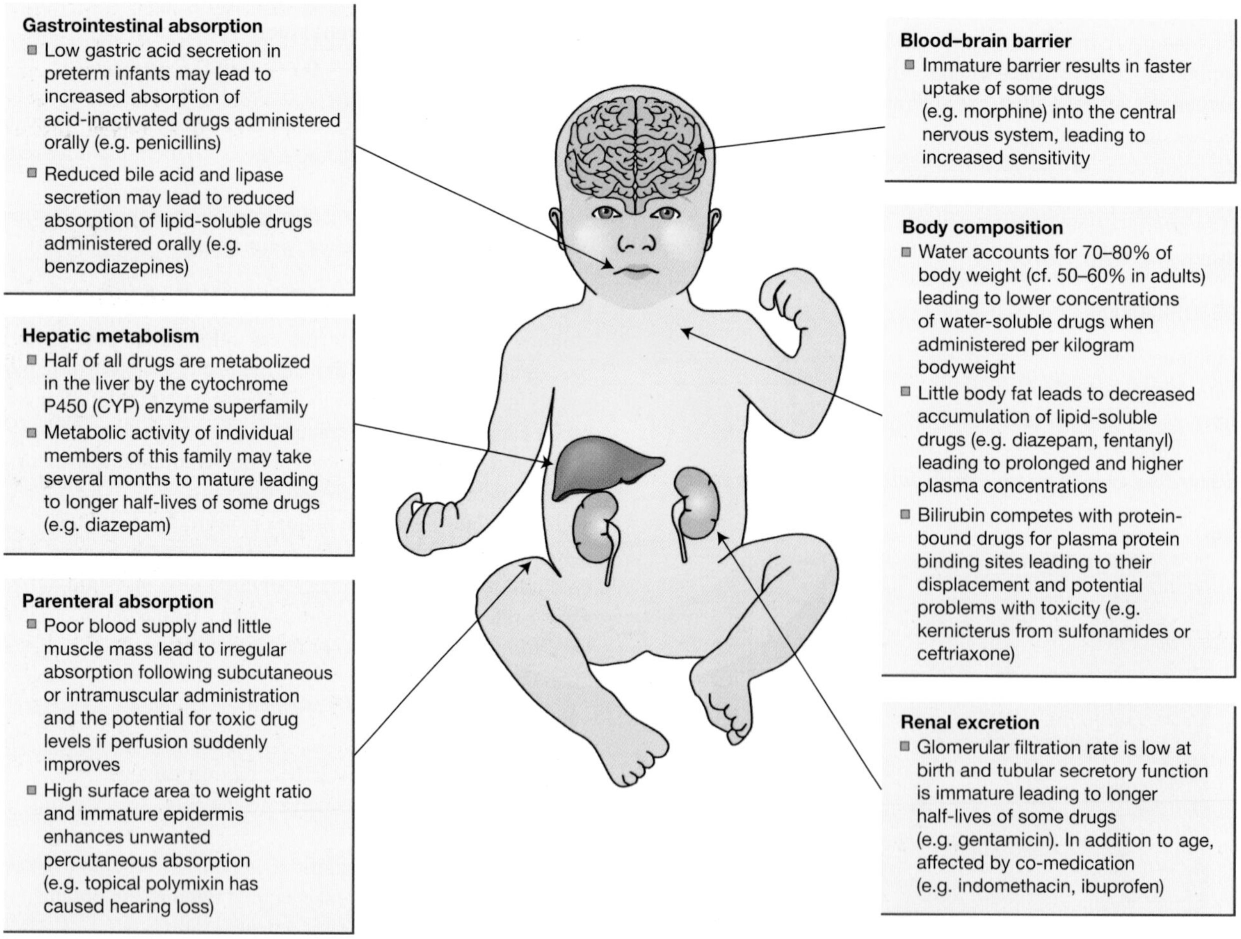

Gastrointestinal absorption
- Low gastric acid secretion in preterm infants may lead to increased absorption of acid-inactivated drugs administered orally (e.g. penicillins)
- Reduced bile acid and lipase secretion may lead to reduced absorption of lipid-soluble drugs administered orally (e.g. benzodiazepines)

Hepatic metabolism
- Half of all drugs are metabolized in the liver by the cytochrome P450 (CYP) enzyme superfamily
- Metabolic activity of individual members of this family may take several months to mature leading to longer half-lives of some drugs (e.g. diazepam)

Parenteral absorption
- Poor blood supply and little muscle mass lead to irregular absorption following subcutaneous or intramuscular administration and the potential for toxic drug levels if perfusion suddenly improves
- High surface area to weight ratio and immature epidermis enhances unwanted percutaneous absorption (e.g. topical polymixin has caused hearing loss)

Blood–brain barrier
- Immature barrier results in faster uptake of some drugs (e.g. morphine) into the central nervous system, leading to increased sensitivity

Body composition
- Water accounts for 70–80% of body weight (cf. 50–60% in adults) leading to lower concentrations of water-soluble drugs when administered per kilogram bodyweight
- Little body fat leads to decreased accumulation of lipid-soluble drugs (e.g. diazepam, fentanyl) leading to prolonged and higher plasma concentrations
- Bilirubin competes with protein-bound drugs for plasma protein binding sites leading to their displacement and potential problems with toxicity (e.g. kernicterus from sulfonamides or ceftriaxone)

Renal excretion
- Glomerular filtration rate is low at birth and tubular secretory function is immature leading to longer half-lives of some drugs (e.g. gentamicin). In addition to age, affected by co-medication (e.g. indomethacin, ibuprofen)

Fig. 64.1 Key physiologic factors affecting neonatal pharmacology.

Neonatology at a Glance, Third Edition. Edited by Tom Lissauer, Avroy A. Fanaroff, Lawrence Miall and Jonathan Fanaroff.
© 2016 John Wiley & Sons, Ltd. Published 2016 by John Wiley & Sons, Ltd.

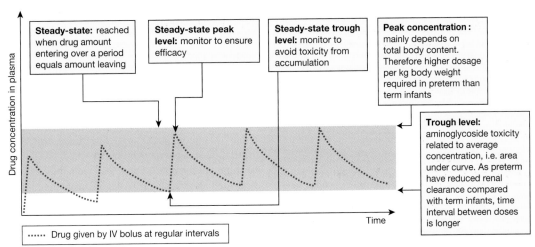

Fig. 64.2 Drug monitoring – steady-state, peak and trough levels.

Table 64.1 Examples of drugs used in breast-feeding mothers that may affect nursing infant. A formulary should always be consulted.

Maternal drug	Effect on infant
Examples of drugs to avoid	
Radioactive iodine	May cause thyroid suppression
Cytotoxic agents	Risk of cytotoxic effect
Diazepam	May cause sedation and may accumulate
Tetracycline	Possibility of permanent staining of teeth
Lithium	Risk of neurologic effects, cardiac malformations

of a drug in breast milk will vary with its concentration in maternal plasma; drugs with a short half-life that may be given after feeding are to be preferred. The majority of drugs are transferred into breast milk in concentrations too low to affect neonatal health; certain drugs must be avoided and general advice should be to avoid the use of any medications wherever possible (Table 64.1).

Drug licensing and neonatalogy

Up to 80% of drugs administered in neonatal intensive care are not licensed by a national licensing body (FDA, Food and Drug Administration, in the US; EMA, European Medicines Agency, in Europe) for use in this population (*unlicensed*), or are used outside their license, e.g. other dosing regimens, other formulation (*off-label*). Doctors can prescribe and nurses can administer unlicensed and off-label medicines, but, it imposes additional responsibility on prescribers to ensure that the use of a particular drug is supported by the best available evidence. Considerable effort and finance are now being devoted to the development, research and licensing of medicines for children.

Question

What lessons in neonatal pharmacology have been learnt from the past?

1886: Aniline dyes used to stamp names on diapers absorbed percutaneously and cause methemoglobinemia.

1956: Sulfonamides displace bilirubin from plasma protein binding sites and cause kernicterus.

1959: Chloramphenicol causes the 'gray baby' syndrome of circulatory collapse due to immature glucuronidation.

1982: Benzyl alcohol, added to intravenous flush solutions as a bacteriostatic agent, accumulates in newborns causing death, intraventricular hemorrhage and the 'gasping baby' syndrome.

1985: Polysorbate 80, a carrier in a parenteral vitamin E preparation, associated with liver failure.

1989: Topical iodine-containing antiseptics noted to be absorbed and may cause hypothyroidism – now used sparingly and excess removed.

Quality assurance

Clinical governance and quality improvement are frameworks for assuring the quality of clinical services and improving them (Fig. 65.1). They are key issues for all who provide care for newborn infants.

Clinical audit

Aims to assess patient care and outcomes through systematic comparison against explicit standards. Change is then implemented and re-audit follows. The audit cycle is shown in Fig. 65.2, and questions about audit are addressed in Table 65.1. More recently neonatal services have been using quality improvement (QI) methodology to implement improvements in care. This uses PDSA (plan-do-study-act) cycles with run-charts to show progress over time. It has the advantage of continuous measurement of outcomes rather than 'snapshots' of data at specific time points as measured by audit. PDSA is described in Fig. 65.3. Changes should be evidence based and action plans should be SMART (specific, measurable, achievable, realistic and timely).

Simulation

Simulation has become an important component of quality assurance in neonatal care. Clinical scenarios are used to train multidisciplinary teams in a safe and educational environment, sometimes using sophisticated models. Widely used in life support courses, e.g. neonatal resuscitation and emergencies, and increasingly for simulated emergencies in the neonatal unit, delivery room and lying-in (postnatal) wards. It can also be used to develop human factor skills in leadership, teamworking and communication. It also allows training in some practical or uncommon procedures before performing them on patients. Simulation can be used to re-create critical incidents identified through risk reporting systems and can also identify latent risks (accidents waiting to happen) that can be fed back into the risk management system of the unit.

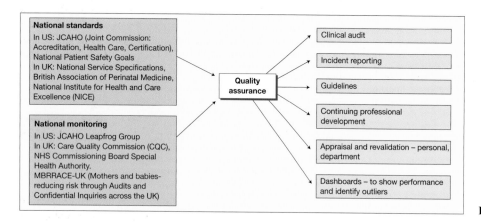

Fig. 65.1 Framework for quality assurance.

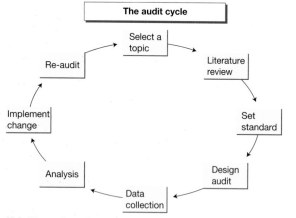

Fig. 65.2 The audit cycle.

Table 65.1 The clinical audit process.

Who should be involved?	All health professionals (multi-disciplinary)
How are topics selected?	Observing current practice
	Clinical incidents, complaints and claims, etc.
Design?	Set or identify standards
	Identify data sample
	Only collect relevant data
Analysis and recommendations	Were standards met?
	Feedback results
	Identify improvements
	Develop an action plan
	Re-audit to check improvement

Neonatology at a Glance, Third Edition. Edited by Tom Lissauer, Avroy A. Fanaroff, Lawrence Miall and Jonathan Fanaroff.
© 2016 John Wiley & Sons, Ltd. Published 2016 by John Wiley & Sons, Ltd.

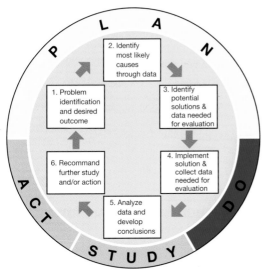

Fig. 65.3 The PDSA cycle to rapidly initiate change in practice and evaluate it.

Question

Are there any quality improvement initiatives specifically for neonatal care?

Many local and national initiatives, but the most comprehensive dedicated to neonatal care is the Vermont-Oxford Neonatal Quality Improvement Collaboratives Program.

It aims to improve the quality and safety of medical care for newborn infants and their families by:

- providing an information resource which also uses material from other disciplines in health-care and other high-reliability organizations, e.g. aviation industry
- providing expert faculty
- promoting four key habits to improve outcome (Fig. 65.4)
- organizing collaborative safety improvement projects, e.g. reducing nosocomial infection, by visits between units or via the internet
- voluntary, anonymous collection of errors on internet.

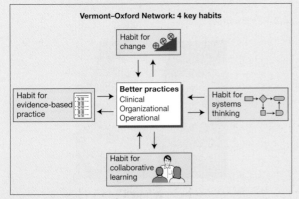

Fig. 65.4 Four key habits for better outcomes promoted by the Vermont–Oxford Network. (Reproduced with permission of J. Horbar, Vermont–Oxford Network.)

Question

How can parents help improve quality in the NICU?

- Offering family-centred care is crucial to support families at a time of high stress and to enable successful bonding with their baby.
- Parent representatives should be involved in the management of neonatal networks and in the development of new services.
- Family integrated care is an innovative program in some units. Pioneered in Canada, parents provide most of the care for their baby, even in the NICU. Nurses and doctors teach and support parents who may provide some highly technical care. This approach has been shown to improve outcomes such as improved weight gain, reduced sepsis and increased rate of breastfeeding at discharge.

Critical incident reporting (Table 65.2)

It is important that the whole neonatal team develops a culture of quality and safety. Reporting critical incidents, not only those that have caused harm but also those that could have caused harm are a key component of quality assurance. The most common and serious critical incidents in neonatal practice and ways to minimize their occurrence are considered in Chapter 66.

Table 65.2 Questions and answers about critical incidents.

What are they?	Unexpected events that cause or could cause harm to the patient. Include near-misses
Who should report them?	Everyone
What should be reported?	The facts
Why report?	To identify causes To develop a strategy to prevent recurrence To act as warning for complaints/litigation To provide information for external monitoring
Who is to blame?	A no-blame culture should be developed – disciplinary action will not follow *except* where acts or omissions are malicious, criminal, or constitute professional misconduct
What level of investigation is required?	Depends on extent of harm to the patient and assessment of likelihood of recurrence by taking the whole circumstance of the event into account, not just the incident itself If risk of harm or recurrence is high, perform root cause analysis
What is root cause analysis?	A structured method used to analyze serious adverse events with the goal of identifying contributing factors
What if major harm has occurred or major damage to the organization?	Because of potential litigation, the hospital risk management group and senior managers should be informed. A more detailed, formal causal analysis (FMEA, failure mode and effect analysis) should be undertaken

66 Critical incidents

A survey in the US showed that medical errors were responsible for 98 000 deaths per year, i.e. more people die in a year in the US from medical errors than from motor vehicle accidents or breast cancer.

In a prospective study of pediatric admissions to hospital, potential adverse events were highest in the NICU (neonatal intensive care unit):

- 91% of admissions had a medication error
- 46% of admissions had a potential adverse event
- 74% of errors involved physician ordering.

Neonatal critical incidents which may relate to fetal or obstetric care will need to be considered in conjunction with maternal–fetal medicine, e.g. hypoxic–ischemic encephalopathy or seizures within 48 hours of birth. Other aspects of quality improvement involving neonatal care are considered in Chapter 65.

The most common critical incidents are medication errors and extravasation injuries, but a selection of frequent or important examples follows. Some approaches to their prevention are given, but each critical incident will need to be considered by the multidisciplinary risk management team.

Prevention of critical incidents requires a culture of safety throughout the unit (Fig. 66.1). Being honest and open with parents is vital.

Medication errors

Why?
- Prescription errors occur as there is a wide range of dosage – varies 10-fold if baby weighs 0.5 kg or 5 kg (unlike adults, where there is usually a standard dose).
- Dilutions often needed – common source of error.
- Use of potentially dangerous drugs – insulin, inotropes, aminoglycosides, digoxin, narcotics, heparin.

Prevention
- Staff training, utilising a pediatric pharmacist.
- Clear formulary.
- Minimize range of drugs used.
- Computer-assisted guidance on dosage and dilutions.
- Avoid abbreviations, e.g. micrograms, not μg.
- Use limited number of standard dilutions, drawn up in pharmacy where possible.
- Clear differentiation between vials, e.g. by color.
- Checking by two trained professionals (but do not rely on this).
- Remove undiluted dangerous drugs, e.g. high concentration KCl.
- Use pre-programmed infusion pumps.
- Pay special attention to potentially dangerous drugs.

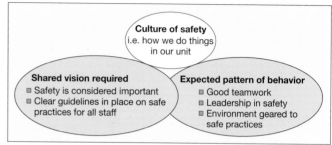

Fig. 66.1 Requirements of a culture of safety in the neonatal unit. (Adapted from J. Horbar, Vermont–Oxford Network.)

Extravasation of intravenous infusions
(Figs 66.2 and 66.3)

Cause
- Fragile tissues.
- Small catheter, difficult to fix securely.
- Movement by infant.
- Irritant infusion – e.g. calcium, high concentration of dextrose, parenteral nutrition.

Prevention
- Expert fixation of catheters.
- Leave potential extravasation area visible.
- Avoid occluding limb with tape.
- Regular checks, pressure-sensitive alarms.
- Give irritant infusions via central lines if possible.

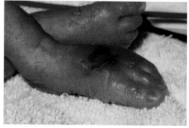

Fig. 66.2 Extravasation injury.

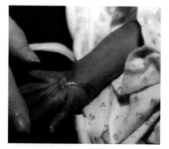

Fig. 66.3 Scarring from extravasation injury.

Neonatology at a Glance, Third Edition. Edited by Tom Lissauer, Avroy A. Fanaroff, Lawrence Miall and Jonathan Fanaroff.
© 2016 John Wiley & Sons, Ltd. Published 2016 by John Wiley & Sons, Ltd.

What to do if extensive extravasation

• Aspirate cannula.
• Flush affected area with saline via several skin punctures. Some centers inject hyaluronidase into extravasation site. Elevate affected limb.
• Consult plastic surgeons if concern about long-term scarring.

Excessive fluid volume infused

Cause

• Incorrect settings on pump.
• Malfunction of pump.

Prevention

• Electronic 'guard-rails' built into pumps (max and minimum rate based on infusion).
• Check and monitor infusion.

Giving wrong breast milk to wrong patient

Cause

• Similar patient names.
• Poor labeling.
• Multiple milk containers kept in same fridge.
• Inadequate checking procedures.

Prevention

• Clear labeling.
• Double-checking.
• Warning mechanism (name alert tags) for staff if babies have similar names.
• Electronic milk storage and dispensing systems.

What to do if occurs

• Inform parents.
• Test donor mother for blood-borne viruses.

Complications of umbilical arterial catheters (UAC)

Incorrect vessel

• Inserted into umbilical vein instead of artery.

Prevention
• Check for presence of arterial pulsation to confirm in artery and arterial waveform on monitor.
• Check position on abdominal X-ray (Fig. 66.4).
  This is important – if in umbilical vein by mistake, excessively high oxygen could be given, which could damage eyes (retinopathy of prematurity, ROP) if preterm.

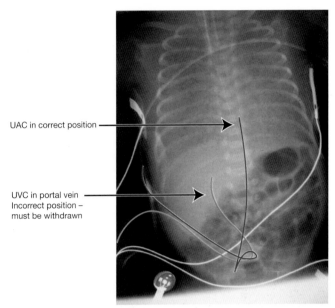

UAC in correct position

UVC in portal vein
Incorrect position –
must be withdrawn

Fig. 66.4 X-ray showing umbilical arterial and venous catheters. Catheter in umbilical artery (red line) – initial course caudally towards groin, then cranially up middle of spine. Catheter in umbilical vein (blue line) – cranial course to right of spine. This catheter is in the portal vein, a potentially dangerous position, and must be withdrawn. In addition, overlapping catheters, as shown here, can easily lead to misinterpretation.

Thrombosis/emboli/vasoconstriction

Consequences
• Occlusion of the artery causes mottling of skin, loss of pulses, cool limb and cyanosis in one or both legs. May result in gangrene/amputation of limb.
• Emboli may affect distant organs.

Prevention
• Regular observation. If skin becomes discolored, reposition or remove catheter.
• Position catheter either high at T6–10 or low at L3–4 to avoid catheter tip near renal vessels to reduce risk of renal artery thrombosis (hematuria, renal failure, hypertension).
• Flush catheter gently, heparin infusion.
• Ensure infant's intravascular volume is adequate.

Blood loss from arterial catheters

Cause

• Disconnection of catheter.

Prevention

• Clear labeling that catheter is arterial.
• Connections screwed together.
• Pressure-sensitive alarm.

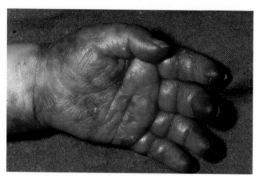

Fig. 66.5 Ischemic damage from radial artery catheter.

Ischemic damage from peripheral artery catheters

Cause

- Small size of vessel.
- Inadequate collateral supply.

Prevention

- Choose suitable artery:
- use radial artery only if ulnar artery shown to be patent (Fig. 66.5) (see Chapter 76 for Allen test).
- avoid superficial temporal artery as can cause ischemia of parietal lobe.
- avoid brachial artery as end artery and occlusion may result in loss of distal limb, and median nerve may be damaged.
- Only use for sampling, not injecting.
- Remove if any significant blanching, other than transient.

Portal vein thrombosis from umbilical venous catheters

Cause

- Catheter in portal vein causing portal vein thrombosis.

Prevention

- Check on X-ray that catheter is in the inferior vena cava and not the portal vein (Fig. 66.4).

Extravasation of parenteral nutrition (PN) from central venous lines

Cause

- Catheters may migrate and PN may be infused into:
  - the tissues, causing swelling and inflammation
  - the lungs, causing pleural effusion
  - the pericardium, causing pericardial effusion and tamponade
  - the liver, causing hepatitis.

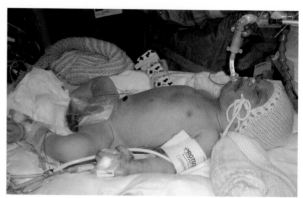

Fig. 66.6 Scalding of skin from excessive heat from radiant warmer after dislodging of skin temperature probe. It resolved within a few hours.

Prevention

- Check catheter tip is in the inferior or superior vena cava, not the right atrium or portal vein.

Burns and scalds

Cause

- Overheating of humidifier in CPAP/ventilator circuit.
- Disconnection of temperature probe or malfunctioning of radiant warmer (Fig. 66.6).
- Failure to move transcutaneous O_2/CO_2 probes regularly.

Prevention

- Temperature alarms.

Scarring of skin

Cause

- Poorly keratinized skin prone to long-term scarring, especially if black ethnicity (keloid formation).

Prevention

- Minimize skin damage:
  - care with adhesive tape, regularly reposition probes and avoid undue pressure from attachments for tracheal tubes, nasal CPAP, etc.
  - if transcutaneous O_2/CO_2 electrodes used, rotate to different skin sites regularly
  - procedures, e.g. chest tube for pneumothorax, avoid breast-bud area (Fig. 66.7).

Nasal damage from tracheal tube

Cause

- Dilatation of nostril or damage to the nasal septum by tube.

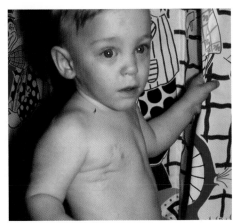

Fig. 66.7 Scarring from chest tubes.

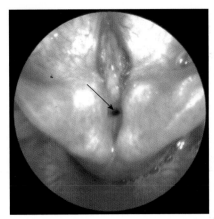

Fig. 66.8 Tracheal stenosis following prolonged mechanical ventilation. The narrowed trachea is shown with an arrow.

Prevention

- Avoid excessively large tracheal tubes.
- Avoid leaving in situ for long periods.
- Fix tube securely to prevent leverage.

Nasal damage from nasal CPAP

Cause

- Pressure on nostrils or nasal septum.

Prevention

- Correct positioning, size and fixing of nasal prongs, avoiding excessive pressure on the nostrils or nose, regular repositioning and monitoring.
- Consider high flow nasal oxygen therapy as causes less nasal trauma.

Tracheal stenosis

Cause

- Damage to subglottic area from tracheal tube (Fig. 66.8).

Prevention

- Avoid excessively large tubes.
- Minimize time left in place.
- Secure to prevent tube movement and irritation.

Infection

Cause

- Nosocomial infection – inadequate hand-hygiene.
- Catheter related – at insertion or subsequently, e.g. breaking of long line and dressing.
- Procedures – infection where skin denuded from monitor probes or tape.

Prevention

- **Meticulous hand hygiene**.
- Sterile insertion.
- Minimize interference of lines.
- Remove lines as soon as possible.
- Care bundles of procedures to minimize infection shown to reduce central line-associated bloodstream infections (CLABSIs).

Aspiration pneumonia from misplaced gavage (nasogastric) feeding tubes

Cause

- Tube inserted into trachea instead of stomach.

Prevention

- Check correct position with pH indicator paper to confirm gastric aspirate is acidic (pH < 5.5).
- If in doubt, X-ray to confirm below the diaphragm and in the stomach to the left of mid-line.

67 Evidence-based medicine

What is evidence-based medicine (EBM)?

It is the conscientious, explicit and judicious use of current best evidence in making decisions about the care of individual patients.

Steps in the practice of evidence-based medicine

See Fig. 67.1.

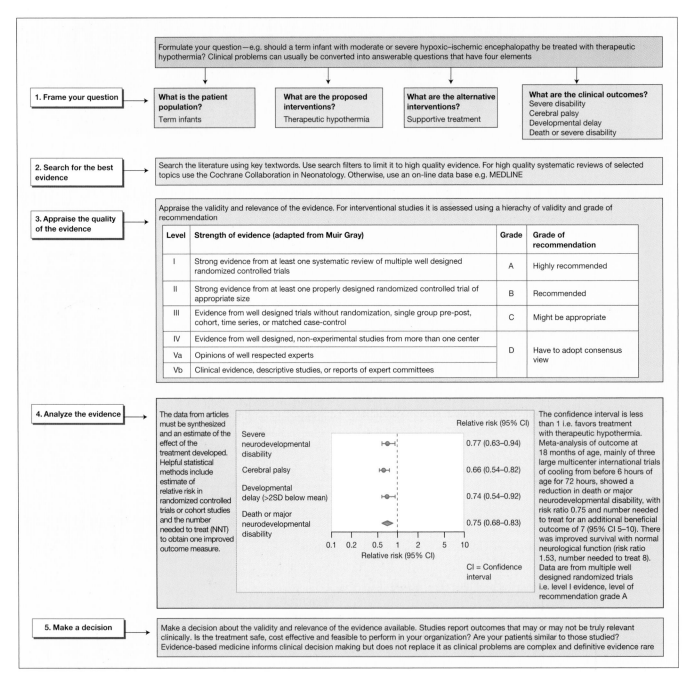

Fig. 67.1 Steps in the practice of EBM (evidence-based medicine). CI=confidence interval. (Data from Jacobs S.E. *et al.* Cooling for newborns with hypoxic ischaemic encephalopathy. *Cochrane Database Syst Rev* 2013; (1): CD003311.)

Neonatology at a Glance, Third Edition. Edited by Tom Lissauer, Avroy A. Fanaroff, Lawrence Miall and Jonathan Fanaroff.
© 2016 John Wiley & Sons, Ltd. Published 2016 by John Wiley & Sons, Ltd.

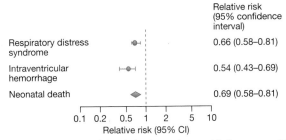

Fig. 67.2 Meta-analysis of prophylactic corticosteroids for preterm birth showing reduction in respiratory distress syndrome, intraventricular hemorrhage and neonatal death. (Data from Roberts D., Dalziel S.R. Antenatal corticosteroids for accelerating fetal lung maturation for women at risk of preterm birth. *Cochrane Database Syst Rev* 2006, (3). CD004454.)

Examples of evidence-based medicine in neonatology

The following are some examples from neonatal medicine of therapy proven to be beneficial or harmful. However, for most decisions in clinical practice, guidance from evidence-based medicine is not available, is inconclusive or may be conflicting. Clinicians have to base their decisions on the best available information, clinical experience and the evaluation of potential benefits and risks for the individual patient.

Beneficial therapies

Examples of therapies shown to be beneficial are:
• Maternal prophylactic corticosteroids for preterm birth (Fig. 67.2).
• Maternal anti-D (Rho) immunoglobulin – to rhesus negative mothers to prevent rhesus disease of the newborn.
• Surfactant therapy in preterm infants.
• Moderate hypothermia for moderate or severe HIE (hypoxic–ischemic encephalopathy) (Fig. 67.1).

Harmful therapies

Examples of therapies shown to be harmful are:
• Uncontrolled oxygen therapy causing blindness in preterm infants. This demonstrates the dangers of the introduction of a new therapy, oxygen, followed by restriction in its use, without evidence from randomized controlled trials (Fig. 67.4).
• Antibiotic side-effects:
  – chloramphenicol (unmonitored) – gray baby syndrome (circulatory collapse)
  – sulfonamides – displacement of bilirubin, resulting in kernicterus
  – tetracycline – yellow staining of teeth and bones.
• Early prophylactic corticosteroids in preterm infants to reduce severity of respiratory distress syndrome and BPD (bronchopulmonary dysplasia) – gastrointestinal perforation, growth failure, hypertension and probable neurodevelopmental deficit.

Question

What is the evidence determining the optimal range for oxygen saturation in preterm infants?

In three international randomized controlled trials (BOOST and BOOST II and SUPPORT trials), oxygen saturation range 85–89% (lower target group) was compared with 91–95% (higher target group). Recruitment to the BOOST II trial was stopped early when an interim analysis of all the results showed an increased rate of death before discharge in the lower target group (23.1% vs 15.9%). The lower target group had a reduced rate of retinopathy of prematurity (10.6% vs 13.5%) and an increased rate of necrotizing enterocolitis (10.4% vs 8%) (Fig. 67.3). There were no significant differences in other outcomes.

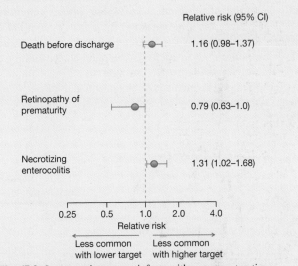

Fig. 67.3 Outcomes in preterm infants with oxygen saturation in lower and higher target ranges. (Data from The BOOST II United Kingdom, Australia and New Zealand collaborative groups. Oxygen saturation and outcomes in preterm infants. *N Engl J Med* 2013; **368**: 2094–2104.)

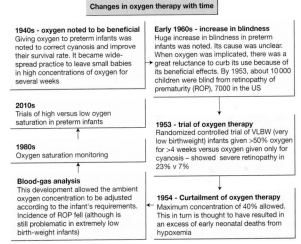

Fig. 67.4 Changes in oxygen therapy with time.

68 Ethics

Sick newborn infants have the same rights to life and access to care as any other person. Their care is dependent on a successful partnership between parents and the clinical team (Fig. 68.1).

Question

What is the role of clinical ethics committees?

Increasingly being developed as a resource for doctors and other health-care professionals and parents facing difficult ethical problems. US hospitals are required to have mechanisms in place to address ethical issues in patient care. Ethics committees are often diverse, including physicians, nurses, lay members, pastoral care, and others. In the US and some centers in the UK, the committee can be rapidly constituted to discuss an individual problem proactively. Ethics committee decisions are generally advisory. In those circumstances where there is continued conflict after ethics committee involvement, referral to court may be required. In addition to assisting with individual cases, institutional ethics committees are becoming more involved in organizational ethical issues such as conflict of interest and the impact of performance incentives on patient care.

Table 68.1 Definitions of the principles of medical ethics.

Beneficence	Do good
Non-maleficence	Do no harm
Justice	Legal justice, respect for rights, fair distribution of resources
Respect for autonomy	Respect for the individuals' right to make informed and thought-out decisions for themselves
Trust	Parents need to develop trust in their physician, who has a responsibility to ensure that this trust is not misplaced

The withholding or withdrawal of life-saving medical treatment

There are a number of situations in neonatal practice where withholding or withdrawal of life-saving medical treatment is considered morally permissible. Their management is influenced by the parents' religious beliefs and cultural background, the laws of the country and national guidelines (e.g. American Academy of Pediatrics, Royal College of Paediatrics and Child Health) (Tables 68.2 and 68.3) These decisions are stressful not only for

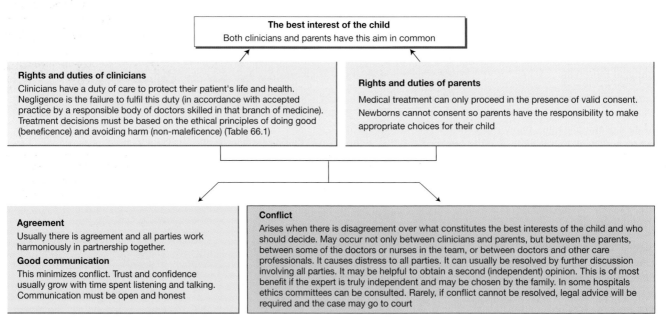

The best interest of the child
Both clinicians and parents have this aim in common

Rights and duties of clinicians
Clinicians have a duty of care to protect their patient's life and health. Negligence is the failure to fulfil this duty (in accordance with accepted practice by a responsible body of doctors skilled in that branch of medicine). Treatment decisions must be based on the ethical principles of doing good (beneficence) and avoiding harm (non-maleficence) (Table 66.1)

Rights and duties of parents
Medical treatment can only proceed in the presence of valid consent. Newborns cannot consent so parents have the responsibility to make appropriate choices for their child

Agreement
Usually there is agreement and all parties work harmoniously in partnership together.

Good communication
This minimizes conflict. Trust and confidence usually grow with time spent listening and talking. Communication must be open and honest

Conflict
Arises when there is disagreement over what constitutes the best interests of the child and who should decide. May occur not only between clinicians and parents, but between the parents, between some of the doctors or nurses in the team, or between doctors and other care professionals. It causes distress to all parties. It can usually be resolved by further discussion involving all parties. It may be helpful to obtain a second (independent) opinion. This is of most benefit if the expert is truly independent and may be chosen by the family. In some hospitals ethics committees can be consulted. Rarely, if conflict cannot be resolved, legal advice will be required and the case may go to court

Fig. 68.1 Ethical framework of clinical practice.

Neonatology at a Glance, Third Edition. Edited by Tom Lissauer, Avroy A. Fanaroff, Lawrence Miall and Jonathan Fanaroff.
© 2016 John Wiley & Sons, Ltd. Published 2016 by John Wiley & Sons, Ltd.

Table 68.2 Situations in neonatal care where withholding or withdrawing life-sustaining treatments may be considered ethically justified if considered not to be in the child's best interest, in the UK (Larcher, V. *et al.* Arch Dis Child 2015; 100(Supp 2)s1–s23).

i) When life is limited in quantity
If treatment is unable or unlikely to prolong life significantly:
- Brain stem death
- Imminent death, irrespective of treatment
- Inevitable death, where prolongation of life confers no overall benefit.

ii) When life is limited in quality
Where treatment may prolong life but will not alleviate:
- Burdens of treatments, which produce sufficient pain and suffering to outweigh potential or actual benefits
- Burdens of the child's underlying condition, which produces such pain and distress as to overcome benefits in sustaining life
- Lack of ability to benefit, where the severity of the child's condition makes it difficult or impossible for them to derive benefit from continued life.

the parents but also for the health-care team, amongst whom consensus and an agreed management plan should be reached. Consent must be obtained from the parents, but the extent to which they may wish to be involved in the decision-making depends on the individual family. Repeated discussion without coercion may be necessary.

If life-saving support is going to be withheld or withdrawn, all aspects of palliative care including symptom management and psychosocial support should be in place (see Chapter 70). Many parents will accept the appropriateness of withdrawal of mechanical ventilation and appreciate the opportunity to spend time with their baby away from the technology of intensive care, but with staff to support them. The baby's comfort should be the priority and pain or distress alleviated. Parents need to know that the infant may continue to breathe for some time after disconnection from the ventilator.

If there is dissent or uncertainty about the best course of action, it is likely to be best to continue to provide full intensive care.

Questions

What is the difference between withholding and withdrawing intensive care?

There is no ethical or legal distinction between them, though emotionally it may be easier not to start treatment than to withdraw it. If there is uncertainty, provide intensive care and subsequently withdraw it after full assessment.

Is euthanasia allowed?

Giving a medicine with the primary intent to hasten death is unlawful in both North America and Europe (though in the Netherlands and Belgium it is accepted on a carefully regulated basis). Giving a medicine to relieve pain, which as a side effect may hasten death (the principle of double effect), is ethically appropriate if its primary purpose is to alleviate distress or suffering.

Table 68.3 Situations where treatment of disabled infants can be withheld in the US – the Baby Doe case.

Legislation regarding the treatment of infants with birth defects was introduced following the case of Baby Doe who was born in 1982 with Trisomy 21 (Down syndrome) and esophageal atresia. Partly on the advice of their obstetrician, the parents refused to consent to life-saving surgery to repair the esophageal defect. They felt that a 'minimally acceptable quality of life was never present for a child suffering from such a condition'. Without the surgery, the infant was unable to eat.

Legal dispute
The hospital disagreed with the parent's refusal to consent and filed in court an emergency petition seeking authorization to perform the surgery. The trial court felt that the parents had a right to choose a medically recommended course of treatment. The obstetrician had recommended against surgery. The court did not give permission for surgery. The hospital appealed the decision, but the baby died when 6 days old.

Political consequences
The case drew widespread media attention, and ignited a national debate over the treatment of infants with birth defects.
President Reagan disagreed with the decision – 'The judge let Baby Doe starve and die.'
The Surgeon General, C. Everett Koop, a pediatric surgeon, became involved in getting Congress to pass the Baby Doe Amendments.

The Child Abuse Prevention and Treatment Act (CAPTA) 1973, reauthorized 2003
This prevents the withholding of 'medically indicated treatment' from disabled newborns with life-threatening conditions.
Five circumstances under which treatment can be withheld are:
1. Chronically and irreversibly comatose
2. Treatment would merely prolong dying
3. Treatment would not be effective in ameliorating or correcting all of the infant's life-threatening conditions
4. Treatment would be futile in terms of survival
5. Treatment would be virtually futile and the treatment itself under such circumstances would be inhumane

69 Research and consent

Research

Health professionals wish to provide the best possible care for newborn infants. This should be evidenced-based, but this is only possible when evidence is available from properly conducted research. It is therefore unethical for properly conducted research on newborn infants **not** to be performed. Failure to do research leads to stagnant and second-rate medical care.

Research may be interventional, e.g. evaluation of a new therapy, or non-interventional, e.g. descriptive or observational (Table 69.1).

There are a number of obstacles to overcome in order to perform research in newborn infants. These are practical and ethical.

Practical difficulties in conducting research in infants

These include:

• The number of newborn infants who are preterm or have a specific problem or condition is small and usually requires trials to be multi-centered, which adds enormously to the complexity and cost of each study. However, a number of networks have been established to facilitate this, such as the Vermont–Oxford and NICHD (National Institute of Child Health and Human Development) Neonatal Research Network and the Canadian, Australian and New Zealand, Italian and other national neonatal networks and many multi-centered trials have been performed throughout the world (see Cochrane neonatal reviews).

• Funding is difficult to obtain as the number of newborn infants with a specific problem is small, making pharmaceutical companies less likely to develop new products or conduct trials.

• In order to proceed with a trial, the information required about a potential new drug or therapy is becoming ever more stringent.

This also applies to pilot studies, making it increasingly difficult to obtain the data required to conduct a larger study.

Table 69.1 Differences between interventional and non-interventional research.

Interventional (therapeutic) research
Research which directly affects the treatment an individual receives. They may receive a new treatment or, in a randomized trial, a new or conventional treatment or placebo. At the start of the project the answer to the question about which treatment is better will not be known (equipoise). Use of a placebo instead of treatment is unethical if there is an accepted treatment. The new and potentially better therapy should be compared with accepted treatment.

Non-interventional (non-therapeutic) research
Research that will *not benefit directly* the person involved. This is observational research – e.g. the normal levels of vitamin A in a particular group of infants. The infants themselves will in no way benefit – so the invasiveness of obtaining the information must be minimal (a small extra volume of blood when venepuncture is required for other reasons, or a single venepuncture, well performed with analgesia).

Table 69.2 Key factors in informed consent for research.

Diagnosis – include description of medical steps leading to the diagnosis
Research – nature and purpose of proposed research
Risks – common risks, less common but severe risks (such as death, brain damage, loss of organ function)
Alternatives – other options, including their risks and benefits. *It is always an option not to participate in a study and to receive standard therapy*

Ethical difficulties in conducting research in infants

All research must be peer-reviewed and sanctioned by an independent ethics advisory committee – Institutional Review Board in North America, appropriate research ethics committee (REC) in the UK.

Parents must be able to make informed choices when asked to give consent for their infant to take part in research. This can be problematic when decisions need to made rapidly, e.g. when a baby suddenly becomes ill, especially immediately after delivery, when parents are emotionally stressed. Key factors of informed consent are outlined in Table 69.2.

Criteria for informed consent for research include:
• **Competence** of the person giving consent.
• **Information** – sufficient for informed choice, including a written information sheet for parents and the use of an interpreter if there are concerns about the parents' understanding of English.
• **Understanding** – parents must have understood the research sufficiently to be able to evaluate choices. In the US and UK, consent can be provided by one parent with parental responsibility; in some countries in Europe both parents must agree.
• **Written consent** should be obtained, with one copy for the parents and another filed in the case record.
• **Voluntary** – parents must be aware that they can decline or withdraw from the research without jeopardizing their baby's care.

All large multicenter trials have a Data Safety and Monitoring Committee which ensures the safety and well-being of the participating subjects. They have the power to terminate enrollment if they have the evidence that the intervention is harmful or if continuing the study cannot demonstrate benefit.

Consent in clinical practice

Health professionals are under pressure to allow parents greater involvement in decision-making and enable them to give consent to treatment.

Parental consent should be obtained for complex procedures or treatment and for all surgical procedures. Documentation about the communication with the parents explaining the basis, benefits and risks of the procedure or treatment is more important than obtaining a signature on a consent form. Consent for a surgical procedure must be obtained by someone familiar with and capable of performing the

Neonatology at a Glance, Third Edition. Edited by Tom Lissauer, Avroy A. Fanaroff, Lawrence Miall and Jonathan Fanaroff.
© 2016 John Wiley & Sons, Ltd. Published 2016 by John Wiley & Sons, Ltd.

procedure. For infants receiving intensive or special care in a neonatal unit, it would be impractical to obtain detailed consent from parents for the multitude of low-risk procedures performed on their baby. However, parents should be given an overview about what the care of their infant involves and what range of procedures will be performed, both verbally and in an information booklet.

In clinical practice, consent is most problematic about the initial resuscitation and immediate management of extremely premature infants at the limit of viability and when withdrawal of treatment is being considered. The former is considered in Chapter 13 on neonatal resuscitation, the latter in Chapter 68 on ethics.

Question – What were the research issues relating to cooling for hypoxic–ischemic encephalopathy (HIE)?

Can research be conducted on infants who become acutely ill at birth?
Yes, the hypothermia studies are a good example.

What was the research question?
Does cooling term infants with hypoxic–ischemic encephalopathy (HIE) reduce death and severe neurodevelopmental disability?

What was the basis?
Studies in adult and newborn animals showed that a reduction of body temperature of 3–4 °C after a cerebral insult is associated with improved histological and behavioral outcome. Pilot studies of cooling infants with encephalopathy showed no complications but the numbers treated were too small to evaluate benefit.

What was the study design?
Several multicenter, prospective, randomized studies of term infants after perinatal asphyxia compared 'intensive care plus cooling for 72 hours' with those allocated to 'intensive care without cooling'. Treatment needed to be started within 6 hours of birth.

What were the results?
Babies randomized to cooling have lower mortality and less neurodevelopmental handicap (see Fig 67.1).

What were the challenges?
Many, including:
• Infants had to be identified, assessed, transferred to a tertiary center and treatment started all within 6 hours of birth.
• Consent had to be obtained rapidly, shortly after parents discovered that their newborn infant was dangerously ill. Many of the mothers were recovering from emergency Cesarean section. A strategy of obtaining consent from all parents prior to delivery was not practicable as HIE needing treatment is very uncommon.
• Parents needed to understand the concept of randomization, i.e. their baby may, but may not, receive the new treatment.
• Clear study inclusion criteria had to be developed, and researchers trained.
• Study infants had to be closely monitored for side-effects.
• Follow-up studies had to be arranged and conducted.
• Difficult to organize and expensive. Only following meta-analysis of several studies in different countries was significant improvement shown (see Fig 67.1).

What questions still need to be answered?
Many, including:
• Must therapy be started within 6 hours?
• What is optimal temperature and duration of cooling?
• Can it be effective in preterm infants?
• Can adjunctive therapy be developed, as 48% of cooled infants with moderate or severe encephalopathy die or have major neurodevelopmental disability at 18 months? Erythropoietin, melatonin and cord blood stem cells are being investigated.
• As the number of large, multicenter clinical trials including long-term follow-up that can be conducted is limited and take many years, are there reliable more immediate markers of neurological damage, e.g. with neuroimaging, that can reliably predict long term outcome?

Question – What issues have arisen relating to randomization?

Issues may arise when infants are in the group which turns out to have a poorer outcome. An example is the SUPPORT trial, where preterm infants were randomized to be cared for with oxygen saturation targeted to low (85–89%) and high (91–95%) ranges. The hypothesis was that the lower range would result in lower rates of retinopathy of prematurity. It was found that infants randomized to the low range did have less retinopathy of prematurity but also had higher mortality (see Fig 67.3). Allegations, both in the press and via social media and legally, have been made that parents were not given sufficient information when consent was obtained and were not fully aware of the implications of being randomized into the low range, and in particular the risk of death. While these allegations have been vigorously disputed, it is likely that they will result in more stringent consent requirements in neonatal clinical trials.

The aim of palliative care is to provide comfort to the baby who is dying or has a life-limiting condition and holistic support for the family. Extreme prematurity, congenital malformations, neonatal encephalopathy and infection account for most neonatal deaths. The decision to offer palliative care may be made antenatally, soon after delivery or later during neonatal care. It should involve the multidisciplinary team caring for the baby, together with the family. National guidelines on end-of-life care are available (see Chapter 68). Discussions should be led by the senior clinician in a private and quiet environment. Parents should be offered the chance to involve extended family or friends. These decisions are difficult and parents must be given time to consider the issues. Involving religious or cultural representatives or a second opinion from an independent clinician may be helpful.

Care Plans

When it becomes clear that the baby is unlikely to survive and treatment aimed at prolonging life is no longer appropriate, a care plan focusing on palliative care should be developed to ensure that the baby dies free of pain or discomfort and with dignity. Pediatric palliative care services may assist.

Regular assessment of comfort, pain and physiological status should be undertaken. Physical care, including positioning, mouth care and skin-to-skin contact, should be offered. Analgesia should not be reduced for fear that it might hasten death; it may need to be increased for pain or distress. Other forms of treatment, such as antibiotics, oxygen, anticonvulsants and antireflux medication, may be required for symptom control. Electronic monitoring is not usually recommended.

The aim of feeding in palliative care is to provide comfort and reduce hunger, not to achieve growth. A baby who can feed orally should do so. Breast-feeding may be comforting even when non-nutritive. Gavage (nasogastric) feeding may be appropriate for a baby who cannot feed orally but shows signs of hunger. Parenteral nutrition is rarely indicated.

Place of care

When death is expected, the baby should be cared for in a private area with the family. This may be in the hospital, their home or a hospice, depending on preference, available support and how long the baby is expected to live. If mechanical ventilation is withdrawn, extremely preterm infants usually die shortly afterwards, but mature infants may live for a considerable period. Parents need to be forewarned, and the place of care may change if the baby survives longer than expected. If parents are taking their baby home for end-of-life care, appropriate support must be in place, including medications not only for current but also potential symptoms, information about who to contact for routine and emergency problems, and what to do after the infant has died.

Support for the parents, siblings and family

The needs of each member of the baby's family should be considered, including parents, siblings, grandparents and extended family. It is now uncommon for people to have experience of death or to have seen a dead person, and many have fears about what will happen around the time of death. This needs to be discussed.

The family should be given the opportunity to create and collect mementoes before the baby dies and siblings can help with this. For example, a 'journey' or 'memory' box can be provided (Fig. 70.1). Mementoes might include antenatal scan pictures, photographs, foot and hand prints, a lock of hair and name tags. Religious ceremonies including blessings and baptisms should be supported.

Care after death

Parents should be encouraged to hold the baby before death and afterwards, if they want to. They may wish to bathe and dress their baby. Give unhurried, sympathetic care of the body after death, and provide unrestricted access for family. Cultural and religious rituals should be respected. Many parents value photographs of them and their baby at this time, especially if this is the first occasion they have held their baby without tubes, lines and monitors. 'Cold cots' can extend the amount of time available for the family to be with their baby after death (Fig. 70.2). Some families may wish to take the baby home and this should be facilitated. Information about registering the death and funeral arrangements should be provided. Inform the family practitioner or pediatrician, health visitor, obstetrician and other professionals involved that the baby has died. Some units have remembrance books and hold memorial services.

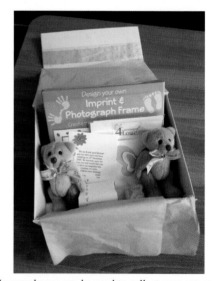

Fig. 70.1 Memory boxes can be used to collect mementoes of the baby's life.

Neonatology at a Glance, Third Edition. Edited by Tom Lissauer, Avroy A. Fanaroff, Lawrence Miall and Jonathan Fanaroff.
© 2016 John Wiley & Sons, Ltd. Published 2016 by John Wiley & Sons, Ltd.

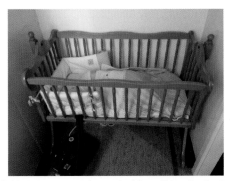

Fig. 70.2 Cold mattresses can be used with traditional cribs (cots) to prolong the time that family can spend with the baby after death.

Grief is a normal response to an infant's death. Parents and staff need to know that it is normal to show emotion and be given the opportunity to express their feelings. Grief may include shock, denial, anger, sadness or relief. There may be physical symptoms of anxiety, depression, tearfulness, loss of appetite, fatigue, insomnia and inability to concentrate. Grief may last years but is highly individual; in many it is most intense in the first few months. Parents may need advice about supporting siblings and other family members. Each parent may have a different pattern of grief and this may place stress on their relationship. Provide information about professional resources and self-help groups for bereavement support and counseling.

Families often find it helpful to have ongoing communication with the health-care team. A meeting arranged a few weeks after the child has died provides an opportunity to discuss the circumstances and to answer any questions and address any unresolved issues. It may be helpful if the obstetrician is also present. Health-care providers must be good listeners, in order to learn how the family is feeling. If there are concerns about abnormal grieving, professional assessment and support are recommended.

Caring for staff

The death of a baby may be distressing for staff, especially after protracted periods of intensive care, during which staff and parents become closely involved. The infant's death may be perceived as a failure. Open discussion between all members of staff is crucial, so that all are fully informed and are able to express their feelings and concerns. Dialogue is especially important when withdrawal of life support is being considered. Many units provide personal psychological support for staff.

Organ donation

Donation of a baby's tissue or organs may provide hope to families in an otherwise hopeless situation. Until recently, neonatal whole organ transplant was not widely available in the UK as guidelines on the diagnosis of death by neurological criteria in neonates had not been published. However, donation of tissues or organs from neonates after circulatory death has sometimes been possible. This includes, but is not limited to heart valves. The US does have

published criteria for the determination of brain death in term infants, and also protocols for donation. This has allowed transplantation of a number of organs, including heart, lung, kidney, liver and small bowel.

Autopsy

Why is it performed?

An autopsy should be offered, even if the cause of death is thought to be known. Advanced imaging and genetic tests mean that clinicians and families sometimes feel that autopsies are unnecessary and the autopsy rate has fallen markedly in the US and UK in the past 20 years. However, autopsy findings differ from the clinical diagnosis in 10–32%. Autopsy can be a legal requirement, e.g. after a sudden unexpected death or recent surgery, or if unnatural causes are implicated. Usually, it is performed to:
- help parents understand why their baby died,
- aid genetic counseling and planning future pregnancies
- help clinicians audit their management
- confirm the diagnosis or identify diagnoses that were missed.
- contribute to medical education and research. It should be performed by a pediatric pathologist.

What is involved in an autopsy?

Imaging:
- Photographs (particularly helpful for dysmorphology).
- X-rays (and MRI if indicated) for skeletal and other pathology not evident on clinical examination.

External and internal examination:
- Involves a full-length incision, which should be invisible when clothed.
- All organs are removed, inspected and weighed. Samples are taken for microbiological and histological analysis.

Organ retention:
- Some organs may need to be retained temporarily for fixing, mainly the brain and heart.
- For teaching or research. This requires explicit consent.

Consent

Detailed consent must be obtained unless the autopsy is legally required. All procedures must be described, and agreement reached about retention and disposal of tissues in a lawful and respectful way, or whether tissues should be returned for burial. Even if autopsy is legally required, parents should be informed about the procedure.

Are there alternatives to autopsy?

Post-mortem MRI, focused autopsy or specific tissue biopsy may be performed, but may miss diagnoses such as infection and metabolic disorders; conventional autopsy remains the gold standard.

Taking home a preterm baby who required intensive care and many weeks in a neonatal unit is often daunting for parents (Fig. 71.1). Their fears are shared by parents of term infants who became seriously ill or have complex problems.

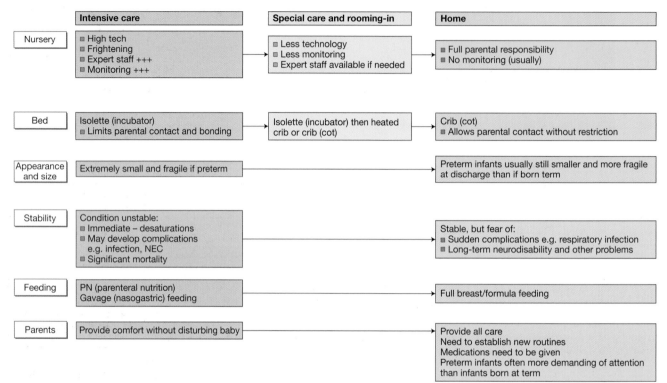

	Intensive care	Special care and rooming-in	Home
Nursery	■ High tech ■ Frightening ■ Expert staff +++ ■ Monitoring +++	■ Less technology ■ Less monitoring ■ Expert staff available if needed	■ Full parental responsibility ■ No monitoring (usually)
Bed	Isolette (incubator) ■ Limits parental contact and bonding	Isolette (incubator) then heated crib or crib (cot)	Crib (cot) ■ Allows parental contact without restriction
Appearance and size	Extremely small and fragile if preterm		Preterm infants usually still smaller and more fragile at discharge than if born term
Stability	Condition unstable: ■ Immediate – desaturations ■ May develop complications e.g. infection, NEC ■ Significant mortality		Stable, but fear of: ■ Sudden complications e.g. respiratory infection ■ Long-term neurodisability and other problems
Feeding	PN (parenteral nutrition) Gavage (nasogastric) feeding		Full breast/formula feeding
Parents	Provide comfort without disturbing baby		Provide all care Need to establish new routines Medications need to be given Preterm infants often more demanding of attention than infants born at term

Fig. 71.1 Transition from intensive care to home.

Questions

When can babies go home?

Most go home when their condition is stable and they have established feeding. Parents must be able to care for the baby and provide health-care needs.

Some babies requiring long-term oxygen therapy, e.g. for BPD (bronchopulmonary dysplasia), or gavage (tube) feeding can be managed at home (Fig. 71.2). Establishing such care at home will depend on the nature of the infant's medical condition, its likely time course and if otherwise stable, the parents, home circumstances and community support available.

Should babies with bronchoulmonary dysplasia have a 24-hour saturation recording done before going home?

This is performed in some units a few days after oxygen therapy is stopped to confirm the absence of significant desaturations. Its value has not been established.

All infants who were preterm should be checked to ensure that they are able to maintain their airway and saturations when placed in a car seat.

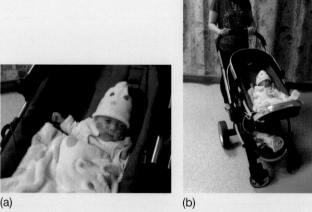

(a)   (b)

Fig. 71.2 (a) Infant receiving oxygen therapy and gavage (nasogastric) feeding at home. (b) Same infant receiving oxygen therapy via an oxygen cylinder in a stroller at home. Long-term oxygen provided via an oxygen concentrator adjusted according to oxygen saturation from a monitor.

Neonatology at a Glance, Third Edition. Edited by Tom Lissauer, Avroy A. Fanaroff, Lawrence Miall and Jonathan Fanaroff.
© 2016 John Wiley & Sons, Ltd. Published 2016 by John Wiley & Sons, Ltd.

Discharge planning

Good discharge planning aims to minimize parental anxiety and ensure seamless transfer of care between professionals in the hospital and community. This can be achieved by:
- having a named nurse with this responsibility
- starting discharge planning as soon as the baby is stable
- considering discharge arrangements (Fig. 71.3) during regular updates with parents and, if necessary, arranging pre-discharge meetings with the parents and other professionals involved, e.g. the family's pediatrician or family practitioner, community nurses, health visitors, therapists, child development team.

Facilities where parents can room in with their baby for several days or longer ('step-down units') before going home are helpful, especially when establishing full breast-feeding.

Some units have specialist nurses who provide care in the family's home and liaise with community-based services. Some of these nurses may also work on the unit and know the baby and family before discharge.

Health promotion
i) SIDS (sudden infant death syndrome) prevention particularly:
- Sleep on back not prone
- Avoid overheating
- Avoid smoking near baby
ii) Resuscitation training:
- Demonstration, may be complemented by video

Medications
What to give, how often, how to give them and for how long

Immunizations
Which have been given, when are the next ones due? Is RSV (respiratory syncytial virus) prophylaxis (palivizumab, a monoclonal antibody) indicated? If so, who will give it and when?

Follow-up arrangements
Who, when and where

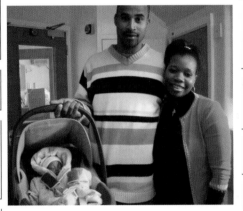

Past and potential medical problems
Check that parents have good understanding
Parents should have a copy of the discharge summary in case professional help is needed

Ongoing or new medical problems
Who to contact and how to manage them
Awareness of most likely problems requiring hospitalization, e.g. respiratory infections, inguinal hernias

Feeding
Is breast milk fortifier or a preterm formula feed required? If so, how can they be obtained and for how long?

Vision and hearing
Have they been checked? Are further checks required?

Parent support group
Would it be helpful, e.g. multiple births, etc? If so, do parents have contact address or is there a helpful internet site?

Fig. 71.3 Parents and their baby leaving the neonatal unit. The items that need to be considered prior to discharge are listed.

72 Follow-up of high-risk infants

Goals

The goals of high-risk follow-up are:
• early identification of disability or developmental or behavior problems
• management of ongoing medical issues
• facilitation of early intervention, with referral if necessary
• family support
• monitoring of neonatal outcomes.

Criteria

High-risk infants include:
• very preterm (usually <1500 g or <32 weeks of gestation)
• neurologic abnormality, including:
  – neonatal seizures
  – hypoxic–ischemic encephalopathy
  – neonatal meningitis
• mechanical ventilation/nitric oxide therapy/ECMO
• severe IUGR (intrauterine growth restriction)
• congenital malformations (significant)
• maternal drug misuse
• significant parental psychosocial problems.

Organization and timing

Timing of visits will vary with different programs and with the extent of pediatric neurodevelopmental expertise available to the family locally. It will also depend on whether neurodevelopmental outcome is being monitored at standard times. A typical program for clinic visits and reason for their timing is shown in Fig. 72.1.

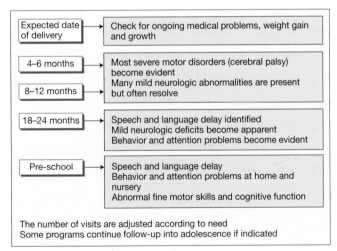

Fig. 72.1 An example of a high-risk follow-up program.

Who should conduct neonatal follow-up?

Many neonatologists provide neonatal follow-up with or without support from other physicians. This has the advantage of continuity of care for the parents. It also gives direct feedback on the sequelae of neonatal care but demands out-of-service referral if specialist help is required.

Good follow-up programs are multidisciplinary and include:
• developmental specialists – particularly for older children, when developmental assessment and management become more specialized and complex; in some programs all follow-up is performed by developmental specialists
• community nursing team – if involved with the family
• dietitian
• therapists
• psychologist
• social services.

The family practitioner/pediatrician provides general pediatric care and other pediatric specialists may be required for specific problems such as pulmonary or ophthalmology.

Components

• Growth monitoring.
• Neurologic and developmental assessment, including behavior.
• Vision and hearing.
• Social/family integration.
• Monitor chronic health conditions.
• School performance.

Outcome measures

Evaluation is tailored to the child's age. Most follow-up programs conduct formal data collection at 18–24 months of age corrected for prematurity, including a disability assessment, neurologic

Table 72.1 Widely used developmental assessments.

Bayley Scales of Infant Development (3rd edition)	Griffiths Mental Development Scales – Revised
Age range: 0–42 months	Age range: 0–24 months (Baby scales) 24–96 months (Extended)
Subscales:	Subscales:
• Fine motor	• Locomotor
• Gross motor	• Personal social
• Receptive language	• Hearing and language
• Expressive language	• Eye – hand coordination
• Cognitive scale	• Performance
	• Practical reasoning (from 2 years)

Neonatology at a Glance, Third Edition. Edited by Tom Lissauer, Avroy A. Fanaroff, Lawrence Miall and Jonathan Fanaroff.
© 2016 John Wiley & Sons, Ltd. Published 2016 by John Wiley & Sons, Ltd.

evaluation and a developmental assessment using a standardized assessment (see Chapter 38).

Widely used developmental assessments at this age are the Bayley Scales or the Griffiths Scales (Table 72.1). They are standardized to a population mean of 100 with a standard deviation of 15 points. Children with scores <55 (−3 standard deviations) have severe developmental impairment likely to persist, children with scores 55–70 have moderate impairment and are highly likely to have low scores at later ages, while children with scores 70–85 have milder impairment and may catch up.

A formal classification of disability at 2 years is shown in Table 38.1. Such definitions are useful for comparing outcomes between centers and for evaluating the results of trials.

Follow up of older children (Fig. 72.2) is outside the remit of most neonatal follow-up programs because it requires formal IQ and behavioral screening. School evaluation by the class teacher is valuable for identifying need for support.

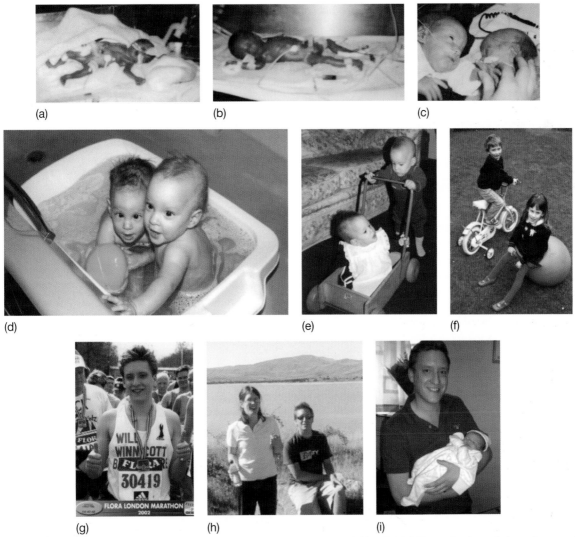

(a)　　　　　　(b)　　　　　　(c)

(d)　　　　　　(e)　　　　　　(f)

(g)　　　　　　(h)　　　　　　(i)

Fig. 72.2 Tiny preterm babies do grow up! Sally and William, from birth at 26 weeks to adulthood. (a) Sally at a few hours in intensive care. (b) William shortly after extubation. (c) Together at last at 4 weeks! (d) At a year. (e) Just walking. (f) At 5 years. (g) At 18 years, William completing the London marathon. (h) At 19 years, Sally and William on vacation in New Zealand. (i) The next generation has arrived, rather larger at birth than her father! (With thanks to Sally and William for permitting the use of these photographs.)

Enormous efforts have been made in many low- and middle-income countries to achieve Millennium Development Goal 4 (MDG 4), a two-thirds reduction in child mortality from 1990 to 2015. The mortality rate for children under 5 years old has declined markedly since 1990, particularly from improved coverage of immunization, early treatment and prevention of malaria and HIV (Fig. 73.1). However:

• Neonatal mortality has declined much more slowly, with 44% of all deaths at age <5 years now in first 28 days of life (Fig. 73.1).

• Progress is slowest in reducing early neonatal deaths (first week of life), when 75% of neonatal deaths occur, 40% in the first 24 hours.

The *Every Newborn Action Plan*, launched in 2014, a global campaign to reduce neonatal mortality beyond the Millennium Development Goal time period, proposes that all countries should reach a target of <10 newborn deaths per 1000 live births by 2035 (compared with current neonatal mortality of 4 per 1000 live births in the US and UK). Through scale-up of known effective interventions, this should be feasible.

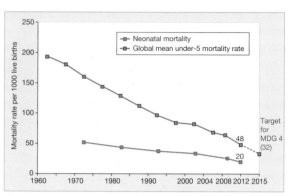

Fig. 73.1 Global progress towards Millennium Development Goal 4 for child survival. (Source: Lawn J.E. Newborn survival in low resource settings – are we delivering? *BJOG* 2009; 116 (Suppl. 1): 49–59; updated 2014 for data to 2012.)

Some resource-poor countries, including Malawi, Bangladesh and Rwanda, have shown that achieving substantial reductions in neonatal mortality rates is possible. However, even when neonatal mortality has been reduced, wealth-related inequity remains a significant problem, with lack of access to skilled birth attendants and adequately equipped facilities being particularly marked in rural compared with urban areas, and in slums in urban areas.

> **Key point**
>
> Globally, every year there are:
> • 135 million births
> • 6.6 million deaths at age <5 years
> • 3 million neonatal deaths (first 28 days).

Geography of newborn deaths

Only 1% of neonatal deaths occur in high-income countries. About three-quarters of all newborn deaths occur in sub-Saharan Africa and South Asia. The same regions have the highest risk and numbers of maternal deaths and stillbirths.

Ten countries account for two-thirds of the world's neonatal deaths (Fig. 73.2). India alone has 0.8 million neonatal deaths per year.

Causes of newborn deaths

The main causes of neonatal death globally are:
• preterm birth
• intrapartum-related conditions (previously more loosely called 'birth asphyxia')
• neonatal infections (including sepsis, pneumonia, tetanus and diarrhea) (Fig. 73.3).

Many infants have growth restriction; mortality is markedly increased in infants who are both preterm and growth restricted.

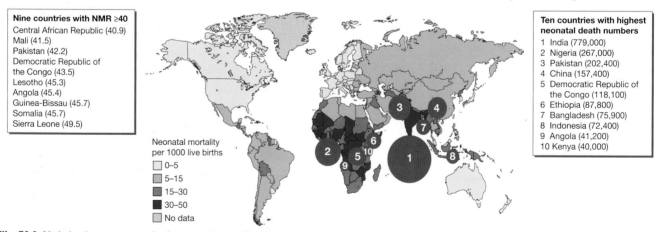

Fig. 73.2 Variation between countries in neonatal mortality rate in 2012. (Adapted from Lawn J.E. *et al*. Every newborn: survival and beyond. *Lancet* 2014; **384**: 189–205.)

Neonatology at a Glance, Third Edition. Edited by Tom Lissauer, Avroy A. Fanaroff, Lawrence Miall and Jonathan Fanaroff.
© 2016 John Wiley & Sons, Ltd. Published 2016 by John Wiley & Sons, Ltd.

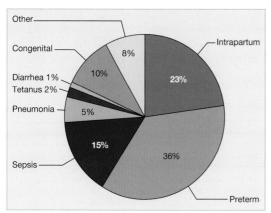

Fig. 73.3 Cause of neonatal death distribution in 194 countries in 2012. (Source: Lawn J.E. *et al*. Every newborn: survival and beyond. *Lancet* 2014; **384**: 189–205.)

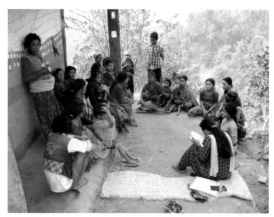

Fig. 73.4 Women's group meeting in Nepal. Participatory women's groups have been shown to reduce neonatal deaths in rural high-mortality settings. (Courtesy of Save the Children. Photographer Joanna Morrison.)

Deaths from neonatal tetanus have declined rapidly due to improved coverage of maternal tetanus toxoid immunization and improved hygiene at birth especially cord care practices. However, slower progress has been made in reducing deaths and disability from other infections, complications of childbirth or preterm birth.

Timing of newborn deaths

The birth of a baby should be a time of celebration, yet all too often it is a time of tragedy. The risk of dying during labor or the first day of life is high. Globally, every year, one million newborns (36% of all neonatal deaths), and 125 000 mothers (nearly half of maternal deaths) die and there are 1.2 million stillbirths during this short time-period.

Birth and the early neonatal period are also a time of high risk for neurologic injury resulting in long-term impairment.

Maternal health and obstetric care

Maternal health and obstetric care have a substantial impact on reducing neonatal morbidity and mortality. The following are priorities to achieve this:
- Before conception:
  - Reduce barriers to family planning – delaying first pregnancy to at least 18 years of age and 3-year birth intervals are proven health strategies for mother and baby.
  - Optimize maternal nutrition – including calories, protein, iodine, folic acid, iron.
  - Optimize prevention and treatment of infections – malaria, tetanus and sexually transmitted diseases such as syphilis and HIV (see Chapter 43, Viral infections).
  - Optimize management of chronic conditions, e.g. hypertension, diabetes.
- During pregnancy:
  - Improve coverage of key interventions, such as mosquito nets and prophylaxis for malaria.
  - Improve quality and uptake of antenatal care.

- Improve detection and management of complications of pregnancy, including maternal infections and hypertensive disorders.
- During labor and delivery:
  - Ensure skilled attendants at all births, including essential equipment and logistical support.
  - Appropriate use of antenatal steroids for preterm labor.
  - Timely management of complications for mother or baby.

Worldwide, 70% of all births are with a skilled birth attendant, but in some countries, such as Ethiopia, Niger, Chad and Sudan, this is not achieved in three-quarters of births. Improved access to skilled attendants and referral pathways to health facilities equipped to deal with obstetric emergencies is urgently required.

Both participatory women's groups offering peer counseling and community mobilization (Fig. 73.4) and home-visit packages by

Question

In HIV infected mothers, what PMTCT (prevention of mother-to-child transmission) interventions should be undertaken in resource-limited settings?

Without intervention, the risk of perinatal transmission is 20–45%. It occurs *in utero*, peripartum and postnatally via breast-feeding.

In 2013, the WHO recommended universal, lifelong combination antiretroviral therapy for all pregnant women or at least until breast-feeding has ceased, aiming to suppress maternal HIV viral load and minimize transmission to the infant.

Countries need to either promote breast-feeding and provide antiretroviral therapy or provide safe nutrition with formula, depending on the degree of increased risk of mortality from gastroenteritis and pneumonia associated with formula.

In resource-poor countries, exclusive breast-feeding in combination with antiretroviral therapy for the newborn (for a minimum of 6 weeks) is recommended for first the 6 months. Thereafter, complementary foods, continuing to breast-feeding until 12 months of age.

Formula-fed infants should also receive antiretroviral therapy for 6 weeks, to prevent transmission from exposure during delivery.

community health workers, during pregnancy and after birth, have been shown to provide an opportunity to empower women to have better outcomes for themselves and for their newborns.

Newborn care in low-resource settings – what works?

It is estimated that over 1 million lives could be saved each year even with simple care that can be provided outside hospitals and does not require intensive care or high-tech machines.

Care around the time of birth

Newborn survival would be improved if:
• Skilled birth attendants were not only present at birth but able to provide care not only for the mother but also for the newborn, including basic resuscitation with a bag and mask and recognition of infants needing additional care.
• Essential newborn care was provided (Table 73.1):
  – Infection control – hand-washing of the birth attendant, clean delivery surface, clean cutting and tying of cord and ongoing cord care (with application of chlorhexidine) to prevent neonatal infections, including tetanus.
  – Adequate thermal care – including drying the baby at birth, keeping warm with skin-to-skin contact, having a warm environment, covering the baby, including the head, and delaying bathing.
  – Early and exclusive breast-feeding – starting within 1 hour of birth and avoiding any formula milk. Exclusive breast-feeding plays a crucial role in prevention of infection and should be strongly encouraged in all countries (Fig. 73.5). Breast milk is especially important for low-birthweight infants.
  – Early detection of problems and appropriate care-seeking. Education of mothers and communities on 'danger signs', but care-seeking may be impeded by cost, distance or, in some cultures, by strong pressure on mothers and newborn babies not to go outside their home for the first 4–6 weeks. In addition, the hospital or health facility must be able to provide quality care for sick babies. When this is not available, home-based treatment may be an alternative. Several studies in South Asia have shown that treatment of infections with antibiotics by injection can be provided at home by community health workers, with reduction of 30% or more in neonatal deaths.

Key point

• Breastmilk offers major health benefits to infants compared to formula milk.
• The promotion and marketing of infant formula milk is restricted by the International Code of Marketing of Breast Milk Substitutes (WHO, UNICEF).

Hospital-based care

Hospitals should be able to provide safe, quality care for sick or small newborns, a key priority for improving newborn survival and health. This includes:
• Health-care professionals specifically trained in providing newborn care.
• Neonatal resuscitation available.
• Up-to-date, evidence based guidelines for common conditions.
• Measures for infection control practiced, e.g. hand hygiene and sterile procedures, equipment cleaned.
• Thermal regulation – warm delivery room, skin-to-skin policy, clothing and hats for babies. Other warming devices such as radiant heaters, incubators or warming mattresses are used appropriately and maintained.
• Feeding support for mothers of preterm babies and supplemental feeding – help for mothers to express milk, cup feeding, gavage (nasogastric) tube feeding if needed.
• Intravenous (IV) fluids, closely monitored.
• Antibiotic treatment for babies at increased risk or signs of infection.
• Management of jaundice.

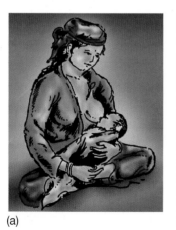
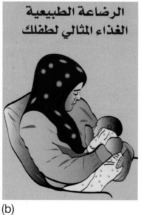

(a)   (b)

Fig. 73.5 Examples of the promotion of breast-feeding: (a) Nepal; (b) Oman. (Courtesy of Dr Saleh Al-Khusaiby.)

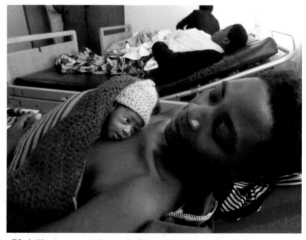

Fig. 73.6 Kangaroo mother care for a preterm newborn. (Photo courtesy of Save the Children, South Africa.)

- Kangaroo mother care – provided continuously by mothers for stable preterm babies (Fig. 73.6). This is a cost-effective intervention which improves thermal care, breast-feeding and bonding and reduces infection and neonatal mortality in low- and middle-income countries. Allows limited staff resources to be focused on the sickest babies. Often limited by lack of space.
- Respiratory support – oxygen, aminophylline or caffeine for apnea, bubble CPAP (continuous positive airway pressure) or other forms of non-invasive respiratory support. Artificial ventilation may be appropriate in some settings with well-functioning neonatal units able to provide basic respiratory support, but requires a high level of resources.
- Supportive care, e.g. control of seizures in hypoxic–ischemic encephalopathy.
- Monitoring, including oxygen monitoring with pulse oximetry – blindness from retinopathy of prematurity has been reported in many middle-income countries affecting relatively mature infants from use of excessively high concentrations of oxygen without appropriate monitoring.

Question

Why is neonatal mortality in resource-poor countries not declining rapidly?

Many reasons, including:
- Improving maternal care – maternal nutrition, health and education, and care antenatally, during labor and delivery, all of which markedly affect the newborn – is complex and takes time.
- Essential newborn care following birth – often not provided; indeed, in some countries, newborn care practices following hone births are harmful, e.g. delay in initiating breast-feeding, early bathing which results in hypothermia, cutting the cord with dirty implements (Table 73.1).
- Early recognition of illness in newborn infants – often difficult and illness progresses rapidly – urgent transfer from home or health center for effective hospital care requires a responsive, integrated health system.
- Inadequate hospital care for sick or preterm infants – health professionals insufficient in number and not trained in neonatology, equipment not available or not maintained, poor facilities that are often hot and cramped.
- Insufficient focus on and investment in newborn-specific nursing skills.

Table 73.1 Summary of survey of newborn care in rural Nepal before 2002, when the neonatal mortality was 50/1000 live births. By addressing these and other issues, neonatal mortality declined to 24/1000 in 2012.

90%	Gave birth at home
6%	Skilled attendant at delivery
11%	Alone at delivery
33%	Cord cut with household sickle
64%	Wrapped baby only at 30 minutes of age
92%	Bathed in first hour (high risk of hypothermia)
99%	Breast-fed

Adapted from Osrin D. *et al.* Cross sectional, community based study of care of newborn infants in Nepal. *BMJ* 2002; **325**: 1063.

- Neonatal care is wrongly considered too 'high-tech' and difficult to provide.
- Many doctors, including some pediatricians, lack interest and experience in newborn care.
- Lack of data on newborn health outcomes; contributes to lower visibility and investment and political will for improvement.

Question

What role can doctors and neonatologists in developed countries play in improving global newborn health?

They can help by:
- Advocacy – promoting newborn care in resource-poor countries.
- Assisting with training courses for health professionals in resource-poor countries e.g. Helping Babies Breathe (neonatal resuscitation), ETAT+ (Emergency Triage, Assessment and Treatment plus Admission).
- Participating in one of the many collaborative programs or partnerships. These need to be appropriate for local conditions, but still retain scientific rigor and be evidence based. Programs must also be aligned to local and national strategy.

Further reading and resources

- The Lancet *Every Newborn* series 2014.
- Health Newborn Network Topic Resources: http://www.healthynewbornnetwork.org/topics

The need for neonatal transport is increasing with centralization of specialist services. Infants must be moved to the right place, by the right team, by the right mode of transport.

Infrastructure

- Specialized trained teams.
- Dedicated equipment (Fig. 74.1).
- A 'transport hotline' – providing efficient referral process, advice and bed locator (if available).
- Contracts and protocols for transport – ambulance, helicopter, fixed-wing airplane.
- Insurance liabilities to cover adverse events.
- Outreach training for less specialized units.

Why transfer?

- Uplift in care level, e.g. extreme prematurity, unstable term infants.
- For subspecialty care – cardiology, surgery, etc.
- Transport back to referral hospital after specialist care.

Equipment

- Transport incubator or lightweight Baby Pod.
- Airways – mask, oro- and nasopharyngeal tracheal tubes.
- Respiratory support – ventilator, CPAP, air, oxygen, nitric oxide.
- Full ICU monitoring.
- IV access – cannulae, syringes, infusion pumps.
- Hand-held blood testing – glucose, electrolytes, hemoglobin, blood gases.
- Power source – available in ambulance, aircraft or hospital. Battery for transfers between power supply.

Equipment is heavy – needs handling skills and special equipment to assist.

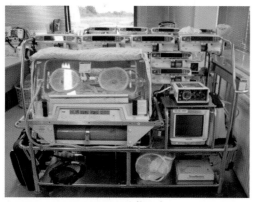

Fig. 74.1 Dedicated, specialized equipment.

Documentation

- Use standardized clinical assessment and treatment records.
- Necessary for debriefing, audit, legal records.

The **ACCEPT** principle is a comprehensive system to ensure that all aspects of the transfer process are managed optimally:

A – Assessment

- Determine the appropriate destination for the identified specialist care needs.

C – Taking **Control** of the situation and **Communication** with all teams involved

These include transport team, receiving unit and subspecialists. Ideally done through central coordinating center using call conferencing facilities.

Initial communication:
- Record all clinical details necessary to plan the retrieval.
- Give appropriate advice for stabilization and ongoing care:
  – ensure that vital signs, laboratory tests and blood gases are up-to-date and appropriate
  – request respiratory support, vascular access, infection treatment, specialist care for cardiac or surgery to be initiated if necessary.
- Ask referring hospital to prepare:
  – full documentation of pregnancy, birth and postnatal course; radiographs; laboratory results; vitamin K status
  – names of baby and parents and contact details
  – maternal blood for cross-match.
- Record exact location of patient, city, hospital, ward.
- Estimate arrival time and inform referring hospital.
- Provide ongoing contact number for clinical advice from specialist if needed.

E – **Evaluation** of the infant to be moved.

On arrival of transport team:
- Ensure detailed handover of patient's condition.
- Review current treatment and management.

Before transport, the infant should have:
- normal temperature (except during therapeutic hypothermia)
- secure airway and breathing
- IV access – two lines preferably if critically ill
- gavage (naso-/orogastric) tube
- optimized blood pressure, circulation, urine output – consider arterial access
- optimized blood results – glucose, electrolytes, complete blood count (CBC), blood gases, etc.
- immediate treatment given, e.g. antibiotics, transfusion, prostaglandin (Prostin), anticonvulsants as appropriate.
- further specialized treatment started if required, e.g. active or passive cooling.

Neonatology at a Glance, Third Edition. Edited by Tom Lissauer, Avroy A. Fanaroff, Lawrence Miall and Jonathan Fanaroff.
© 2016 John Wiley & Sons, Ltd. Published 2016 by John Wiley & Sons, Ltd.

P – Preparation by transport team

Prepare emergency medications, including fluid boluses, and emergency equipment, e.g. airways, endotracheal tubes. IV lines that may be needed en route.

P – Packaging

- The infant's clinical status needs to be rechecked after transfer to the transport incubator, ensuring that all transport equipment is functioning, i.e. ventilator, monitors, infusion pumps.
- Check that all lines, endotracheal tubes, catheters, etc. are secure.
- Make baby as comfortable as possible.
- Secure infant in the transport incubator with harnesses. The incubator, monitors and infusion pumps must be well secured to the transport trolley.

T – Transfer

- Transport trolley must be secured in ambulance (Fig. 74.2).
- Continuous monitoring, record vital signs regularly as in ICU.
- Avoid all unnecessary interventions.
  On arrival at receiving hospital:
- Hand over to receiving staff.
- Ensure stable transfer to ICU monitoring and therapy.
- Complete documentation.

Key points

- Remember parents – they need information, support, transport, accommodation, finance, child care and counseling.
- Ideally should be offered the opportunity to travel with their baby.
- They will remember this experience for the rest of their lives.

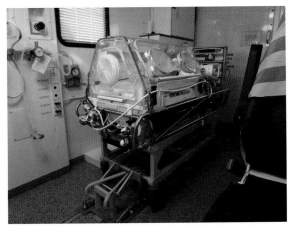

Fig. 74.2 Securing trolley in ambulance.

Aeromedical considerations (Figs 74.3 and 74.4)

- May be faster if ground transport takes more than 2 hours.
- Helicopter maximum distance is about 300 miles, then use fixed-wing airplane. Local conditions will determine the choice. Problems:
- Expensive.
- Multiple transfers between vehicles.
- Cramped space/difficult access to baby.
- Noise and vibration.
- Decreased barometric pressure – fixed-wing airplanes are pressurized at about 8000 ft (2500 m), so, for example, 50% FiO_2 at ground level will require 67% at 8000 ft (2500 m). There will be expansion of closed air-filled cavities:
  - Ensure gavage (naso-/orogastric) tube on free drainage and aspirated regularly.
  - Air leaks may worsen.
  - Blood pressure cuffs may cause occlusion of blood vessels.

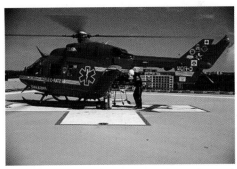

Fig. 74.3 Helicopter transfer in Northern Canada.

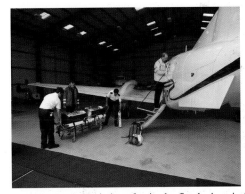

Fig. 74.4 Long distance repatriation of twins by fixed wing airplane.

Pitfalls for all modes of transport

- Extreme weather.
- Vehicle failure.
- Equipment failure.
- Battery or medical gas failure.
- Accidents.
- Travel sickness.
- *Be prepared!*

Endotracheal intubation

Indications

- Neonatal resuscitation (see Chapter 13) to aspirate meconium or in advanced resuscitation.
- Mechanical ventilation for respiratory failure:
  - prolonged/recurrent apnea, not responding to non-invasive respiratory support
  - increasing respiratory distress or inadequate oxygenation (hypoxemia) and/or carbon dioxide elimination (hypercarbia) on CPAP or high-flow nasal cannulae.
- To replace a blocked or dislodged tracheal tube.
- For administration of surfactant (**see video: INSURE technique**).
- Upper airway obstruction – to provide a secure airway.
- Congenital diaphragmatic hernia – to avoid bowel distension.
- Prior to surgical procedures/general anesthesia.

Procedure

- Ensure you have assistance and prepare equipment in advance.
- Premedicate, e.g. with propofol or a combination of fentanyl, suxamethonium and atropine unless an emergency.
- Ensure good oxygen saturation but avoid hyperoxia. Monitor oxygen saturation and heart rate continuously.
- Place head in the midline in a slightly extended position. Pressure on the cricoid by an assistant can be helpful to visualize vocal cords.
- Insert laryngoscope with left hand to just beyond base of tongue and epiglottis.
- Lift entire blade (Fig. 75.1). Suction to clear secretions if needed.
- Insert tracheal tube with right hand into right side of infant's mouth and pass through the vocal cords (Fig. 75.2) to the level

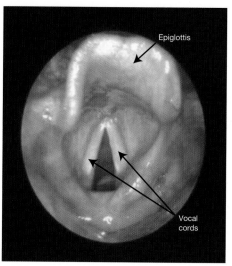

Fig. 75.2 View of vocal cords at intubation.

Table 75.1 Guide to endotracheal tube size.

Weight (kg)	Gestation (weeks)	ET tube size (mm)	Depth of insertion oral tube (cm from upper lip)
<1	<28	2.5	6–7
1–2	28–34	3.0	7–8
2–3	35–38	3.5	8–9
>3	>38	3.5–4	9–10

of the black line near the tube tip. A stylet may help stiffen the tube but must not protrude beyond the end as it may cause trauma.
- Note depth of insertion from the lips (see Table 75.1).
- Verify correct tube placement by:
  - observing symmetrical chest rise and an improvement in heart rate and oxygen saturation
  - observing color change in a CO_2 detector (this shows the tube has passed into the trachea, but it may still be malpositioned)
  - auscultation: hearing air entry over upper lungs and none over the stomach. If air entry is greater on right side than left, tube is in right main bronchus; withdraw until breath sounds equal.
- Secure tube and confirm position with chest X-ray.
- Limit attempts to 20–30 seconds and avoid bradycardia.
- Mask-ventilate and oxygenate infant between attempts.

Nasal intubation gives better stability of the tracheal tube but can be more difficult to insert and can cause nasal trauma. A lubricated ET tube is passed through the nostril to back of throat; once the cords (and tube) are visualized with the laryngoscope, the tube is lifted into the airway using McGill forceps if necessary and then advanced.

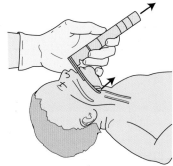

Fig. 75.1 Technique of laryngoscopy for endotracheal intubation. Place tip of blade at base of epiglottis or lift epiglottis. Lift the entire blade to visualize the vocal cords. Do not tilt blade upwards, as it may damage gum or palate. Cricoid pressure may help.

Neonatology at a Glance, Third Edition. Edited by Tom Lissauer, Avroy A. Fanaroff, Lawrence Miall and Jonathan Fanaroff.
© 2016 John Wiley & Sons, Ltd. Published 2016 by John Wiley & Sons, Ltd.

Chest tubes (chest drain)

Indications

- Pneumothorax.
- Pleural effusion.

Technique

The Seldinger technique (insertion over a guidewire) has largely replaced open dissection (**see video: Chest drain insertion**).
- Site: preferably lateral – third to fifth intercostal space, anterior axillary line or otherwise anteriorly, second intercostal space, mid-clavicular line. Just above rib to avoid neurovascular bundle.
- Avoid nipple and breast bud.
- Sterile technique.
- Local anesthesia – 1% lidocaine.
- Seldinger technique – insert needle into chest, aiming apically and anteriorly for pneumothoraces and posteriorly and basally for fluid, and aspirate small volume of air or fluid.
- Insert guidewire into needle (Fig. 78.3); then remove needle over wire.
- Thread chest tube (8 or 10 FG) over the guide wire (Fig. 75.4). Some chest tubes change color on entry into the pleural space. Remove guidewire.
- Connect tube to three-way tap and underwater seal, observe air bubbles and swinging with respiration.
- Fix to chest wall with sterile strips and adhesive dressing. Avoid suturing round the tube as it may leave scars (see Fig. 66.7).
- X-ray to check tube position and lung re-expansion (Fig. 75.5).

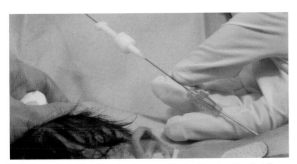

Fig. 75.3 Insertion of guidewire into needle (red) using the Seldinger technique.

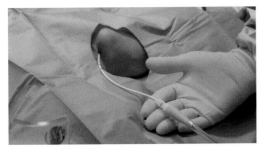

Fig. 75.4 Chest tube has been threaded over guidewire, which has been withdrawn and attached to underwater seal.

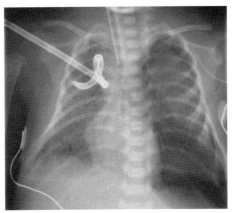

Fig. 75.5 X-ray showing a right chest tube (pigtail) to drain a pneumothorax. There is also a left pneumothorax with mediastinal shift.

Complications

- Hemothorax.
- Infection.
- Surgical emphysema.
- Scarring of skin or breast tissue.

Needle thoracotomy (chest needling)

Indication

- Immediate treatment of tension pneumothorax.

Technique

- Quickly confirm by auscultation and transillumination.
- Site – second or third intercostal space, mid-clavicular line.
- Approach – upper edge of rib to avoid neurovascular bundle.
- Insert butterfly needle. Create underwater seal or aspirate air from chest with syringe via a three-way tap.
- Usually followed by chest tube insertion.

Pleural tap

Indications

- Pleural fluid, e.g. chylothorax, pleural effusion.

Technique

- Sterile technique.
- Use ultrasound to identify fluid.
- Local anesthesia – 1% lidocaine.
- Insert a 22G cannula just above the rib.
- Attach to three-way tap and aspirate fluid.
  If pleural fluid reaccumulates, insert a chest drain.

Complications

- Pneumothorax or hemothorax.

Neonatal care involves a large number of practical procedures. Each has specific advantages and risks. Team training and preparation are the key to success and avoiding complications. Minimize pain with sucrose, gentle wrapping and positioning. Optimize timing from the baby's perspective in relation to feeds and other procedures. Ensure appropriate consent is obtained. For all these procedures meticulous attention to asepsis is important – both to avoid the risk of introducing infection and to prevent contamination of sterile samples, leading to overuse of antimicrobials. Skin preparation with cleansing agents should be used to clean the skin. Dispose of all sharps safely directly into a sharps bin. Some common procedures are shown in Table 76.1.

Table 76.1 Some common procedures.

Procedure	Preparation and equipment	Comments	Technique	Advantages	Potential complications
Capillary blood sampling (heelstick)	Clean procedure Gloves, sterile alcohol swab, automatic mini-lancet, tubes, gauze	Autostylets less painful than stylets inserted by hand. Avoid undue squeezing of heel, as painful and gives misleading results. Catch drops in bottle. Stop bleeding with gauze	**Fig. 76.1** Shaded areas show sites for capillary sampling.	Simple technique for blood glucose, hematocrit, complete blood count, electrolytes and blood gases	If results are abnormal, confirm with venepuncture Bruising Infection Rarely osteomyelitis
Venous blood sampling	Clean procedure Gloves, sterile alcohol swab, needle, tubes for blood sample, gauze	Use venepuncture needle. Avoid potential central line sites	**Fig. 76.2** Venous blood sampling from back of the hand.	Good flow of blood – avoids hemolysis of sample	Bruising Infection Difficult access in some infants Loss of veins for cannulation
Peripheral venous cannulation	Clean procedure Gloves, sterile alcohol swab, cannulae, flushed T-piece, stopper, syringe, tape, clear dressing, splint if necessary	Avoid potential central line access sites Fiber-optic light may facilitate visualization of veins Dress with sterile clear adhesive dressing, with entry site visible	**Fig. 76.3** Peripheral venous cannulation. When blood flows back, advance cannula over and withdraw stylet.	Usually achieved relatively quickly Best method for blood culture	Bruising/ Hemorrhage Inflammation Infection Extravasation injury

Neonatology at a Glance, Third Edition. Edited by Tom Lissauer, Avroy A. Fanaroff, Lawrence Miall and Jonathan Fanaroff.
© 2016 John Wiley & Sons, Ltd. Published 2016 by John Wiley & Sons, Ltd.

Table 76.1 (*continued*)

Procedure	Preparation and equipment	Comments	Technique	Advantages	Potential complications
Peripheral arterial cannulation	Clean procedure Gloves, sterile alcohol swab, cannulae, flushed T-piece, stopper, tape, dressing	Use limited by potential complications Identify artery by pulse and transillumination. Hand: radial artery; check for collateral circulation (Fig 76.4) Foot: posterior tibial, dorsalis pedis Never use temporal, brachial or ulnar artery Infuse heparinized saline Clearly mark as arterial Sample and flush slowly	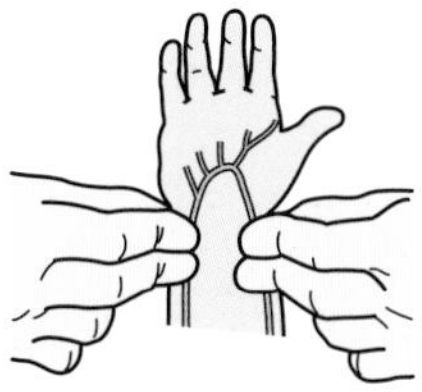 **Fig. 76.4** Peripheral arterial cannulation. Check for collateral circulation (Allen test) – hand blanches when both arteries occluded; color returns when occlusion of one artery is released.	Access for repeated blood sampling Invasive BP measurement unless poor peripheral circulation	Short functioning time (hours to few days) Variable success at insertion Blood loss if line disconnected If poor perfusion of fingers/toes –**REMOVE** Rarely ischemia or gangrene
Urinary catheter	Sterile procedure Gloves, sterile towel, cleaning fluid, lubricated urinary catheters 4 or 5 FG	To obtain sterile urine Treatment of urinary retention Monitor urinary output		Simpler More reliable to obtain sterile specimen than suprapubic aspirate and no needlestick	Urethral damage Hemorrhage Contaminated urine sample Infection
Suprapubic aspirate (bladder tap)	Sterile procedure Gloves, sterile alcohol swab, needle, syringe, sterile pot, gauze	To obtain sterile urine sample Higher success rate if ultrasound abdomen to check if bladder is full In an infant the bladder extends into the abdomen.	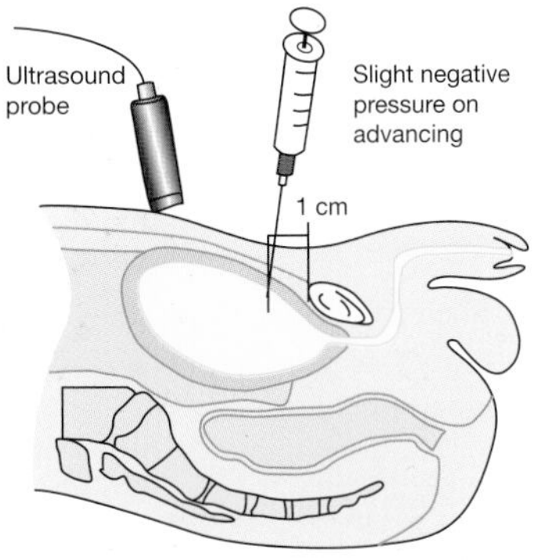 **Fig. 76.5** Suprapubic aspiration under ultrasound guidance. (Adapted from Lissauer T. and Clayden G. *Illustrated Textbook of Paediatrics*, Elsevier, 2012.)	Sterile sampling for reliable diagnosis of urinary tract infection	No urine obtained Rare – hemorrhage or needlestick injury to bowel
Lumbar puncture	Sterile procedure Gown, mask and sterile gloves. sterile towels, cleaning fluid, gauze, LP needles, containers for CSF samples	Position infant lying on side or sitting with spine flexed Minimize discomfort; topical analgesia Prepare sterile field Slowly advance needle with stylet in direction of umbilicus. May feel a "give" when pierce dura and enter subarachnoid space. Remove stylet and check for CSF. Collect 5–10 drops into each of 3 sterile containers and glucose bottle. Replace stylet, remove needle, apply sterile adhesive dressing.	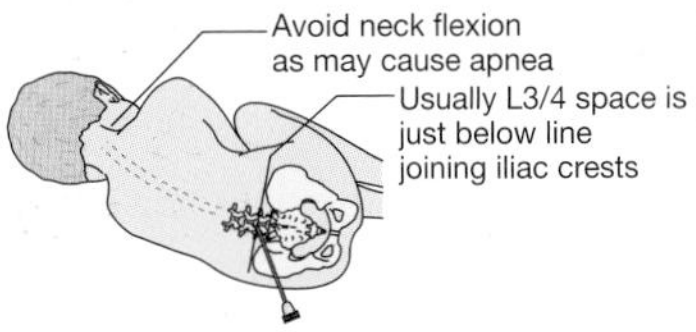 **Fig. 76.6** Lumbar puncture (**see video: Lumbar puncture**). Back curved. Skilled assistance required. Infant may also be held upright.	Identifies meningitis Withdrawal of CSF in treatment of post-hemorrhagic hydrocephalus Rarely, identification of metabolic disorder	No CSF obtained. Blood-stained CSF – trauma or hemorrhage (intraventricular or subarachnoid) Contraindicated: • bleeding disorder, e.g. thrombocytopenia • cardiorespiratory instability • Local skin infection

Umbilical catheters

Umbilical artery catheter (UAC)

Indications
- Continuous measurement of arterial blood pressure.
- Frequent blood gases or other blood samples.
- Exchange transfusion – to remove blood.

Contraindications
- Vascular compromise in the lower extremities or gluteal area.
- Necrotizing enterocolitis, peritonitis.
- Omphalitis (infection of the umbilical cord).
- Omphalocele.

Insertion (see video: Umbilical catheter insertion (arterial and venous))
Easiest on first day, possible within first 3–4 days.
- Wear gown, mask and sterile gloves, prepare sterile field.
- Prime catheter with saline.
- Clean the umbilicus and skin with chlorhexidine 2%/70% isopropyl alcohol swabs (ensure no pooling under baby).
- Place nylon tape around the base to control bleeding, then cut umbilical cord 1–2 cm from skin.
- Identify artery (Fig. 77.1). Dilate the artery with fine forceps or a dilator.
- Insert gently a 3 or 4.5 French gauge catheter to predetermined length (Table 77.1). There is gentle resistance from the muscular wall of the artery. Check that blood can be withdrawn (Fig. 77.2).
- Secure catheter (Fig. 77.2).
- Check position with X-ray (Figs 77.3 and 77.4) or ultrasound.
- Flush with heparinized saline.
- Label line as arterial or use red three-way tap.

Complications
- False track by catheter.
- Poor perfusion of lower limbs. If ischemic immediately **REMOVE** catheter.
- Blood loss if line disconnects.
- Aortic thrombosis and emboli.
- Infection (remove line as soon as no longer needed).
- Anemia from repeated excess blood volume sampling.

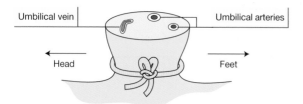

Fig. 77.1 Two arteries and one vein in umbilicus. The arteries are small, circular and have a muscular wall; the vein is larger, thin-walled and irregular.

Table 77.1 Formula to calculate length of umbilical lines.

Type of line	Length (cm) – add on the length of the umbilical stump
Umbilical artery catheter (UAC) (high position)	3 × weight (kg) + 9 cm
Umbilical vein catheter (UVC)	Half the UAC length + 1 cm

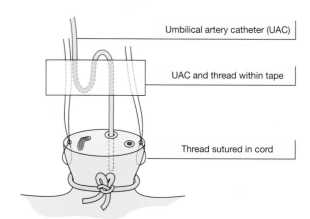

Fig. 77.2 Insertion and fixation of umbilical artery catheter. Transverse cutting of cord as shown here or cut down onto artery. Dilate with fine forceps or dilator. Magnification may be helpful. The umbilical cord is tied to a strip of tape to avoid tape on the skin. In some units, tape is placed in an H-shape on the abdominal wall and incorporates the catheter and thread suture from the cord.

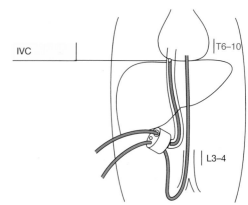

Fig. 77.3 Position of catheters. For an arterial catheter (red), the high position (T6–10) is above the diaphragm, avoiding the celiac axis (T12), superior mesenteric artery (T12–L1) and renal arteries. This is the ideal position with less vascular complications. The low position (L3–4) is below the inferior mesenteric artery but above the aortic bifurcation. IVC, inferior vena cava. The position of the venous catheter is shown in blue.

Neonatology at a Glance, Third Edition. Edited by Tom Lissauer, Avroy A. Fanaroff, Lawrence Miall and Jonathan Fanaroff.
© 2016 John Wiley & Sons, Ltd. Published 2016 by John Wiley & Sons, Ltd.

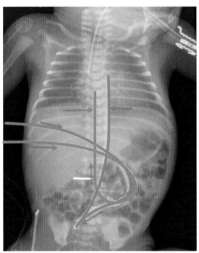

Fig. 77.4 X-ray to confirm position of the umbilical artery (red) and umbilical vein (blue) catheters, which need to be withdrawn. The artery first goes towards the groin before going towards the head just to the left of the vertebral column. Also check position of tracheal tube (satisfactory) and gavage (nasogastric) tube (missing).

Umbilical vein catheter (UVC)

Indications
- Resuscitation – for urgent venous access.
- Inotropes.
- Parenteral nutrition.
- Exchange transfusion.

Contraindications
- Omphalitis.
- Omphalocele (exomphalos).
- Peritonitis.

Insertion
- Insert umbilical arterial catheter first if also required.
- Prepare sterile field and clean stump as for UAC.
- Select single- or double-lumen catheter.
- UVC can sometimes be inserted several days after birth.
- Prime catheter with saline and insert to required length (see Table 77.1).
- Check position with X-ray (Fig. 77.4) or ultrasound. Tip should lie in the inferior vena cava 1 cm below the diaphragm.
- Label clearly that it is a venous line.

Complications
- Thrombosis or emboli.
- Extravasation of fluid (e.g. PN) into liver.

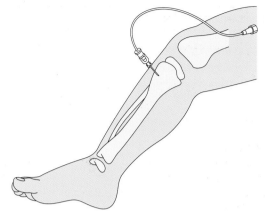

Fig. 77.5 Intraosseous infusion into tibia.

- Infection.
- Pleural or pericardial effusion (if in right atrium).
- Remove as soon as no longer essential.

Intraosseous cannulation

Indication
- Emergency infusion of fluids and drugs when no venous access possible.

Preparation
- Clean the skin and prepare sterile field.
- Position infant with knee flexed and supported.

Insertion
- Proximal tibia 1–3 cm below tibial tuberosity – medial flat surface (Fig. 77.5).
- Use neonatal intraosseous needle.
- Insert needle at 10–15° from vertical towards foot (avoids growth plate).
- Use twisting motion or use drill device.
- Place dressing around base to secure needle.
- Aspirate marrow to confirm position.
- Infuse drugs using syringe.

Complications
- Fracture.
- Extravasation causing cellulitis.
- Osteomyelitis.

Central venous catheters (CVC)

In neonatal practice, central catheters are usually peripherally inserted, but sometimes a surgically placed subclavian or internal jugular catheter is required for long-term management, or if venous access is very difficult.

Peripherally inserted central catheters (PICC lines)

Indications
- Parenteral nutrition.
- Inotropes (due to vasoconstriction).
- Hyperosmolar infusions, e.g. glucose >12.5%.
- Prolonged administration of antibiotics.

Site
- Common veins – brachial, saphenous, sometimes scalp.

Insertion (Figs 78.1–78.3)
- Prepare infant – optimize position, minimize discomfort (see Chapter 63), temperature control, monitoring.
- Measure length of insertion from cannulation site to inferior or superior vena cava as appropriate.
- Prepare equipment – gauze, polyurethane catheter, cannula or needle for insertion, T-piece and connection, dressing, saline flush.
- Sterile procedure – wear gown and mask and two sets of gloves – remove outer gloves once the area is cleaned and sterile.

Quality improvement care bundles to reduce central line-associated bloodstream infection (CLABSI) have markedly reduced late-onset sepsis rates. Achieved through practical training and improving procedures to optimize infection control, root cause analysis of positive blood cultures, feedback and use of results to further improve guidelines.

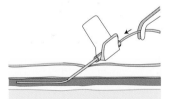

Fig. 78.1 An example of placing a peripherally inserted central catheter (PICC line). Needle is inserted into vein. The central line is threaded through the cannula. Non-toothed forceps may be used. (Figs 78.1 and 78.2 Courtesy of Dr Sunit Godambe.)

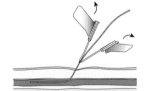

Fig. 78.2 The cannula is removed and then split, leaving the long line in place.

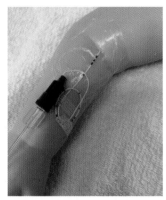

Fig. 78.3 Securing the line using sterile strips followed by clear adhesive dressing, incorporating loops of the central line. Ensure that insertion site is visible, that the infant is comfortable and that the dressing is not constricting the line or arm.

Line tip position and management
- Ideal position of the tip is in the inferior or superior vena cava *outside* the right atrium.
- Position of the long line should be checked by X-ray or ultrasound (Fig. 78.4) to ensure it is not in the right atrium. If position in doubt, inject sterile intravenous contrast and X-ray.
- If line inserted in upper arm, perform X-ray with arm abducted.
- If line inserted in lower limb, ensure it has passed superior to the lumbar venous plexus.
- Line management – usually last several weeks. They must be handled aseptically.

Complications
- Infection.
- Thrombus and emboli.
- Extravasation – pleural effusion, pericardial effusion (tamponade), tissue edema.
- Superior vena caval obstruction.
- Blockage.
- Leakage at connection sites.
- Line breaking off on removal.

Surgically tunneled subclavian or jugular line

Indications
- Long-term central access.
- Peripheral insertion not successful.

Insertion
- Usually by a pediatric surgeon or interventional radiologist under general anesthetic in operating theater.
- Tunneled under skin.
- Tip position in superior vena cava.

Neonatology at a Glance, Third Edition. Edited by Tom Lissauer, Avroy A. Fanaroff, Lawrence Miall and Jonathan Fanaroff.
© 2016 John Wiley & Sons, Ltd. Published 2016 by John Wiley & Sons, Ltd.

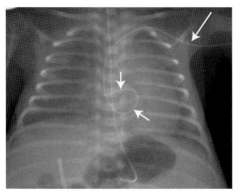

Fig. 78.4 X-ray demonstrating the importance of confirming catheter position. Central line may be radiopaque or need contrast flushed into it. The central venous catheter inserted into a vein in the left arm (arrow) is in the right atrium (arrows) and must be withdrawn.

Complications
- Pneumothorax.
- Surgical scar.
- Superior vena caval obstruction.
- Blockage or extravasation.
- Infection.

Exchange transfusion

Indications

- Severe hyperbilirubinemia – exchange with fresh blood, 2 × blood volume (i.e. 2 × 90 mL/kg).
- Severe polycythemia (hematocrit >0.75 or symptomatic) – exchange with normal saline to reduce hematocrit to 0.55 (usually ~ 20 mL/kg).

Exchange transfusion is performed infrequently for hyperbilirubinemia since the introduction of routine anti-D antibody to rhesus-negative mothers, better phototherapy and intravenous immunoglobulin for severe jaundice.

Technique (see video: Haemolytic disease of the newborn)

- Use fresh, CMV-negative, irradiated, whole blood or plasma reduced red cells (not packed red cells), ideally with hematocrit 0.5–0.6.
- Prepare sterile field. Ensure operator will not be disturbed during procedure.

Blood withdrawn via umbilical or peripheral arterial line; infused via umbilical or peripheral vein
- Infuse blood at a constant rate through the vein via a blood warmer.
- Withdraw blood from arterial line in aliquots (5 mL extremely preterm, 20 mL term).

Via umbilical venous catheter (Fig. 78.5)
- Alternate between withdrawing and infusing aliquots (5–20 mL) of blood. Use a closed system, designed for exchange transfusion, to reduce the risk of error.

Monitoring

- Heart rate, blood pressure, temperature throughout.
- Volume infused and withdrawn (separate observer).
- Glucose, electrolytes, calcium, acid–base.
- Allow time for equilibration – perform over several hours for double volume exchange.
- No feeds during procedure.

Complications

- Technical problems (e.g. loss of access).
- Air embolization or thrombosis.
- Volume overload or depletion.
- Electrolyte imbalance – hyperkalemia, hypocalcemia, acidosis or alkalosis.
- Hypoglycemia.
- Infection.
- Hypothermia.
- Mortality – possibly up to 1%.

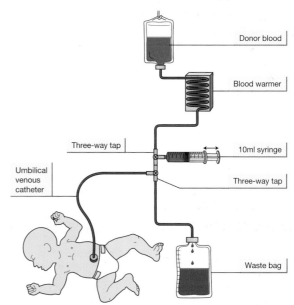

Fig. 78.5 An example of exchange transfusion via umbilical vein with 10 ml aliquots. 1. Withdraw 10 mL of baby's blood into syringe. 2. Inject baby's blood into waste bag. 3. Draw 10 mL of donor blood into syringe. 4. Inject 10 mL of blood into baby. Repeat to replace calculated blood volume.

The anterior fontanel provides a window through which the brain can be visualized using ultrasound (**see video: Cranial ultrasound**). This allows the identification of a range of brain lesions in newborn infants. The examination is non-invasive and can be safely performed at the bedside with minimal disturbance to the infant. It allows injuries to be timed. Serial imaging allows monitoring of progression or resolution of lesions. It provides prognostic information, and may assist in decision-making about continuation or withdrawal of intensive care.

The appearance of the brain varies with gestation and age. At 23–25 weeks, the cortex is relatively smooth with few cerebral fissures, sulci and gyri and the ventricles are prominent. By term, the surface of the cortex appears convoluted and sulci and gyral patterns are well developed with slit-like ventricles. These changes can also be seen on MRI scans (see Chapter 81).

Indications

- Infants <1500 g birthweight or <32 weeks' gestation.
- Infants requiring mechanical ventilation.
- Neurologic abnormality – abnormal tone, seizures, encephalopathy.
- Antenatally detected neurologic abnormality.
- Suspected genetic syndrome.
- Major congenital anomaly.

Lesions that can be identified

Preterm infants

- Hemorrhage (in germinal matrix, ventricles or parenchyma).
- Ventricular dilatation.
- Parenchymal infarcts and porencephalic cysts.
- Periventricular leukomalacia.

All infants

- Structural brain malformation.
- Ventricular dilatation.
- Cerebral edema.
- Calcification from congenital infection.
- Basal ganglia lesions in hypoxic–ischemic encephalopathy.
- Stroke (e.g. middle cerebral artery infarction).
- Hematoma (see below).

Standard views for scans

Coronal views (Fig. 79.1)

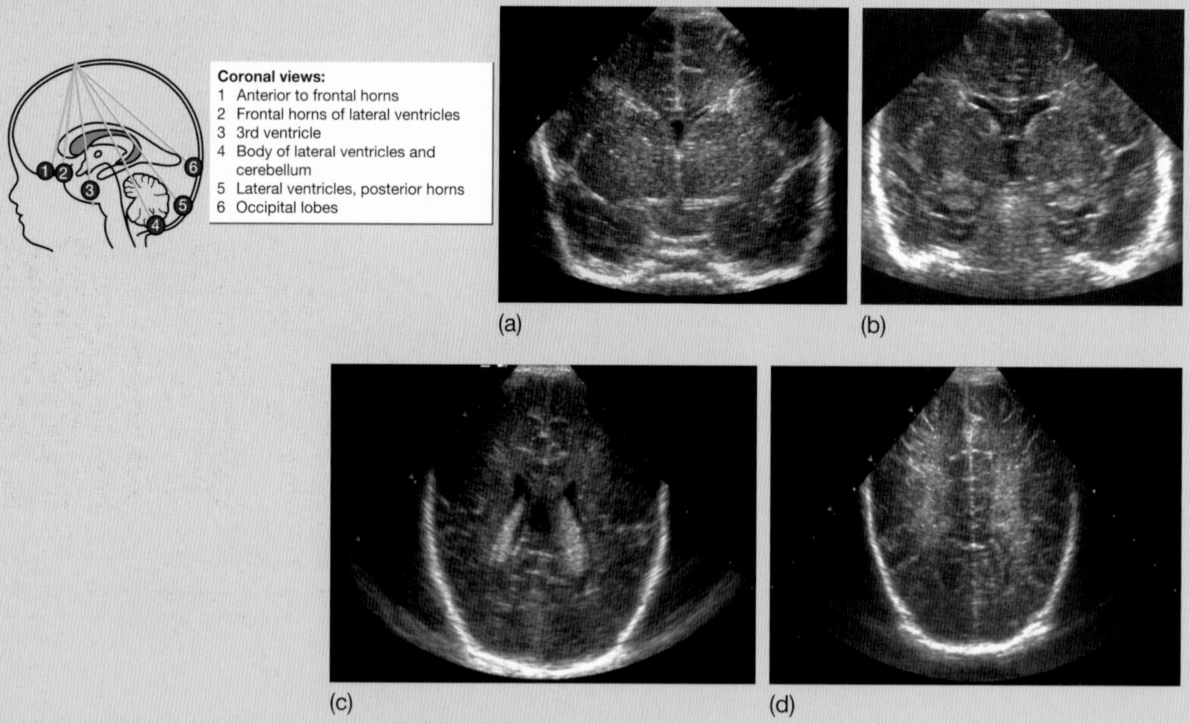

Coronal views:
1 Anterior to frontal horns
2 Frontal horns of lateral ventricles
3 3rd ventricle
4 Body of lateral ventricles and cerebellum
5 Lateral ventricles, posterior horns
6 Occipital lobes

(a) (b) (c) (d)

Fig. 79.1 Coronal views. (a) Frontal horns, view 2. (b) Third ventricle, view 3. (c) Lateral ventricles, posterior horns view 5. (d) Periventricular white matter, view 6.

Neonatology at a Glance, Third Edition. Edited by Tom Lissauer, Avroy A. Fanaroff, Lawrence Miall and Jonathan Fanaroff.
© 2016 John Wiley & Sons, Ltd. Published 2016 by John Wiley & Sons, Ltd.

Sagittal views (Fig. 79.2)

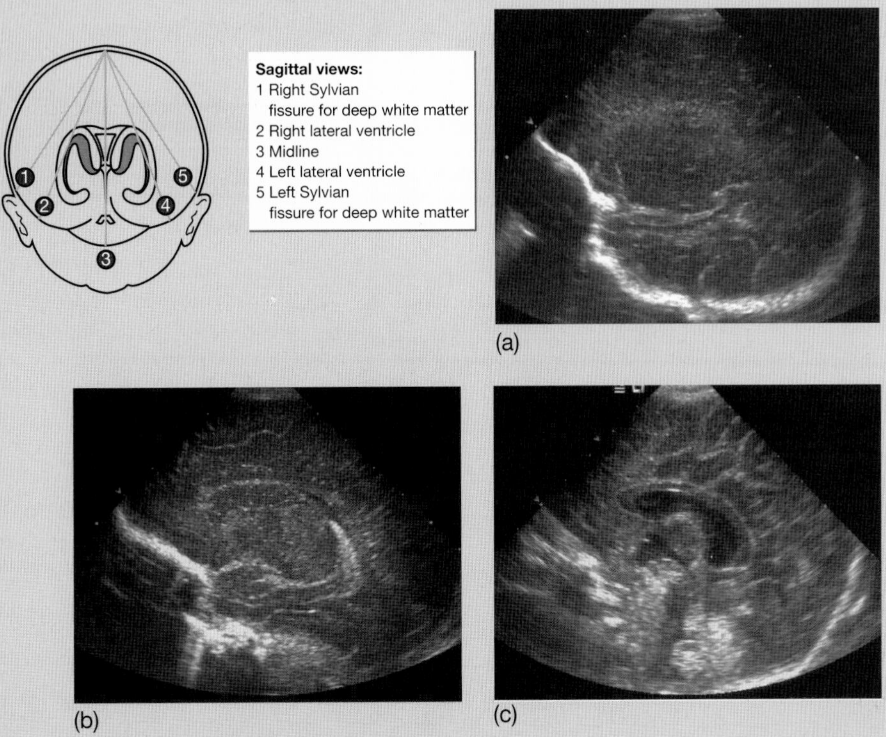

Sagittal views:
1 Right Sylvian
   fissure for deep white matter
2 Right lateral ventricle
3 Midline
4 Left lateral ventricle
5 Left Sylvian
   fissure for deep white matter

(a)

(b)

(c)

Fig. 79.2 Sagittal views. (a) Sylvian fissure for deep white matter, view 1 and 5. (b) Lateral ventricle, view 2 and 4. (c) Midline, view 3.

Hemorrhage

Germinal matrix hemorrhage, GMH (Grade I) (Fig. 79.3)

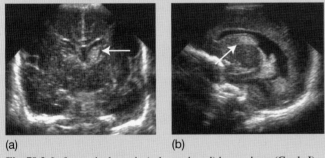

(a)   (b)

Fig. 79.3 Left germinal matrix (subependymal) hemorrhage (Grade I).
(a) Coronal view. (b) Sagittal view.

Intraventricular hemorrhage, GMH-IVH (Grade II – no ventricular dilatation) (Fig. 79.4)

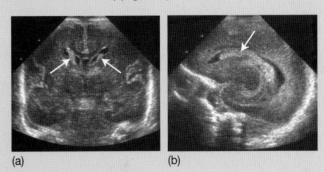

(a)   (b)

Fig. 79.4 Bilateral intraventricular hemorrhage, GMH-IVH (Grade II).
(a) Coronal view. (b) Sagittal view.

(continued)

Intraventricular hemorrhage, GMH-IVH with dilatation (Grade III – ventricular dilatation) (Fig. 79.5)

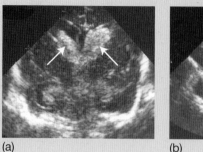
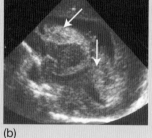

(a) (b)

Fig. 79.5 Bilateral intraventricular hemorrhage, GMH-IVH with ventricular dilatation (Grade III). (a) Coronal view. (b) Sagittal view.

Hemorrhagic parenchymal infarct (Grade IV) (Fig. 79.6)

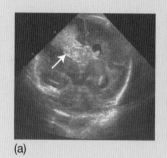
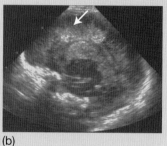

(a) (b)

Fig. 79.6 Right hemorrhagic parenchymal infarct (Grade IV). (a) Coronal view. (b) Sagittal view.

Porencephalic cyst (Fig. 79.7)

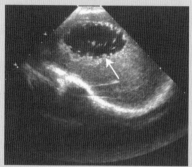

Fig. 79.7 Porencephalic cyst at site of a unilateral hemorrhagic parenchymal infarct.

Post-hemorrhagic ventricular dilatation (PHVD) (Fig 79.8)

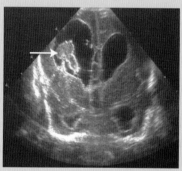

Fig. 79.8 Marked bilateral post-hemorrhagic ventricular dilatation (PHVD) and hemorrhage in right ventricle on coronal scan (arrow). Regular ultrasound and head circumference monitoring is indicated. If symptoms of raised intracranial pressure develop or head circumference rapidly crosses centiles, a ventricular access device or ventriculo-peritoneal shunt will need to be inserted to remove CSF.

Ventricular index (Figs 79.9–79.10)

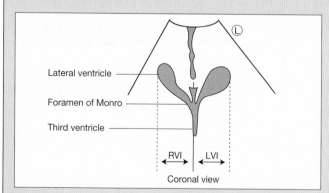

Fig. 79.9 Ventricular index, measured from the midline to the lateral border of the ventricle on a coronal scan in the plane of the third ventricle to aid monitoring of ventricular dilatation. Other indices can be used. (LVI, left ventricular index; RVI, right ventricular index.)

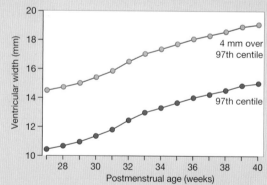

Fig. 79.10 Centiles for ventricular index showing 97th centile. Used to monitor progression or resolution of ventricular dilatation. See Chapter 59, Neural tube defects and hydrocephalus. (Source: Levene M.I., *Arch Dis Child* 1981; **56**: 900–904.)

Echodensities (Fig. 79.11)

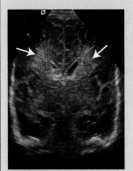

Fig. 79.11 Bilateral echodensities on coronal view.

Cystic periventricular leukomalacia (PVL) (Fig. 79.12)

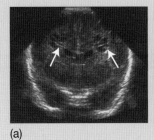

(a)   (b)

Fig. 79.12 Widespread periventricular cysts on day 55 in (a) coronal and (b) sagittal views. Initial scans were normal and then showed some increased periventricular echogenicity evolving into cystic PVL.

View from additional window (Fig. 79.13)

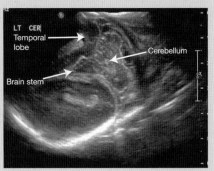

Fig. 79.13 Mastoid fontanel view showing cerebellum.

Color Doppler flow velocity measurements

Cranial ultrasound can be combined with color Doppler flow velocity measurements to distinguish vascular from non vascular structures and to ensure that the blood flow is normal. Abnormalities in flow after severe HIE may guide prognosis.

Additional windows

Other fontanels may be used to provide additional views, if indicated:
• Posterior fontanel – occipital and temporal horns of lateral ventricles, occipital and temporal parenchyma and posterior fossa.
• Temporal window, positioned above ear – brain stem and cerebellum.
• Mastoid fontanel, at junction of temporal, occipital and posterior parietal bones – posterior fossa and mid-brain (Fig. 79.13).

Limitations of ultrasound

Poor sensitivity in identifying:
• cerebral white matter injury
• cerebral edema
• subdural, subgaleal (subaponeurotic) hemorrhage
  Cannot reliably distinguish between hemorrhage and infarction.
MRI imaging is more sensitive in identifying these lesions.

Question

When can brain injury in preterm infants be identified on ultrasound?
Shortly after birth – identifies antenatal and early injury – small cysts, periventricular flare, hemorrhage.
During first week – hemorrhage, early ventricular dilatation, periventricular flare.
At 3–4 weeks old – ventricular dilatation, evolving PVL cysts, progression of lesions.
Discharge or term – prognosis is good if ventricles are normal, there is no cerebral atrophy, no cystic lesions and head circumference is increasing along normal centile.

Practical issues

• Sonographer should be specially trained.
• Probe must be cleaned before and after use with each infant.
• Ensure the probe marker is on the right hand side of the baby's head and that the screen is correctly labeled.
• Images are recorded digitally for review and storage.
• Abnormality should be visible on both coronal and sagittal views.
• Written report by experienced neonatologist or radiologist or radiographer into patient record.

Amplitude-integrated electroencephalography (aEEG) is a bedside tool for continuous monitoring of changes in the amplitude of the electroencephalogram using a cerebral function monitor (CFM). It compares well with standard EEG when used to assess the severity of neonatal encephalopathy, but a standard EEG is still required to provide additional important information about changes in frequency and in the synchrony, distribution and other characteristics of cerebral cortical activity.

Use of aEEG in neonates

Term infants

- To assess the severity of hypoxic–ischemic encephalopathy (HIE).
- For prediction of neurologic outcome following HIE.
- For seizure detection.
- To monitor response to anticonvulsant therapies.
- To select infants for clinical trials of neuroprotection.
- To monitor and assess etiology of neonatal encephalopathy.

Preterm infants

- To detect complications such as intraventricular hemorrhage and posthemorrhagic ventricular dilatation.
- To predict neurodevelopmental outcome following preterm delivery.

Cerebral function monitor

The CFM records one or two channels of EEG from scalp electrodes; the signal is filtered and the signal amplitude is displayed. Frequencies <2 and >15 Hz are selectively filtered to reduce artifacts caused by movement, ECG and other electronic equipment. The speed is usually set at 6 cm/hour, making every major division equal to 10 minutes.

Interpretation

The standard CFM display appears as a band of activity moving slowly across the display screen. The lower edge of the band indicates the lowest peak-to-peak amplitude reached by the filtered EEG over a period of time, whereas the upper edge is related to the highest levels. The width of the band indicates the variability of the EEG amplitude. In term infants the aEEG trace can be classified according to voltage or pattern of trace (Fig. 80.1).

Normal

The upper margin of the trace is above 10 μV and the lower margin is greater than 5 μV. The width of the band fluctuates between

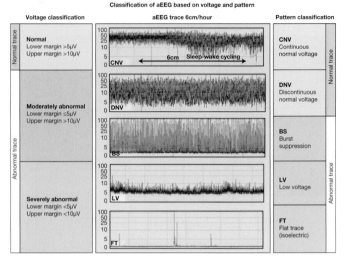

Fig. 80.1 Classification of aEEG. This is based on voltage (upper and lower margins of the trace), shown on the left, or on pattern of the trace, shown on the right. They overlap.

10 and 50 μV, changing with the sleep–awake state of the infant (sleep–awake cycling), and is called a continuous pattern.

Moderately abnormal

The upper margin is > 10 μV and the lower margin is < 5 μV. Hence the band appears wider and is called a discontinuous pattern. This is seen in infants with moderately severe encephalopathy. It may also be seen immediately after administration of anticonvulsants and sedatives. The aEEG should therefore not be used for assessing severity of encephalopathy during the first 30–60 minutes after therapy with these medications. A discontinuous pattern may be normal in preterm infants.

Severely abnormal

The upper margin is < 10 μV and lower margin is usually < 5 μV. Hence the band appears narrow and is called a low-voltage pattern. Rarely, the lower margin may be raised above 5 μV because of interference from ECG.

This low-voltage pattern may be accompanied by brief bursts of higher voltage spikes, which appear as single spikes above the background activity. This is called 'burst suppression'. A severely abnormal trace is usually seen with severe encephalopathy and is often accompanied by seizure activity.

Isoelectric EEG

Absent cerebral electrical activity is seen as a flat line or narrow band of activity with very low voltage.

Neonatology at a Glance, Third Edition. Edited by Tom Lissauer, Avroy A. Fanaroff, Lawrence Miall and Jonathan Fanaroff.
© 2016 John Wiley & Sons, Ltd. Published 2016 by John Wiley & Sons, Ltd.

Seizure detection and response to anticonvulsants

• Seizures are characterized by a sudden rise and narrowing of the trace, reflecting the increase in EEG voltage. The trace returns to the previous appearance or is depressed when the seizure activity stops (Fig. 80.2).
• Very frequent or continuous seizure activity (status epilepticus) may result in a 'sawtooth' appearance or in an elevated narrow band of activity.
• Inspection of the underlying EEG helps to confirm seizures suspected from the CFM trace.
• Since the aEEG is usually displayed at 6 cm/hour, brief seizures less than 1–2 minutes will not be seen.
• A standard EEG is needed to document the electrographic characteristics and distribution of seizures.
• aEEG is often used to monitor the response to treatment with anticonvulsants (Fig. 80.3).

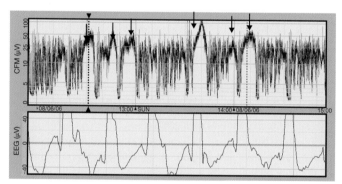

Fig. 80.2 aEEG showing seizures (arrows), with rise in baseline and lack of variability in voltage. The corresponding raw EEG with high amplitude spikes is shown in the lower panel.

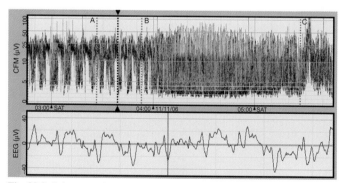

Fig. 80.3 Seizures and response to anticonvulsants. Point A: phenobarbitone was given followed by a second dose at point B, resulting in termination of seizures. Seizure activity is seen again at point C.

Artifacts on an aEEG trace

• Poor contact with electrodes causes high amplitude artifact.
• An artifact from electrical activity of the heart may result in elevation of the band of activity even in the absence of cerebral activity.
• Muscle or movement artifact can result in an artificially broad band or sudden changes in the band of activity.
• The underlying raw EEG should always be inspected if artifact is suspected.

aEEG as a prognostic tool in HIE

• The aEEG, in conjunction with other neurophysiologic investigations and imaging is helpful in predicting neurodevelopmental outcome following neonatal HIE. Combining clinical assessment with the aEEG trace further improves prognostic accuracy.
• Hypothermia improves neurologic outcomes when started within the first 6 hours of age in infants with HIE with a moderately or severely abnormal aEEG trace. As normalization of the aEEG occurs later in cooled infants, it should not be relied upon as the sole prognostic factor before 48h of age.
• In cooled infants, normal background amplitude or recovery of background amplitude within 6 hours of birth is associated with a likely normal outcome.
• Many infants with recovery to normal EEG activity within 36–48 hours of birth go on to make a good clinical recovery.
• A burst suppression pattern or depressed trace persisting beyond 48 hours or absence of sleep–awake cycling by 96h indicates a high probability of abnormal neurodevelopmental outcome
• It is not clear whether the occurrence of seizures in HIE alters the prognosis in infants with a suppressed EEG.

Use of aEEG in preterm infants

• There are well-characterized developmental changes in the EEG of preterm infants; the EEG is discontinuous at 24–25 weeks' gestation and gradually becomes less discontinuous with increasing maturity.
• Sleep–awake cycles begin to emerge from about 30 weeks, but remain incomplete until about 37 weeks' gestation.
• A semiquantitative scoring system of maturity based on sleep–awake cycling pattern, continuity and bandwidth has been described and shown to correlate with subsequent neurologic outcome, although its reliability is not proven.

81 Perinatal neuroimaging

The human brain follows a highly programmed sequence of organization and maturation, which begins in the first few weeks of fetal life and continues to young adulthood. Neuroimaging provides detailed characterization of brain development and can provide accurate biomarkers with which to quantitatively study particular clinical states and therapies. Magnetic resonance imaging (MRI) is ideal, as images with high spatial resolution can be acquired without ionizing radiation, even in the fetus and extremely preterm infant. MRI brain scans are increasingly used in neonatology as MRI has high sensitivity for detecting adverse neurologic outcome, particularly cerebral palsy.

Early in human gestation, the brain is relatively lissencephalic (smooth surface), with subsequent gyrification following a clearly defined sequence, starting with the large interhemispheric fissure (10–15 weeks post-menstrual age, PMA) and sylvian fissure (14–19 weeks PMA). The secondary and tertiary sulci (such as the central sulcus, which separates the primary motor and somatosensory cortices) are not visible until approximately 20 weeks PMA, when neuronal migration from the ventricular zone is completed. As the brain matures through the third trimester (Fig. 81.1), there is an exponential increase in surface area through the formation of gyri and sulci, compared with a slower linear increase in whole brain volume; deviation from this relationship in preterm infants predicts adverse cognitive outcome later in childhood.

In addition to developmental changes in the structure of the brain, marked maturational changes in the contrast of specific tissues can be visualized, particularly in the periventricular white matter (Fig. 81.2). They represent underlying changes in tissue composition and water content.

Functional mapping of the brain

Diffusion MRI can be used to delineate axon fiber bundles accurately and thus provide a detailed map of the structural 'connectivity' of the neonatal brain (Fig. 81.3). Functional MRI (fMRI) can provide information about the brain's activity through rapidly sampling changes in the localized MR signal that result from differences in the magnetic properties of hemoglobin when bound to oxygen (Fig. 81.4). Through the combination of such techniques, it may be possible to characterize accurately a detailed 'connectome' of the neonatal brain, in which all of the structural and functional connections of the developing brain are mapped.

Practical and safety considerations

There are drawbacks to MRI scanning:
- it is expensive
- long time required to acquire good-quality images (minimum 20 minutes with head kept still); some infants can be 'fed and wrapped' but others need general anaesthesia

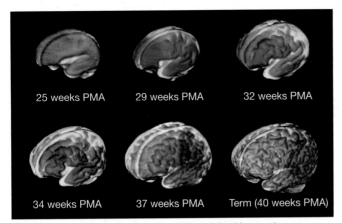

Fig. 81.1 Three-dimensional rendered T2-weighted images in preterm infants at different gestation showing the dramatic evolution of cortical folding up to term. (PMA – post-menstrual age.)

25 weeks PMA   29 weeks PMA   32 weeks PMA
34 weeks PMA   37 weeks PMA   Term (40 weeks PMA)

Fig. 81.2 Tissue-specific changes during brain maturation. Early in the third trimester, myelin is not seen in the periventricular white matter, and concentric 'bands' of tissue can be seen, including migrating cells and an important structure called the subplate which acts as a 'waiting area' for branching axons (white arrow). Myelination is not clearly seen until term (40 weeks PMA), first in the posterior limb of the internal capsule (PLIC) (yellow arrow), proceeding in a caudal to cephalic direction, with the frontal white matter the last to myelinate. Myelination continues through to young adulthood, when it can be seen throughout the white matter.

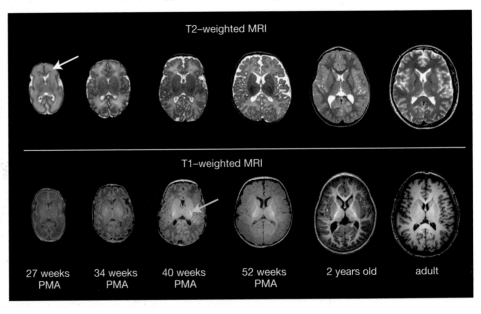

T2–weighted MRI

T1–weighted MRI

27 weeks PMA   34 weeks PMA   40 weeks PMA   52 weeks PMA   2 years old   adult

Neonatology at a Glance, Third Edition. Edited by Tom Lissauer, Avroy A. Fanaroff, Lawrence Miall and Jonathan Fanaroff.
© 2016 John Wiley & Sons, Ltd. Published 2016 by John Wiley & Sons, Ltd.

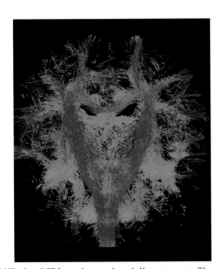

Fig. 81.3 Diffusion MRI can be used to delineate axon fiber bundles accurately and thus provide a detailed map of the structural 'connectivity' of the neonatal brain. In this example, the brain of an infant at term is shown in the coronal plane, with the delineated connections shown by color for their directionality; those running superior–inferior (or vice versa) in blue, those left–right in red, and those anterior–posterior (or vice versa) in green. (Reproduced and adapted with permission from Pandit A.S. *et al.* Diffusion magnetic resonance imaging in preterm brain injury. *Neuroradiology* 2013; **5S** (Suppl 2): 65–95.)

- possible distress from transfer and being inside scanner
- metal-containing objects/implants are contraindicated in the MRI scanner due to the powerful magnetic field.

There are only a handful of neonatal units worldwide with dedicated MRI facilities, but standard MRI scanners can increasingly produce faster and motion-tolerant image acquisition sequences, and MR-compatible equipment (e.g. incubators) is now available.

Prognostic information

Cranial ultrasound and MRI have similar high specificity for predicting later cerebral palsy; a normal cranial ultrasound allows confident prediction of normal motor outcome. Therefore, although MRI scanning has a clear role in particular infants where accurate delineation of a pathologic lesion can provide diagnostic and prognostic information (such as HIE and stroke), in standard neonatal care it is complementary to cranial ultrasound. However, MRI is providing important information about early brain development and the pathophysiology of neonatal brain injury and potentially the evaluation of the effectiveness of new therapies.

Key point

MRI neuroimaging provides:
- high resolution images for detecting brain injury
- prognostic information following HIE

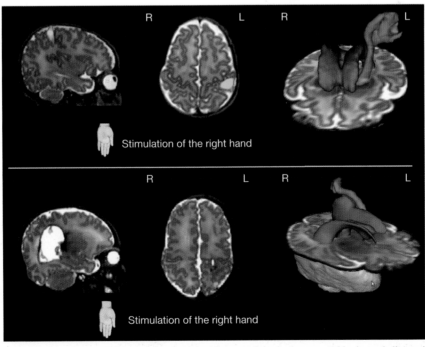

Stimulation of the right hand

Stimulation of the right hand

Fig. 81.4 MRI can accurately characterize patterns of functional and structural connectivity in the neonatal brain, and allows visualization of neuroplasticity following brain injury, as demonstrated in these two infants born prematurely and scanned at term equivalent PMA. Top row: following passive motor stimulation of the right hand, in a normal infant fMRI has identified a cluster of functional brain activity (red/yellow) in the contralateral (left) hemisphere, which is structurally connected to the thalamus via a nerve fiber bundle (top right, yellow) that has been delineated with diffusion MRI. Bottom row: this infant has a large right-sided porencephalic cyst following grade IV intraventricular hemorrhage. Following stimulation of the right hand, the induced functional activity has been displaced posteriorly by the cyst, while the structural connections have similarly grown to circumvent the damaged area.

82 Echocardiography for the neonatologist

Targeted neonatal echocardiography (functional echocardiography) provides physiologic information in real time in order to support clinical decision-making. It enhances clinical judgment, provides a better understanding of active physiologic processes and allows monitoring the response to treatment. It enables one to:
- assess the hemodynamic impact of a PDA (Chapter 33)
- assess cardiac function in hypotensive neonates to determine the need and efficacy of inotropes and volume support
- identify the position of umbilical and central venous lines
- exclude major cardiac defects
- identify pulmonary hypertension (PPHN), its severity and impact on right ventricular performance and cardiac output
- exclude pericardial effusion.

It may be performed by a pediatric cardiologist or trained neonatologist working in close collaboration with a pediatric cardiac center. However, echocardiography of complex congenital heart disease is the responsibility of the pediatric cardiologist.

Views (see videos)

The standard views (Figs 82.1 and 82.2) are:
- four- and five-chamber views from the apex
- parasternal short-axis view
- parasternal long-axis view
- subcostal view.
  High-quality images must be obtained.

Four-chamber view

- Confirms (Fig. 82.3a and b) that:
  – there are four chambers, and allows evaluation of their size
  – there are normal mitral and tricuspid valves, and that tricuspid is offset, i.e. nearer the apex
  – ventricular septum is intact.
- Quantifies the degree of tricuspid regurgitation – useful for estimating pulmonary artery pressure.
- Detection of thrombi or vegetations in the atria or valves.

If the probe is angled more anterior to the four-chamber view, the five-chamber view is obtained, which allows direct visualization of the left ventricular outflow tract. This allows indirect measurement of left ventricular output.

Short-axis view

This view (Fig. 82.4a and b) allows the identification of:
- patent ductus arteriosus and flow direction
- perimembranous ventricular septal defect (VSD)
- PPHN (persistent pulmonary hypertension of the newborn)

Echocardiography

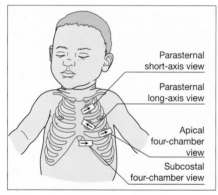

Fig. 82.1 Positions of probe and views obtained.

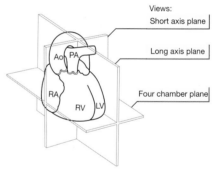

Fig. 82.2 The planes of the long-axis, short-axis and four-chamber apical or subcostal views. The five-chamber view is obtained by aiming the probe anterior to the subcostal view to visualize the left ventricular outflow tract.

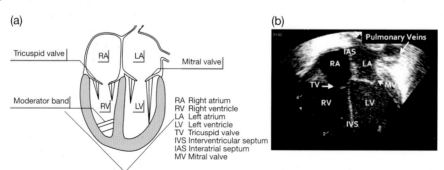

Fig. 82.3 (a) Four-chamber view. The right ventricle can be identified from a band of tissue, the moderator band. (b) Ultrasound showing four-chamber view.

Neonatology at a Glance, Third Edition. Edited by Tom Lissauer, Avroy A. Fanaroff, Lawrence Miall and Jonathan Fanaroff.
© 2016 John Wiley & Sons, Ltd. Published 2016 by John Wiley & Sons, Ltd.

(a) 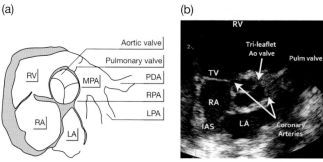 (b)

Fig. 82.4 (a) Short-axis view. (b) Ultrasound of short-axis view. RA, Right atrium; RV, Right ventricle; LA, Left atrium; PDA, Patent ductus arteriosus; MPA, Main pulmonary artery; RPA, Right pulmonary artery; LPA, Left pulmonary artery.

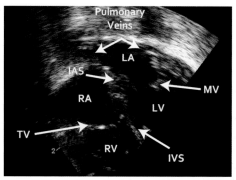

Fig. 82.6 Ultrasound showing subcostal atrial view.

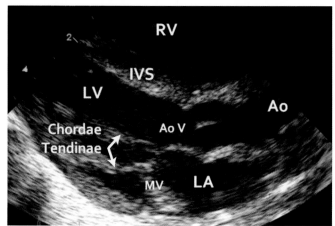

Fig. 82.5 Ultrasound showing long-axis view. (RV Right ventricle, LA Left atrium, LV Left ventricle, AoV Aortic valve, MV Mitral valve, IVS Interventricular septum)

- usual arrangement of pulmonary artery and aorta
- structural defects, e.g. transposition of the great arteries, pulmonary stenosis.

Long-axis view

This view (Fig. 82.5) is used to:
- identify correct position of pulmonary artery and aorta
- assess myocardial performance using shortening fraction.
- detect structural defects, e.g. tetralogy of Fallot
- assess volume overload in a patent ductus arteriosus (left atrial: aortic root ratio).

Subcostal view

This view (Fig 82.6) is used to:
- assess shunting at atrial level
- check liver on right and aorta on left side, i.e. situs solitus
- obtain high-quality images if other views are affected by lung hyperinflation or high-frequency oscillation (HFOV)
- check position of central lines in inferior vena cava or aorta.

Assessment of left ventricular function in critically ill neonates

Targeted neonatal echocardiography can determine if there is poor myocardial performance or volume depletion better than clinical examination alone, by:
- Subjective assessment of myocardial performance from the variation in left ventricle size.
- Estimation of systolic function from the left ventricular shortening fraction.
- Intravascular volume estimation from inferior vena caval filling – it is collapsed with hypovolemia; however, assessment of cardiac volume loading is particularly difficult in the first few days of life, when the transitional circulation is present.
- Calculating left ventricular output – to determine whether impaired systolic performance, hypovolemia or increased left ventricular afterload is leading to compromised systemic blood flow.

Assessment of PPHN

Echocardiography allows the diagnosis of increased pulmonary artery pressure and its impact on right and left ventricular performance. Right ventricular systolic pressure may be estimated if tricuspid regurgitation is present. A flat interventricular septum (or one that bows into the left ventricle) indicates elevated pulmonary pressures. The magnitude of the pulmonary hypertension may also be estimated from the direction of blood flow across the ductus arteriosus:
- pure right-to-left (from pulmonary artery to aorta) flow implies suprasystemic pulmonary artery pressure (Chapter 33)
- bidirectional ductal flow (right-to-left during systole and left-to-right during diastole) implies that pulmonary artery pressure approximates systemic arterial pressures
- left-to-right transductal flow implies pulmonary artery pressure less than systemic arterial pressure.

Calculation of right and left ventricular output allows rational use of therapies such as nitric oxide and milrinone.

83 Gestational age assessment, BP, severity of illness scores, jaundice treatment chart

Gestational age assessment: Ballard exam

The most accurate gestational age estimate is usually by first trimester ultrasound. Gestational age can also be assessed clinically (±2 weeks) from the changes in neuromuscular and physical maturity with gestation. The most widely used scoring systems are the revised Dubowitz and the somewhat shorter new Ballard score shown in Fig. 83.1 and Table 83.1.

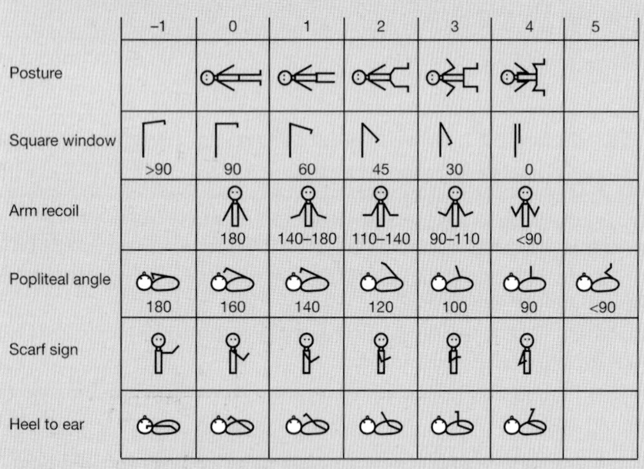

Fig. 83.1 Neuromuscular maturity.

Calculating an estimated gestational age

The exam is most accurate when performed between 30 and 42 hours of life. Add up the individual neuromuscular and physical maturity scores for the 12 categories, then obtain the estimated gestational age from Table 83.2. The neuromuscular maturity score may be unreliable if the infant is sedated or ill.

Table 83.2 Gestational age estimated from summed neuromuscular and physical maturity scores.

Total score	Gestational age (weeks)
−10	20
−5	22
0	24
5	26
10	28
15	30
20	32
25	34
30	36
35	38
40	40
45	42
50	44

Table 83.1 Physical maturity scores.

Sign	−1	0	1	2	3	4	5
Skin	Sticky, friable, transparent	Gelatinous red, translucent	Smooth pink, visible veins	Superficial peeling and/or rash, few veins	Cracking, pale areas, rare veins	Parchment, deep cracking, no vessels	Leathery, cracked, wrinkled
Lanugo	None	Sparse	Abundant	Thinning	Bald areas	Mostly bald	
Plantar creases	Heel-toe 40–50 mm = −1 < 40 mm = −2	Heel–toe >50 mm, no creases	Faint red marks	Anterior transverse crease only	Creases over anterior 2/3	Creases over entire sole	
Breast	Imperceptible	Barely perceptible	Flat areola, no bud	Stippled areola, bud 1–2 mm	Raised areola, bud 3–4 mm	Full areola, bud 5–10 mm	
Eye and ear	Lids fused loosely = −1, tightly = −2	Lids open, pinna flat, stays folded	Slightly curved pinna, soft with slow recoil	Well-curved pinna, soft but ready recoil	Formed and firm, with instant recoil	Thick cartilage, ear stiff	
Genitalia, male	Scrotum flat, smooth	Scrotum empty, faint rugae	Testes in upper canal, rare rugae	Testes descending, few rugae	Testes down, good rugae	Testes pendulous, deep rugae	
Genitalia, female	Clitoris prominent, labia flat	Prominent clitoris, small labia minora	Prominent clitoris, enlarging minora	Majora and minora equally prominent	Majora large, minora small	Majora cover clitoris and minora	

Neonatology at a Glance, Third Edition. Edited by Tom Lissauer, Avroy A. Fanaroff, Lawrence Miall and Jonathan Fanaroff.
© 2016 John Wiley & Sons, Ltd. Published 2016 by John Wiley & Sons, Ltd.

Blood pressure charts (Fig. 83.2)

There is no consensus either on the definition of hypotension or on when low blood pressure should be corrected. Blood pressure spontaneously increases in preterm infants during the first 24 hours. Infants hypotensive by gestational age criteria but with clinical evidence of good perfusion have as good an outcome as normotensive patients. When there is severe hypotension or it is associated with poor perfusion, treatment includes fluid bolus, inotropes and corticosteroids, in a stepwise approach (see Chapter 24, Stabilizing the sick newborn infant). Functional echocardiography can provide information on cardiac contractility and intravascular volume (see Chapter 82, Echocardiography for the neonatologist).

Severity of illness scores

Scores have been devised in order to be able to compare and predict morbidity and mortality while allowing for severity of illness. They incorporate measures of physiologic instability in the first 12 postnatal hours. Clinically, these scoring systems are not helpful to guide care decisions for individual patients, but provide a method to compare outcomes between various centers and countries.

The most widely used in neonatology are:
- SNAP-PE II score
- CRIB II score.

The SNAP-PE II (Score Neonatal Acute Physiology Perinatal Extension) is based on the physiologic derangement in a number of organ systems (urine output, mean blood pressure, worst PaO$_2$/FiO$_2$ ratio, lowest serum pH, occurrence of seizures) in the first 12 hours after admission to the NICU, birthweight, Apgar score at 5 minutes and whether there is IUGR.

The CRIB II (Clinical Risk Index for Babies) score is for very low birthweight (VLBW) infants and is based on birthweight, gestation, maximal base excess in the first 12 hours of life and temperature on admission.

The use of the SNAP-PE is limited by the complexity of the data required and the CRIB score by the overwhelming effects of birthweight and gestational age on outcome.

Jaundice treatment chart

The recommended bilirubin levels for treatment with phototherapy and exchange transfusion in the UK for infants ≥ 38 weeks gestation are shown in Fig 83.3. Charts at earlier gestational ages are publishes in NICE guidelines.

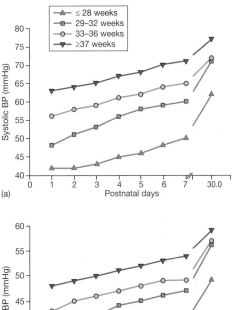

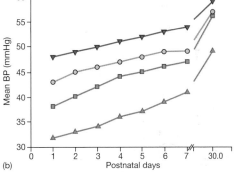

Fig. 83.2 Increase in (a) systolic and (b) mean blood pressure measured oscillometrically in hemodynamically stable infants during the first month of life. (Source: Pejovic B. *et al.* Blood pressure in non-critically ill preterm and full-term neonates. *Pediatr Nephrol* 2007; **22**: 249–257.)

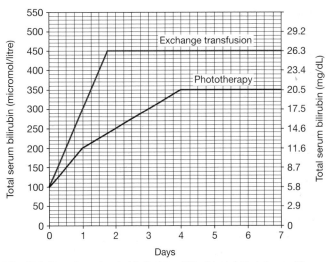

Fig. 83.3 Treatment thresholds for hyperbilirubinemia in infants ≥ 38 weeks in the UK. (NICE Clinical Guideline 2010).

Index

Neonatology at a Glance, Third Edition. Edited by Tom Lissauer, Avroy A. Fanaroff, Lawrence Miall and Jonathan Fanaroff.
© 2016 John Wiley & Sons, Ltd. Published 2016 by John Wiley & Sons, Ltd.

Trust Library
Central Manchester University Hospitals
Education South
Oxford Road
Manchester M13 9WL

Trust Library
Central Manchester University Hospitals
Education South
Oxford Road
Manchester M13 9WL